Group Therapy in Clinical Practice

Group Therapy in Clinical Practice

Edited by

Anne Alonso, Ph.D.

Associate Clinical Professor of Psychology, Department of Psychiatry, Harvard Medical School; Director, Postgraduate Fellowship in Psychodynamic Psychotherapy, Massachusetts General Hospital, Boston, Massachusetts; Faculty Member, The Fielding Institute, Santa Barbara, California

Hillel I. Swiller, M.D.

Associate Professor of Psychiatry, Mount Sinai School of Medicine; Director, Division of Psychotherapy, Department of Psychiatry, Mount Sinai Hospital, New York, New York

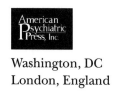
American Psychiatric Press, Inc.

Washington, DC
London, England

Copyright © 1993 American Psychiatric Press, Inc.
ALL RIGHTS RESERVED
Manufactured in the United States of America on acid-free paper
96 95 94 93   4 3 2 1
American Psychiatric Press, Inc.
1400 K Street, N.W., Washington, DC 20005

Library of Congress Cataloging-in-Publication Data

Group therapy in clinical practice / edited by Anne Alonso, Hillel
  Swiller.
      p. cm.
    Includes bibliographical references and index.
    ISBN 0-88048-323-7 (alk. paper)
    1. Group psychotherapy. I. Alonso, Anne. II. Swiller, Hillel,
  1939–   .
    [DNLM: 1. Psychotherapy, Group. WM 430 G8837]
  RC488.G733 1993
  616.89′152—dc20
  DNLM/DLC   92-10416
  for Library of Congress   CIP

British Library Cataloguing in Publication Data

A CIP record is available from the British Library.

Contents

PART III
Special Populations in Group Therapy

PART IV
Special Considerations

PART V
Gender Issues in Groups

PART VI
New Applications of Group Theory and Technique

PART VII
Research

PART VIII
Teaching and Training

Contributors

Anne Alonso, Ph.D.
Associate Clinical Professor of Psychology, Department of Psychiatry,
Harvard Medical School; Director, Postgraduate Fellowship in
Psychodynamic Psychotherapy, Massachusetts General Hospital, Boston,
Massachusetts; Faculty Member, The Fielding Institute, Santa Barbara,
California

Lawrence J. Bader, Ph.D.
Faculty Member, Massachusetts School of Professional Psychology,
Dedham, Massachusetts

Howard S. Baker, M.D.
Associate Clinical Professor of Psychiatry, University of Pennsylvania;
Senior Attending Psychiatrist, Institute of Pennsylvania Hospital,
Philadelphia, Pennsylvania

Margaret N. Baker, Ph.D.
Assistant Clinical Professor of Psychology, Widener University, Chester,
Pennsylvania

David W. Brook, M.D.
Associate Professor of Psychiatry; Director, Division of Drug Abuse
Research, Prevention, and Treatment, New York Medical College,
Valhalla, New York

Kathleen Whiteman Carroll, M.S.W., L.C.S.W.
Mental Health Clinician, Kaiser Permanente, Department of
Psychosocial Services, San Diego, California

Arnold Cohen, Ph.D.
Group Consultant, South Shore Mental Health Clinic and Boston
Evening Clinic, Boston, Massachusetts

Robert R. Dies, Ph.D.
Professor of Psychology, University of Maryland, College Park, Maryland

Patricia Doherty, Ed.D.
Instructor in Psychology, Department of Psychiatry, Harvard Medical
School; President, Boston Institute for Psychotherapy, Boston,
Massachusetts

Pamela L. Enders, Ph.D.
Clinical Instructor in Psychology, Department of Psychiatry, Harvard
Medical School; Clinical Psychology Associate, Massachusetts General
Hospital; Associate Director of Training, Postgraduate Center, Boston
Institute for Psychotherapy, Boston, Massachusetts

Allen Fay, M.D.
Assistant Clinical Professor, Department of Psychiatry, Mount Sinai
School of Medicine, New York, New York

Joel C. Frost, Ed.D.
Instructor in Psychology, Department of Psychiatry, Harvard Medical
School; Associate in Psychology, Department of Psychiatry, Beth Israel
Hospital, Boston, Massachusetts

Sarah Golden, Ph.D.
Clinical Instructor in Psychology, Department of Psychiatry, Harvard
Medical School at The Cambridge Hospital; Chief Psychologist, William
James Unit, Metropolitan State Hospital, Waltham, Massachusetts

Kurt Halliday, Ph.D.
Clinical Instructor in Psychology, Department of Psychiatry, Harvard
Medical School at The Cambridge Hospital; Doctoral candidate in
Clinical Psychology, New School for Social Research; Research Associate,
Harvard Cocaine Recovery Project, Cambridge, Massachusetts

David A. Halperin, M.D.
Associate Clinical Professor of Psychiatry, Mount Sinai School of
Medicine, New York, New York

Sylvia Hutchinson, B.Sc.
Coordinator of Training, Clinical Psychologist, Institute of Group
Analysis; Supervisor, Westminster Pastoral Foundation, London, United
Kingdom

Priscilla F. Kauff, Ph.D.
Assistant Clinical Professor of Psychology, Department of Psychiatry, Cornell University Medical Center, Payne Whitney Hospital; Senior Supervising and Training Analyst, Postgraduate Center for Mental Health, New York, New York

Lawrence L. Kennedy, M.D.
Director, Partial Hospitalization Services, C. F. Menninger Memorial Hospital, Topeka, Kansas

Edward J. Khantzian, M.D.
Associate Clinical Professor of Psychiatry, Harvard Medical School at The Cambridge Hospital; Principal Psychiatrist for Substance Abuse Disorders, Department of Psychiatry, The Cambridge Hospital; Associate Medical Director, Danvers State Hospital, Danvers, Massachusetts

Howard D. Kibel, M.D.
Associate Professor of Clinical Psychiatry, Cornell University Medical College; Coordinator of Group Psychotherapy, New York Hospital–Cornell Medical Center, Westchester Division, White Plains, New York

Steven Krugman, Ph.D.
Instructor in Psychology, Department of Psychiatry, Harvard Medical School; Director of Training, Trauma Clinic, Massachusetts General Hospital, Boston, Massachusetts

Enid A. Lang, M.D.
Assistant Clinical Professor of Psychiatry, Mount Sinai School of Medicine, New York, New York

Arnold A. Lazarus, Ph.D.
Distinguished Professor in the Graduate School of Applied and Professional Psychology, Rutgers University, Piscataway, New Jersey

Marguerite S. Lederberg, M.D.
Clinical Associate Professor of Psychiatry, Cornell University Medical College; Associate Attending Psychiatrist, New York Hospital; Associate Attending Psychiatrist, Memorial Sloan Kettering Cancer Center, New York, New York

Maria T. Lymberis, M.D.
Assistant Clinical Professor of Psychiatry, Department of Psychiatry and
Biobehavioral Sciences, University of California, Los Angeles, Los
Angeles, California

K. Roy MacKenzie, M.D., F.R.C.P.C.
Professor of Psychiatry, University of British Columbia, Vancouver,
British Columbia

Beryce W. MacLennan, Ph.D.
Clinical Professor, George Washington University School of Medicine
and Behavioral Science, Washington, D.C.

William E. McAuliffe, Ph.D.
Associate Professor of Psychiatry, Department of Psychiatry, Harvard
Medical School at The Cambridge Hospital; Lecturer, Department of
Behavioral Sciences, Harvard School of Public Health; Principal
Investigator, Harvard Cocaine Recovery Project, Project Outreach, and
the Rhode Island Prevention Project, Cambridge, Massachusetts

Samuel Osherson, Ph.D.
Faculty Member, The Fielding Institute, Santa Barbara, California

Malcolm Pines, M.D.
Founder Member, Training Group Analyst, Institute of Group Analysis,
London, United Kingdom

Kenneth Porter, M.D.
Assistant Clinical Professor of Psychiatry, Columbia College of Physicians
and Surgeons; Faculty Member, Supervisor, National Institute for the
Psychotherapies, New York, New York

Cecil A. Rice, Ph.D.
Director, Postgraduate Center, Boston Institute for Psychotherapy;
Director, Training Board of the American Group Psychotherapy
Association, Boston, Massachusetts

Albert E. Riester, Ed.D.
Professor and Director, School Psychology, Department of Education,
Trinity University; Psychologist and Consultant, SouthWest
Neuropsychiatric Institute, San Antonio, Texas

J. Scott Rutan, Ph.D.
Associate Clinical Professor of Psychology, Department of Psychiatry,
Harvard Medical School; Director, Center for Group Therapy,
Massachusetts General Hospital, Boston, Massachusetts

Melvin J. Stern, M.D.
Clinical Professor of Psychiatry, George Washington University School of
Medicine, Washington, D.C.

Walter N. Stone, M.D.
Professor of Psychiatry, University of Cincinnati College of Medicine,
Cincinnati, Ohio

Hillel I. Swiller, M.D.
Associate Professor of Psychiatry, Mount Sinai School of Medicine;
Director, Division of Psychotherapy, Department of Psychiatry, Mount
Sinai Hospital, New York, New York

Bessel A. van der Kolk, M.D.
Chief, Trauma Clinic, Massachusetts General Hospital; Lecturer in
Psychiatry, Harvard Medical School, Boston, Massachusetts

Acknowledgments

This book was compiled and completed with the support and encouragement of a number of colleagues and friends whom we would like to acknowledge here.

First are those who inspired us to enter and explore the field of group psychotherapy, especially the late Aaron Stein and Elvin Semrad. We also wish to acknowledge our contributors, all experts in their areas. Their scholarship, erudition, and zestful cooperation inspired and guided us toward the completion of the work.

Other colleagues offered helpful suggestions along the way, as well, including Drs. Jerome Gans, Carol Nadelson, Kenneth Arndt, Anne Arndt, Henry Weinstein, and Morton Siegel.

Our sincere thanks go to Jane Waldman, Josh Swiller, and Lucille Luciano, who edited, typed, managed, and toiled long into the night to keep us all organized. Similarly, we appreciated the splendid editorial and managerial talent that was made available to us through the American Psychiatric Press, Inc.

The generosity and forbearance of our spouses, Ramon and Willa, allowed us to stay relatively sane and calm in the face of the magnitude of the task. For this and all their many gifts, we are greatly indebted.

But most of all, we are appreciative of the years we have spent working with our patients in groups. They have taught us, healed us, and this book belongs to them as well.

Anne Alonso, Ph.D.
Hillel I. Swiller, M.D.

Preface

J. Scott Rutan, Ph.D.

Fueled by the extraordinary psychological needs of World War II soldiers, group therapy was suddenly elevated to a primary treatment modality in the 1940s. The group therapists of those days typically had little formal training, and they did the best they could through trial and error and by incorporating their dyadic psychotherapy skills in a group setting. These early group therapists soon became aware that there was something especially healing about therapy groups, and from that point serious thinking went into establishing a theoretical base for group therapy.

The first group therapists tended to be drawn from the ranks of psychoanalytically oriented individual therapists. Debates erupted among analysts as to the ultimate effectiveness of this new treatment. The debate usually reduced itself to those who practiced group therapy and those who did not. Those who worked with analytic theory in individual therapy or analysis tended to view group therapy as a supportive but fundamentally shallow treatment. They argued that transference was diluted by the multiperson field, thus severely limiting the potential of groups to truly effect character change. Those who actually ran the groups, however, noted that transference thrived and indeed was perhaps enhanced in groups. They pointed out that groups offered an opportunity to observe many types of transference (e.g., to parents and to siblings) at the same time.

Over time group therapy demonstrated its effectiveness to the point that the scholarly debates occurred *between* group therapists. Should the leader focus on group-as-a-whole interactions or on the individual within the group? Should the leader primarily use the group process as a healing factor, or should the members of the group best be used as an audience while a single individual works with the therapist? Should the leader encourage or discourage group members from speaking about events outside the life of the group itself?

In the late 1960s and early 1970s, groups reached fad proportions as the general population became aware of the power of the model to help individuals experience affect, alter self-image, and learn more about "belonging." Despite the continuing ascendance of groups as therapy, support, and training vehicles, there remained a dearth of literature on the theory and technique of group therapy. Although some excellent books were written, such as *The Group in Depth* by Durkin (1964) and *Psychoanalysis in Groups* by Wolf and Schwartz (1962), they received little attention among the general mental health community. It was left to *The Theory and Practice of Group Psychotherapy* by Yalom (1970) to excite both the general mental health community and the lay public about group therapy. The unprecedented sales of Yalom's book demonstrated the need for such a book and the widespread interest in group therapy.

In fact, however, Yalom's theoretical bent was atypical of that of most group therapists. He presented an existential, "here-and-now" approach to group therapy. The book was so popular and well written that it altered the focus of group therapy for a decade. Recently more balanced books have appeared, but there is still a great need for books presenting concise modern psychodynamic approaches to group therapy. Further, in recent years group therapy has been incorporated by clinicians from theoretical positions heretofore not involved in groups, including cognitive-behaviorists and humanistic theorists. In addition, a great number of homogeneous groups were formed to treat populations such as patients with eating disorders, substance abusers, adult children of alcoholics, and others. Group therapy in inpatient settings has become central to hospital treatment.

Research continually documents that group therapy is at least as effective as individual psychotherapy. In this era of the escalating cost of health care, the relative economy of group therapy makes it more and more attractive. Clearly it is time for a new and comprehensive work on the state of group therapy today.

Alonso and Swiller have accomplished that task by assembling a stellar group of authors presenting a comprehensive view of group therapy in the 1990s. The authors, each widely known for his or her contributions to group therapy, systematically cover the important aspects of group therapy today.

The Plan of the Book

The goal of long-term psychodynamic psychotherapy is the reorganization of the personality structure through the process of character analysis and the resolution of unconscious conflict.

The book begins, as did the field of group therapy, with a review of psychoanalytic contributions to the model. The authors in Part I take the position that training in psychodynamics is the foundation for the development of a competent group therapist. From this base the clinician can go on to practice in a variety of settings and with a wide range of patients. The authors here write from the perspectives of the major psychoanalytic theories. In Chapter 1, Kauff puts forth the classical psychoanalytic group therapy position. Pines and Hutchinson then cover the group-as-a-whole school, often associated with the British school of Melanie Klein and of Wilfred Bion. Margaret and Howard Baker apply the tenets of self psychology—the work of Heinz Kohut and his students—to group psychotherapy in Chapter 3.

Part II finally offers in print substantive information on groups in hospital settings, where so many actual therapy groups occur. The adaptations of technique and the expansion of theory that have emerged from working in these settings are put forth by authors with specialized expertise in these settings. In Chapter 4, Stone presents a model that applies the basic principles of group psychotherapy to the most profoundly and chronically psychiatrically ill of our patients. Kibel applies these principles to the most acutely ill of our patients in Chapter 5, and Rice looks at work with these patients and the professionals who care for them in the context of the community meeting in Chapter 6. In Chapter 7, Kennedy writes about group therapy with a partially hospitalized population that combines certain aspects of those populations covered in the three preceding chapters. Brook then describes medication-focused work with a related population. Shifting to medically ill patients, Lederberg looks at the needs of medical professionals who care for the severely ill in Chapter 9, Stern examines the rehabilitation of medical patients in Chapter 10, and Whiteman Carroll considers how group therapy can aid in meeting the needs of the patients' families in Chapter 11.

Part III introduces the reader to the world of homogeneously formed groups, and the authors examine how special populations can be helped by group psychotherapy. The advantages and compromises that ensue with the clustering of homogeneous groupings of patients are the focus of these chapters. Riester examines the application of group psychotherapeutic principles to adolescents in Chapter 12, and MacLennan addresses work with those at the other end of life in Chapter 13. Frost and Golden and her co-authors cover work with two specific populations that present major public heath issues in Chapters 14 and 15: patients who have tested positive for the human immunodeficiency virus (HIV) or have acquired immunodeficiency syndrome (AIDS) and patients who abuse substances, respectively. Completing this section, van der Kolk explores the use of group psychotherapy with patients who have posttraumatic stress disorder in Chapter 16.

Part IV explores three special situations not commonly covered in volumes on group therapy. It deals with some pragmatic issues that surround the practice of group psychotherapy. In Chapter 17, Porter discusses the advantages and the problems of combining group and individual psychotherapy, as well as the indications for and implementation of such a treatment plan. Lymberis then writes about the legal and ethical concerns surrounding the practice of group therapy, and Cohen offers a practical chapter on how to add groups to a practice that is focused on individual treatment.

Part V examines new advances in theories of gender development, with special regard to how these have an impact on work with patients in group therapy. Doherty and Enders cover women's development in Chapter 20; Krugman and Osherson write about men in group therapy in Chapter 21.

Part VI looks at some of the ways group therapy is practiced beyond the more traditional long-term or inpatient models. In Chapter 22, MacKenzie writes about time-limited group theory and technique. Fay and Lazarus then explain the theory and practice of cognitive-behavioral group therapy.

Part VII offers a splendid and extensive review of current research on group therapy by Dies in Chapter 24.

Part VIII moves to the training needs of the group practitioner. This section is of particular relevance to the teacher of group therapy. In Chapter 25, Alonso proposes models of training and how they relate to the current clinical climate. Swiller and coauthors then address the question of process (experiential) groups in the training of group clinicians in Chapter 26. Finally, in Chapter 27, Bader offers guidelines for conducting a training event, such as a workshop for teaching aspects of group therapy to other clinicians.

The reader is invited to sit back and enjoy a cornucopia of knowledge about a truly fascinating and powerful treatment opportunity for our patients.

References

Durkin HE: The Group in Depth. New York, International Universities Press, 1964
Wolf A, Schwartz ED: Psychoanalysis in Groups. New York, Grune & Stratton, 1962
Yalom ID: The Theory and Practice of Group Psychotherapy. New York, Basic Books, 1970

Introduction:
The Case for Group Therapy

Anne Alonso, Ph.D.
Hillel I. Swiller, M.D.

Philosophical Considerations

People thrive best in a community that values their participation and protects their dignity. The essential capacity of the infant to delight and engage potential caregivers through smiling, gurgling, and eye-to-eye contact is built into the fabric of human attachments. So too are the instinctual responses to the infant that comprise the foundations of caregiving behaviors. In this psychological birth of the child, biological patterns unfold within the context of a unique interpersonal matrix and a shared cultural environment. The child's impact on the important others in his or her world and their influence on the child interact synergistically to form a maturational environment that either supports or frustrates healthy development. Ultimately, mature mental health is characterized by mutually enhancing interdependence.

This integration of mind, body, and social context is vulnerable to assault from problems in any one of these dimensions. When problems occur, people suffer and seek our help for their suffering. Group psychotherapy offers the opportunity for purposefully created, closely observed, and skillfully guided interpersonal interaction. Such interactions can positively influence the countless varieties of human distress and malfunction. Distorted perceptions of others, inefficient communications, inadequately discharged affects, stereotyped behaviors, impulsive actions, alienation, and so on, can all be addressed and modified within the therapeutic group.

Theoretical Underpinnings

A broad range of theories informs the practice of group psychotherapy. In the psychodynamic spectrum, the classical analytic emphasis on libido and aggression finds expression in the unconscious forces that propel the group as a whole along its epigenetic trajectory. Object relations theory finds in groups a natural environment for the projections of internal part-objects onto the other members and the gradual reintrojection of the split-off aspects of the self within the containment of the group envelope. Self psychologists recognize the mirroring and empathic possibilities among committed members who can serve as selfobject functions for one another. Sullivanians and other interpersonal psychologists stress the healing that comes from the real relationships among the members, and the feminists see in groups an opportunity to examine the impact of gender on environment and vice versa, as do others interested in the specifics of gender development along the life-span. Cognitive-behaviorists see in the group model the opportunity to rethink and learn about cognitive distortions from trusted colleagues, and biologically oriented theorists are beginning to validate the benevolent synergy between physical healing and psychological healing in groups.

What Happens in the Therapy Group?

Multiple efforts have been made to isolate and name the curative factors in group therapy. Taken together, these factors can be integrated into the following description of the healing process in group therapy:

1. *Vital enactment of the characterological dilemmas of the members.* In the group, every member is bound to *have* his or her problems, not just to talk about them. Difficulties and distress are not simply recounted; they are enacted and experienced. Members can feel their own authenticity, their powerful affects, the tolerable exposure of their injured selves, and the support of others. They can learn how they are experienced by others and how their own perceptions may be distorted. Group members have the opportunity to observe the interpersonal skills and deficiencies of others and to experiment with methods of interaction that are new to them. They can learn both the universality of human anguish and the uniqueness of the potential value of every individual.

2. *Exposure and the resolution of shameful secrets.* Exposure is universal in groups. Many individuals who seek treatment are initially reluctant to join a group for fear of exposing their "secrets" and their pathology to strangers. Many clinicians harbor this same fear for their patients and for themselves and may be reluctant to recommend such treatment. On the

other hand, a distressed patient's shame and doubt almost always lead to self-judgments that are more severe than external reality warrants. Patients in groups experience enormous relief when they find that others who are clearly their peers have similar secret fears and act in similarly ignoble ways, and yet can make compassionate responses to one another. Shame and guilt flourish best in the darkness of isolation. Pathological shame and guilt are best healed by being exposed to light in a carefully monitored empathic interpersonal environment in which one is surrounded by others who are concerned for that person's and their own well-being.

3. *Support around the universality of the members' wishes, fears, and distress.* The kind of therapeutic exposure available in group therapy includes the patient in the universality of human pain. Group therapy is a source of unique support. Patients and referring clinicians frequently ask for a supportive group. Of course, no treatment is useful unless the patient feels respected. Any group that is to be effective must be supportive in that manner. But there are other dimensions of support that may ultimately be even more useful. Support means much more than simple positive regard. Candor and nonjudgmental containment of primitive affects are every bit as healing. The greed, envy, and hatred that are locked within our patients also seek expression in a setting that can tolerate and confront the dark sides of the soul.

4. *Reintegration of split-off aspects of the self.* As the split-off and unconscious parts of the self emerge in the group, they can be viewed first in the mirrored response of the others and finally take on the scale of ordinary human failings, capable of being dealt with, forgiven, and resolved.

Technical Applications

The clinical case for group therapy is the main concern of this book. We are dedicated to the position that the treatment of patients in group therapy is a primary option for the definitive treatment of human suffering and psychopathology.

In the decades since its inception with Dr. Joseph Pratt in Boston, group psychotherapy has established itself as a clinical field of astonishing vigor, scope, and validation. A vast array of professionals have embraced its principles and methods. Psychiatrists, psychologists, social workers, psychiatric nurses, and pastoral counselors are its practitioners. So are other medical professionals not directly involved in mental health, as well as experts from organizational development and education. When a theory or method enjoys such broad-based support, it is reasonable to deduce that it touches on some fundamental and universal truths in the human experience.

The needs of patients and their capacities to use help vary enormously depending on their pathologies and their strengths. Unremarkably, the techniques of group therapists also vary greatly, but a single fundamental resource unites them all: the presence of the group. The ideas and the techniques of group therapists vary greatly, but all group therapists, by the very nature of their work, believe in the healing, educational, and growth potential of other human beings.

Benefits for the Group Therapist

In addition to its therapeutic effectiveness for patients, group therapy presents the clinician with a number of advantages. Anyone who has observed an individual patient begin to work in a group is familiar with the amazing gains in the therapist's understanding of this patient that were not available in the individual hour. Beyond what the clinician can learn about the patient, there is much to learn about oneself when conducting a group. Caught in those same group processes of resonance and amplification, the clinician has the advantage of observing his or her own character and countertransference reactions afresh and of continuing the work of self-understanding and personal growth.

Among the many gratifications of being a group therapist is that group therapy is artistically and scientifically fascinating. If storytelling is the first art, then directly observing the interdigitating of several human stories as they unfold is a privilege of the highest order. Group therapists are the beneficiaries of the generosity of patients who open their lives and their selves to their therapists. The unconscious processes that unfold in a group deepen the awareness of the interpersonal dimensions of health and pathology, as well as the impact of the system on intrapsychic experience. The clinician is free to step back and to make space for the personal and the "tribal" stories to emerge. Groups offer the clinician a perspective from which he or she can step back and observe without disengaging from the empathic bond, as might happen if he or she were to take this kind of distance in the dyadic hour with the patient.

A pragmatic reality confronts patients and their healers. The finances of mental health care delivery are stretched drastically. The economics of group psychotherapy are obvious and cannot be ignored in this era of limited resources, cost containment, and managed care.

One of the most important advantages of group psychotherapy is its ability to extend optimal mental health services to more of those in need of treatment. It is incumbent on all of us to make the best care available to a population who are underserved by the private sector because of limited financial resources. Many patients who cannot afford individual therapy, or who can afford it only through subsidized public clinics, can afford group psychotherapy with the most senior clinician.

To Whom Is This Book Addressed?

This overview of the field is offered as a guide for the novice as well as a review for the more experienced clinician. The reader will find that some of the chapters are basic and some assume more sophistication in the field, yet they all have a clinical focus, with the exception of the in-depth review of the research in the field. Many clinicians who have never specialized in group therapy are now finding themselves interested for a variety of reasons. Some wish to add a new option to their own practice. Others find themselves administering group programs in a health maintenance organization or an inpatient unit. Some may wish to refresh their knowledge with a look at what's new in the field. Clinical faculty may wish to use some of these chapters for part of their curriculum.

In the words of one reviewer, the book is designed as "a warm companion to any student in the field." The broad range of readers to whom we address ourselves parallels the breadth of the field of group therapy and theory. Finally, the group stands as a strong statement of all the ways that group therapists help people help one another to learn, to grow, and to heal.

PART I

Long-Term Psychodynamic Therapy Groups

CHAPTER 1

The Contribution of Analytic Group Therapy to the Psychoanalytic Process

Priscilla F. Kauff, Ph.D.

> "Most of us have just one story in us; we live it and breathe it and think it and go to it and dance with it; we lie down with it, love it, hate it, and that's our story."
>
> Carolyn See, *Golden Days*

Introduction

It is commonly believed that personality change and concrete alteration in the course of one's life is the intended outcome of psychotherapy, of whatever variety. Although there is truth in this belief, the ultimate task of psychoanalytic treatment is not change, per se, but rather to *set the conditions* for change and further growth. The process is fundamentally one of inquiry; the overall goal is to articulate as much as possible and to understand what can be understood. The psychoanalytic process aims at telling the "story in us" as clearly and completely as possible in order to *maximize the individual's control* over that story, both during the treatment and long after it has terminated.

Forces originating within both the individual and the treatment situation conspire with external factors to complicate the analytic process. When the forces are intrapsychic, they are understood to reflect in part the patient's resistance to treatment and as such constitute a specific expression of the pathology targeted for treatment. The same is true to

3

the extent that intrapsychic forces find their expression in transference resistance, a part of the fiber of the relationship between therapist and patient. Again, such factors become a critical target of the treatment process.

The evolution of the dyadic treatment modality (including the role of the analyst and the specific techniques he or she uses) has been shaped by the goal of successfully dealing with the transference and resistance of the patient. Although some specific techniques have had rather humble beginnings, they have survived over time because of their (sometimes unexpected) contributions to this effort. The use of the couch, for example, a technique initiated by Freud as much to circumvent his own self-consciousness as to facilitate his patient's regression and free association, has endured in large measure because of its effectiveness in encouraging the emergence of transferential feelings that might otherwise have remained inhibited.

Similarly, the use of the dyad, the traditional patient-doctor mode of consultation, has consistently exhibited certain features that appear to be therapeutic in and of themselves. For example, the dyad has been likened to the mother-child unit; the dyad, merely by being a continuous, dependable interaction, serves a "holding function" (Winnicott 1965) for the patient, with its own positive therapeutic consequences. The safety, security, constancy, and privacy of the dyad, coupled with the presumed undivided attention of the therapist, are unquestionably conducive to the rigorous self-examination of which the psychoanalytic process largely consists. These factors in turn, combined with the intense emotional ties that such an intimate, persistent relationship generates, facilitate self-revelation and the emergence of the transference.

On the other hand, the dyad has both intrinsic limitations and some disadvantages as the sole modality for treatment. For example, the secondary gains of the recapitulation of the mother-child unit can, particularly in a long-term treatment, engender exaggerated dependency on the therapist, which may in turn take on a pathological life of its own. The "undivided attention of the analyst" is at best an approximation, and the patient unwittingly competes with the internal life of the analyst for that attention. The privacy of the dyad, helpful though it may be in encouraging the patient to share his or her inner life, depends on a structure in which only one other person is listening and only one other person is responding to the patient's communications. And that one person brings to the dyad his or her own limitations, which affect communication and understanding—sometimes in critical ways. Beyond the countertransferential pitfalls to which any therapist may be subject, the requirements of proper analytic behavior (e.g., neutrality and abstinence) can become liabilities because they prohibit certain kinds of responses from the therapist that may be necessary to the ultimate success of the treatment. Similarly, the regression that the intense emotional climate and the use of the couch can generate may itself become a serious pitfall for patients whose ego strength is less consistent than it appeared at the start.

Analytic group therapy originally developed in the hands of practitioners who, most often for practical reasons, ventured out of the security and privacy of the dyad into the more hectic world of the group to carry on treatment. These pioneers, among them Henriette Glatzer, Helen Durkin, Alexander Wolf, and Wilfred Bion, typically did not arrive at the use of a group modality in a deductive way based on a metapsychological rationale. Nor did they, at a more concrete level, initially turn to the group to circumvent the technical or operational limitations of the dyad mentioned above. A fuller awareness of the advantages of the group has been a long, largely post hoc process.[1] Articulating the logic that supports the use of the group modality and explaining the clinical effectiveness that it has consistently demonstrated have required a continuing effort, of which this chapter is a part. To that end, the significant contributions of the analytic group to the analytic process generally are considered in detail, both in terms of the group's capacity to exceed the limitations that may be encountered in the dyad and in terms of the therapeutic power that it independently generates.

---

[1] Over the course of its development, there have been some serious metapsychological arguments offered as a rationale for group treatment, among them the impressive discussions by Foulkes and Anthony (1965) and by Bion (1959), each of whom suggested that a multiperson modality for treatment more closely fits the intrapsychic and developmental realities of human existence as they conceptualized it. At the far more practical end of the spectrum, Durkin (1964) argued that group members benefit ipso facto from sharing the treatment stage, because "all members share the same basic drives and the same mental structure, albeit in different proportions. They have lived through the same epigenetic phases and experienced analogous conflicts at each level of development. That each member has found his own effective or pathological resolution of his conflicts . . . merely serves to enrich their communications and provide opportunity for acquiring wider horizons while arriving at a more complete personal determination" (pp. 3–4).

Basic Theoretical Considerations

Group therapy was originally developed by clinicians schooled primarily in the use of the dyadic modality. Most students today follow the same route (i.e., training in the traditional patient-therapist modality precedes training in group). Psychoanalytic concepts of pathology and treatment are also typically first learned in a dyadic framework. Transforming the treatment context from one to many requires more than the expansion of the treatment boundaries; it simultaneously requires altering some fundamental concepts to accommodate both the new data that the group modality will yield and the unfamiliar forms that some of the old material will assume. Similarly, some group treatment techniques differ significantly from those appropriate to the dyad, and the relevant technical changes need to be absorbed and understood by the prospective group practitioner. Such changes in concept and technique, to say nothing of changes of treatment modality, must be set within a comprehensible overall framework. Techniques without a theoretical substructure are like unguided missiles. There is little point in arguing the legitimacy, clinical validity, or ultimate usefulness of group therapy as a mode of psychoanalytic treatment without clarifying its place within the overall conceptual framework of which it is a part.

All clinicians evolve belief systems—personal theories, as it were, whether articulated or not—as to the nature of psychopathology and how it is meant to be treated. Such belief systems typically reflect those theoretical frameworks that best fit one's personal conceptual proclivities. They are also intimately connected at a practical level, whether or not the connection is immediately obvious; that is, our theoretical assumptions spotlight the material to which we attend, guide our understanding of it, and largely determine how we intervene or respond in the treatment setting.

Students of Freudian theory are familiar with the relevance of theoretical framework to the specifics of technique. Each of the five major models of mental functioning that have characterized the theory (i.e., the topographic, economic, genetic, dynamic, and structural models) has made its own particular contribution to the understanding of the nature and/or origins of psychopathology. Even more to the point, each model has built into it some more or less complete notion of how that psychopathology is best treated. The topographic model, for example, postulates that the contents of the mind are layered into strata differentiated by their proximity to conscious awareness. These strata, appropriately enough, are designated "conscious," "preconscious," and "unconscious." Within this model of psychic functioning, psychopathology is understood to result both from the amount and kind of mental contents residing in ("repressed in") the unconscious. The impulses associated with such mental contents continuously attempt to penetrate the successive barriers through the preconscious into conscious awareness. The pressure generated by these intruding impulses gives rise to anxiety, symptom formation, and other defensive maneuvers. To properly treat the resulting pathology, an appealingly simple, logical track dictates that one must make the unconscious conscious, clearing the paths and exorcising the dybbuk, so to speak. It is presumed that in doing so, the fallout consequent to the pressure generated by the buried contents will be relieved and the pathology alleviated.

With the advent of the structural model, emerging much later in Freud's work (1923), both the nature of psychic functioning and psychopathology as well as the prescription for its treatment changed. The model no longer proposed vertical stratification of mental processes but postulated instead three definable mental structures, the ego, the id, and the superego, each of which in turn had conscious and unconscious components. Within this model, psychopathology was no longer conceptualized as a function of buried mental contents pushing their way into consciousness but was defined in a more complex way (i.e., as a disequilibrium between the three psychic structures). Psychopathology resulted from the ego's failure to mediate adequately between the pressures of the instinctual drives and the superego's prohibitions against their gratification, succumbing instead to the conflicts in which it became embroiled. Typically, the ego also proved insufficient in dealing with the reality tasks of which it is meant to be in charge. Just as the motto "make the unconscious conscious" summed up treatment within the topographic model, the appropriate treatment of psychopathology within the structural model is summed up in the phrase "where id was, ego shall be." The guideline, in other words, is to restore equilibrium between the psychic structures such that the ego is able to maintain a comfortable compromise among instinctual life, superego requirements, and reality demands.

In the past several decades, as ego psychology has become increasingly prominent, the nature and quality of the ego's functioning have become increasingly significant as both a diagnostic parameter and a focus for treatment. In the most general sense, the ego is appraised in terms of the appropriateness of its responses and the effectiveness of its long-term solutions to the variety of developmental and adaptive tasks that fall within its provinces. Likewise, it is to the ego's deficiencies or failures that treatment is increasingly addressed. Within the framework of treatment, psychopathology manifests itself in its "purest," most accessible form in the transference process evolving during the course of therapy. Both the transference and the resistance mobilized against its exploration embody the individual's specific pathology; in other words, they are at once the product and the in vivo expressions of the ongoing difficulties or deficiencies of ego functioning. Thus it has been the hallmark of "psychoanalytic" technique that the focus of analytic intervention and exploration be on the resolution of resistance and transference, with relief of psychic distress expected as a consequence of such resolution.

Because ego psychology postulates that psychopathology is a function of inadequate, disturbed, or otherwise defective ego functioning, the sources of data as to that pathology need not be limited to treatment phenomena such as resistance and transference. Ego disturbances are expected to appear in the patient's behavior generally, in more or less obvious form, depending on the nature of the setting in which the behavior is observed. Whether reporting a dream or a primitive fantasy or functioning at top tilt in one's profession, *the same ego is in operation* and will show itself to be subject to the same difficulties. Of course, the degree to which pathology dominates experience or behavior will vary from case to case, but careful observation will reveal signs of its presence in every aspect of the individual's life, in or out of the treatment setting. Traditional indicators of psychopathology, such as its dystonic manifestations (active anxiety, outright symptoms, rigid defenses, cognitive or drive disturbances, and impaired object relations), will be ubiquitous, if in varying degrees. Moreover, it is understood within the ego psychological framework particularly that psychopathology is not limited to dystonic manifestations but will also appear in *ego-syntonic* forms such as enduring character traits, patterned or repetitive response to similar stimuli, fixed body postures or other physical characteristics, and the whole range of more active but nonverbal behaviors.

In this context, it is no accident that analytic group psychotherapy has flourished along with the shift to ego psychology as a prominent conceptual framework. The larger the window into the ego in action is, the more varied the opportunities to observe and the richer and more productive the data collection can be. Analytic group therapy as a treatment modality provides just such an expanded window through which to view ego functioning from its most glorious to its sorriest moments. (For a treatise on the impact of object relations theory to group therapy, see Chapter 2.)

Analytic Group Therapy and the Psychoanalytic Treatment Process

The fundamental techniques of psychoanalysis apply equally to individual and group treatment. The focus on the analysis of transference and resistance to improvement of ego functioning, as well as on expanding ego dominance over experience and behavior, characterizes psychoanalytic treatment in any form. In both group and individual treatment, resistance must be dealt with so that the transference is available for analytic scrutiny. When the resistance is characterologically determined and appears in combination with the transference (i.e., when it is incorporated into the syntonic, patterned, enduring behaviors and attitudes of the patient), the group modality is often more effective in facilitating the analytic process than is the dyad modality.

Although the overall technical approach and the goals of psychoanalytic treatment in both the group and the dyad are basically the same, there are some differences that should be considered. These include the sources of data, the question of regression, and the overall use of the group as a context for treatment.

Sources of Data

The primary data in analytic treatment are basically what the patient says, what he or she does, and how he or she "characteristically" is. No "id," "superego," or "defense mechanism" presents itself in an observable or tangible form. These are hypothetical constructs whose presence we deduce from the behavioral data (e.g., words, actions, and body communications) that are empirically available to us. It is from these immediate behavioral data that we derive our explanatory notions of unconscious material and defensive operations. Clearly, the more such data we have, the better. *The more we can see of our patient in action, the more we can understand about our patient and the more he or she can understand about himself or herself and alter what is potentially alterable.*

Although it is impractical in most instances to observe patients conducting their everyday lives (except in inpatient settings), it is advantageous to have as much opportunity as possible to observe patients under a variety of conditions. Observing patients in a psychoanalytic setting, in which there is some control over and some consistency to the stimuli, will in turn lend clarity to, or reduce confusion about, that which is observed.

Such observation created in the dyad is both enriched and limited by the carefully controlled stimulus condition that it offers. Although the dyad has the distinct advantage of there being only one other person in the room with the patient, thus more or less focusing the transference process on only one object, this very dimension generates its own problems (some of which are mentioned above). The sources of data that are available to the treatment are limited to patient reports, to the working relationship and the real relationship between therapist and patient (as observed by the therapist), and finally to the transference manifested in the treatment. Although the therapist can, of course, observe the body language of the patient and—over longer periods of time—the patterning of his or her responses to certain repetitive stimuli, the primary mode of communication is verbal. Verbal reports by a patient, whether in the form of free association, response to the therapist's interventions, or re-telling of experiences from outside the therapy room, per se, clearly require that the patient supersede his or her own resistance in order to provide a full account. In the traditional mode of analytic work, much effort is required to work through that resistance in the first place, a process that generates valuable data but also lengthens the treatment.

Although the group does not allow for the privacy and reduced stimuli of the dyad, it does allow for virtually all the same data to be gathered. What is sacrificed in terms of the "purity" of the transference (if such a thing exists) is more than compensated for by the direct observation of the patient's actual functioning and/or dysfunctioning. The group not only allows for the patient's own reporting of internal and external experience and for his or her perceptions of and responses to the therapist, but it also provides more people to whom he or she can respond and more people to react to him or her. The data are active, not passive. The arena for transference is extended from its traditional vertical axis to a horizontal one involving many different objects and even, on occasion, to the group as a whole.

Furthermore, because the stimulus conditions in the group setting are not generally subject to the patient's control, his or her responses are likewise less controlled. Although we may not get as "pure" a picture of the transference, we do get a much more complete picture of the patient's character pathology in action. The patient's spontaneous, unedited responses and his or her enduring behavior patterns in response to both constant and occasional stimuli can be observed not only by the therapist but also by other patients and by the patient himself or herself. This far more complex portrait of the patient with all his or her strengths and weaknesses—this kaleidoscopic view of the person—is a direct function of a multimodal treatment situation.

The Question of Regression

Regression has long held a revered position in the psychoanalytic domain, both as a clinical phenomenon and as an important feature of treatment. One of its primary functions is to facilitate the exposure or clarification of fixation or other adaptive failures to which later psychopathology can be linked. Many aspects of the dyadic treatment situation coupled with traditional technique such as the frequency of meetings, the dependency on the analyst, the use of the couch, and analytic abstinence encourage the development of prolonged and intense regression.

It is unquestionably true that the group does not foster such regression; indeed, within the group context it is neither encouraged nor deemed necessary. In fact, with the exception of the sickest patients for whom only modified analytic group treatment would be appropriate in any case, prolonged regression almost never occurs. On the other hand, short-lived, intense, and sometimes very primitive regressions will indeed occur in the group, even within the least pathological patients (Durkin and Glatzer 1973). Such regressions are usually simultaneous with the emergence (often for the first time) of primitive, negative transference. These regressions often surprise the patient and the analyst alike because the dyadic situation tends to exclude such "outbursts" from otherwise extremely well-functioning patients.

The differences in regression as it occurs in the dyad and in the group raise some interesting questions. First, in the context of an ego-psychological view of psychopathology, regression may be far less critical in the treatment process than had been assumed earlier in the history of psychoanalysis when the vicissitudes of the libido were carefully tracked to locate psychopathological fixations. Rather, as the ego and its defenses have become more focal for understanding and treating psychopathology, the process and content of regression become *less* important than the *ego's capacity to deal with such regression* and its possible consequences. This is not to suggest that contemporary psychoanalytic treatment is interested only in structure and not in content. Certainly regression has been and continues to be a useful vehicle for revealing the specific content—usually primitive—of which the transference consists and which, of necessity, defines the topics discussed in treatment. But content is revealed in a variety of ways and in the group setting is often increased because the patient responds to so much. And because sporadic regressions do occur, the ego's ability to deal with and recover from them is also clarified.

Regression can be thought of in terms of the linear, chronological course that it takes (i.e., backwards in time developmentally). It also can be thought of in terms of the level of experience and the breadth of the emotional component it involves (i.e., a process in which the more primitive but still active layers of experience are exposed in their emotional context). Insight in the absence of emotion is of little value therapeutically; the contribution of regression in terms of the intensified emotional context that it generates cannot be underestimated. Indeed, transference as a primary vehicle of analytic treatment is crucial precisely because it provides an opportunity for understanding in an intensely emotional context.

To the extent that regression or a regressive process plays a part in transference, its contribution can be equally influential in both individual and group settings despite the different forms that it takes. In the dyad, it can best be understood as the prime vehicle for the release of primitive emotion and its associated content, which might otherwise be inaccessible in the more controlled two-person medium. In the group, because of the intense emotional climate that develops naturally among members, regression as a vehicle for emotional release is far less critical. When it does occur, it tends to be a sign that particularly primitive or sensitive material that far exceeds the ego's defensive capacities has been touched, thereby highlighting both important content and the vagaries of certain aspects of ego functioning.

The Analytic Group as a Context for Treatment

In the initial phases of dyadic analytic treatment, the most important aspect of the analyst's role is to establish the conditions necessary for the work to proceed. This task generally involves the delineation of the contract, the beginning of the working alliance, and the development of a trusting, dependable, uncritical environment. (For a more complete discussion of the working alliance, see Glatzer 1978.) The desired outcome is for the patient to be able to access his or her internal process and report that process to the analyst with minimal inhibition, including, of course, feelings and fantasies about the analyst. In other words, the intent is to establish the condition that is most conducive to free association and that will involve the least amount of resistance and maximize the potential for the transference to develop and unfold.

Similarly, in the group setting, it is the initial task of the group leader to help develop and maintain a method of functioning that will provide the conditions necessary for the analytic work to proceed most efficaciously. In the group, too, both the working alliance and the contract among the members regarding confidentiality, the parameters of the treatment, and the behavior expected from both patient and therapist must be established in the beginning phase of treatment. The contract is renegotiated whenever necessary throughout the life of the group. However, because the group is a multiperson modality, the goal is not simply to foster the association process in each individual involved. Transference and resistance are not limited to the patient-analyst dyad. The situation becomes more complex in the group, where there are many individuals interacting and reacting. The increased sources of data provide the analyst with a multitude of options and challenges. Relevant and important material can come from the individual alone, from members, from the individual interacting with member(s), and from the group as a whole unit.

Analytic group therapy is no more monolithic than psychoanalytic theory as a whole. All the available data can potentially provide the analyst and patient with rich material, but the focus of the therapist's attention varies significantly from leader to leader. The many approaches to the specific use of the analytic group modality as a vehicle in the overall analytic process are differentiated primarily by the preferred sources of data and the processes deemed necessary to collect data. These differences among analytic practitioners become clear when their underlying theoretical assumptions are articulated.[2]

It is equally true of group and individual therapists that one's view of psychopathology and what is required to treat it will dictate the chosen treatment approach. When we add the therapist's concept of the *role of the group* in that treatment process, the source and kinds of data that he or she will seek and the nature of the interventions that he or she will make will logically follow. Three major orientations can be identified.

---

[2] The material that follows has been presented in much greater detail in an earlier publication (Kauff 1979).

First, the group can be used primarily as a *setting* for treatment, in which the most important interaction is that between the analyst and patient at any one moment. Pathology is seen as originating and located within the individual, and it is the individual who is the primary object of treatment. Second, the group itself can be seen as the *object* of treatment. In this orientation, psychopathology is understood to be located in the group as a whole. Treating the psychopathology requires treating the whole group. Third, the group can be used as a significant or even the sole *agent* of treatment. Although pathology in this orientation is generally viewed as located in the individual, the designated object of the treatment, it is the therapeutic power of the group that is mobilized to treat pathology.

The group as a setting.   The use of the group as a setting for treatment is best exemplified in the work of Wolf and Schwartz (1962). As rigorous adherents of the earlier models of psychoanalysis (topographic, genetic, and economic), they understood psychopathology to be located intrapsychically, a function of repressed, conflictual material, the specifics of which were expected to emerge into consciousness during treatment. The role of the analyst was to "take the lead in the search for unconscious processes by promoting free association, the analysis of dreams, resistance and transference" (Wolf and Schwartz 1971, p. 250). Because the growth and differentiation of the individual was a major goal of treatment, these practitioners tended to be quite wary of any involvement with the group or so-called group processes, which they considered to be mythical. Rather, they viewed the group as merely a collection of mutually interested individuals who could contribute to the treatment of a fellow member in any number of ways, all auxiliary. They could listen and give support, empathy, and suggestions. They could also act as alternate objects of the transference but were not expected to be involved in that transference or its interpretation, a job reserved for the analyst. For the analyst to attend to "group phenomena" or the "group process" was considered by Wolf and Schwartz to be sabotage to the goals of treatment.

In the actual practice of group therapy, this model most resembles individual analysis in a group setting. Although it requires little revision of technique, it also does not take advantage of the power of the group as a therapeutic agent. On the other hand, it does retain some of the particularly therapeutic aspects of the dyad, especially the opportunity to focus exclusively on one individual's unconscious process and to pursue it in depth, while making treatment available to many patients at once. This was clearly desirable because individual unconscious processes were, for Wolf and Schwartz, the source of pathological perception and behavior in adults and therefore the most appropriate targets for treatment.

The group as an object.   The view of the group as the object of treatment, a model that has come to be known as the "group as a whole," owes its origins to the early work of Bion (1959). Bion's metapsychology, largely governed by the object relations theory of Klein (1968), led him to a basic principle quite the opposite of that of Wolf and Schwartz, namely, that the individual cannot truly be understood outside of his or her group membership. From an object relations point of view, that is, psychological life is shaped by the development of and the interaction among internal objects and the impact of the internal object world on perception and reality testing. Following Klein's lead, Bion held that pathology is largely preoedipal in origin, that the anxieties that lie at the root of most adult psychopathology are quite primitive, and that a rather major regressive process is required for those anxieties to be revealed in treatment.

Furthermore, Bion held that group participation, per se, functions to revive these anxieties, which in turn trigger precisely the regressive process needed. Bion called these group regressions "basic assumptions," defined by attitudes, fantasies, and emotions clustering around and defending against primitive (psychotic, in Bion's framework) anxieties. They represent a collective effort of the group to resist the emergence of early psychotic material underlying the psychological life and pathology of each member. Thus the group, for Bion, is required at once to expose and to treat pathology. The only appropriate target for treatment in Bion's model is the commonly shared anxieties and defenses of the group as a whole (although the individual remained the presumed beneficiary of the treatment).

According to Bion, the role of the group leader is to understand and interpret the group resistance. This role dictates the peculiar technique of leadership that has come to be known as the *Tavistock method,* named for the clinic in which Bion developed and wrote about these techniques. The leader's task is to abstain from interventions of any kind except those directed toward the psychotic anxieties of the whole group as they manifested themselves during group meetings. To address the individual or his or her anxieties apart from the group is a technical error viewed by him with the same gravity as Wolf and Schwartz viewed the notion of the mythical "group," that is, as a sabotage of treatment.

The group as an agent.   Most contemporary analytic group therapists do not subscribe to either of the rather extreme positions outlined above. Rather, as might be expected, techniques that focus on the individual at times and on the group at others tend to be more common. Indeed when the group is seen as a potentially powerful agent of treatment, focus shifts back and forth from the group to the individual quite freely. The direction of the intervention is toward the source of the resistance to treatment at any moment in time (i.e., individual or group resistance) and is guided generally by an intent to facilitate the processes ongoing in the group. Although this tradition began partly with Foulkes and Anthony (1965), it was developed in the United States during the many decades of the work and writing of Durkin and Glatzer (1973).

The notion of group process is critical to the understanding of an orientation that deliberately cultivates the group as a therapeutic tool. The term *group process* refers to the product of the spontaneous verbal and nonverbal interaction among the group members and the group leader. In a metapsychological extension from individual to group dynamics, Foulkes and Anthony (1965) described a process that he called "group association" as follows:

> In the group, the minds of strangers with a totally different individual conditioning are reacting and responding to each other. . . . Their responses, verbal or non-verbal, conscious or unconscious, to each other's productions, can be used as quasi-associations to a common context. . . . We now treat associations as based on the common ground of unconscious instinctive understanding of each other. . . . We accept that ideas and comments expressed by different members have the value of unconscious interpretations. (p. 29)

Group process is the closest analogue in the group setting to the free-association process in the dyadic setting, and the leader is dedicated to facilitating this process throughout group treatment. The unfolding of the group process resembles that of free association but exceeds intrapsychic boundaries and moves both to a horizontal plane (among members) and to a vertical plane (member or members to therapist). It involves the whole array of transference and resistance, ego function and dysfunction, and symptoms and character defenses that we would hope to see revealed in the intensive individual setting. The working assumption in this model of group therapy is that if the group process operates at full tilt (i.e., if the resistances, group or individual in origin, are consistently and successfully addressed), the many mutative forces of the group will also operate at maximum capacity to the benefit of each individual member. In this sense, the group process is both a product and an agent of the analytic process as it is carried out in the group. It ultimately becomes the medium through which the group can serve an interpretive function and make a wide variety of other mutative interventions. Thus the group process has a curative force of its own while serving as a condition for individual growth.

The Group Process as an Agent of Treatment: Clinical Example

Group therapists frequently inherit patients with character pathology that has proven partly or wholly resistant to prior treatment. Such patients may return to therapy many times over and, in fact, are often referred to a group therapist by colleagues as a "last resort." Chronic character pathology is infamous for such resistance, especially when its origins are developmentally early (as in oral character pathology).[3] The problem becomes even more severe when the character pathology has as one mode of expression the tendency to act out.

Treating character pathology in the dyad has proven to be a hard row to hoe. Anna Freud (1966) was certainly correct in claiming that it is " . . . responsible for most of the technical difficulties which arise between analyst and patient." She contended that both the syntonicity of character pathology and the fact that it enters the transference primarily as a defense make it uncommonly hard to reach in analytic treatment. Certainly the entrenchment of character pathology, its "life-or-death quality," is well known to clinicians, who so often feel frustrated if not defeated by it. However, treatment problems should be looked at not just from the point

---

[3] Character pathology, as used here, refers to enduring, repetitive perceptions and responses that become a part of the individual's behavioral repertoire over a long period of time. These behavior patterns may be verbal or nonverbal. They may appear only in response to certain situations or develop a life of their own, becoming typical of the individual's style. Character pathology is ego syntonic, anxiety free, and experienced as part of the self, and it is most elusive from a treatment point of view. It is a manifest product of the ego's early attempts to solve developmental problems in a less-than-successful way, becoming (in Anna Freud's words [1966]) "permanent defense phenomena." In treatment, character pathology will present in the patient's behavior and as a part of the transference resistance.

of view of the pathology, per se, but also from the perspective of the modality that is enlisted for its treatment. For example, the combination of intractable patient resistance with the constraints on the analytic therapist can prove lethal when character pathology is treated in a dyad. The analyst is required to be neutral, objective, and in control of his or her countertransference even in the face of the profoundly negative transference and rage that so typically accompany this kind of character pathology. As such, the analyst is prohibited from many kinds of responses that are open to members of a therapy group and that have proven to be exceptionally helpful to patients under these circumstances.

Acting out,[4] on the other hand, can present some serious challenges to the therapy group, challenges that are circumvented in the dyad. Group therapy is, by definition, a more active-reactive modality than is individual treatment. Observable behavior is part of the modus operandi of the group: "Action," in the sense of active interacting with others, is considered one of the group's assets compared with the more exclusively verbal dyad. Understandably, action is an asset only when it is in the service of the treatment; the line between expressing oneself nonverbally and acting out is a thin one at best. Clearly the group as a multiperson modality may be highly vulnerable to contagion when one member acts out. The therapist, too, is more vulnerable to provocation when faced with a potentially serious threat to the group while his or her own behavior is being scrutinized. The likelihood for countertransferential episodes is thus increased, and the potential for the therapist to unconsciously provoke or collude with acting out is likewise greater.

On the positive side, however, when properly facilitated, the group process can be extremely effective in containing and dealing with acting out for many of the same reasons that it is so uniquely effective with character pathology in general. The following example, involving a case of acting out in a masochistic character, illustrates both the unique power of the group modality and the specific function of the group process in dealing with this particularly knotty psychopathology in an analytic framework.

---

[4] *Acting out* as used here refers to behavior by the patient that substitutes for the verbal communication of material in treatment in such a way that the material as presented is not accessible to analytic intervention. The motivation for such behavior is unconscious or not otherwise in the patient's control and is governed by the repetition compulsion. The patient is aware of his or her actions but not of their origin or meaning. Such behavior is typically irrational and inappropriate, yet it is experienced by the patient as reasonable and syntonic.

Case 1

The following events[5] occurred in a training group conducted quite far from the participants' homes. During the initial phase of the group, issues of trust, confidentiality, and so forth were raised, and a preliminary working contract was evolved. During this process, Ms. A expressed her conviction that the leader would turn out to be a "good, strong, analytic type," a feeling that she said pleased her though she did not know why.

Early on in the group Ms. A shared her anger at the airline for overbooking her flight, thereby casting doubt on her previously "guaranteed" passage home. She had had a heated interchange with the airline's manager, who apparently had then complained to the organizers of the training program about the "intolerable" behavior of one of their participants. The organizers, in turn, feared that the problem was escalating and might threaten the entire program. The leader was brusquely put "on alert."

When the group resumed after a break, the leader waited to hear the members' response to the airline situation. Many of the members had actually had the same problem with the airline and were therefore readily able to commiserate with Ms. A's plight. Their empathy encouraged Ms. A to continue with her story, which now revealed her growing indignation and some rather alarming fantasies. Specifically, she told the group that she was planning to avenge herself against the airline by joining forces with other similarly abused participants and launching a retaliatory offensive. She had thoughts, for example, of "leaking the story to the press," "going into court," and so on.

When the leader tried to question why Ms. A's reaction should be so much stronger than the reactions of other group members to essentially the same situation, Ms. A responded with anger. She declared that the therapist could not possibly understand the humiliation she had suffered nor was her "healthy and assertive response" to the situation being credited. The group reacted quite quickly and accurately to the self-destructive component in the seemingly "healthy" picture that Ms. A was presenting. They understood the meaning of the therapist's original comparison between Ms. A's intense reaction and their own more moderate one to the same situation. They understood that an irrational component was at work in Ms. A, causing her to overreact, and set about gently but persistently questioning her as to the lengths she was prepared to take her case. In so doing they were able to raise a doubt in Ms. A's mind as to the appropriateness of this heavily rationalized behavior, a doubt that the therapist could not even suggest. Ms. A seemed so vulnerable to narcissistic insult from the

---

[5] Some of the material to follow has appeared in an earlier publication (Kauff 1978).

therapist's comments that it was clearly the better course to let the group take over. The therapist also felt relieved at this effective mobilization of the group process in a situation where the acting out was threatening not just Ms. A and the group but virtually the whole program.

As the group progressed and Ms. A. began to feel more comfortable with the other members, she shared with them some of her other feelings that were being disguised by her ubiquitous anger. Being away from home seemed to intensify feelings of loneliness and vulnerability, which in turn led to fantasies of being persecuted by the airline, which was "preventing" her access to her own home. As the group members shared similar feelings, Ms. A. opened up even more. She had threatened the airline manager, she told them, and he responded by a counterthreat to have her arrested and sued for libel. Again, the group gently challenged her behavior. This time, however, Ms. A. shifted into a defensive mode, demanding that the group not challenge her in any way. She had a fantasy, she said, that they were part of the underground in a Third World country. Would they, she wondered, reveal each others' names (especially hers!), even under torture? Needless to say, the group was rather taken aback by this fantasy and especially by the extent of her demand for loyalty. There were only two choices in this dichotomized world view: absolute loyalty or total abandonment. At this point, the leader intervened, suggesting that Ms. A's persistent hostile in-teraction with the airline had been, at least in part, a test of the group's loyalty all along; in other words, would they "rip her off" and betray her as she felt the airline had or would they stand by her?

The group picked up on the leader's suggestion that Ms. A was acting out an unconscious plot, carrying the interpretation one step further by comparing her behavior with that of Mr. B, another member. Mr. B had been dealing in the group with a long-standing belief that people never identified him as separate from his twin brother. However, it quickly be-came apparent that he himself almost compulsively raised the subject of his twin. Often in relating events to the group he made it very unclear as to whether he was talking about himself or his brother. When he finally slipped and called himself by his brother's name, Ms. A was among the first to see that Mr. B was masochistically ensuring the very confusion with his brother that he consciously found so painful and wished to avoid. The group was quick to use this opportunity to point out to Ms. A that her sensitivity to Mr. B's behavior was a signal of its similarity to her own uncon-scious, equally self-defeating behavior. They began to help her explore the difference between what she consciously feared and what she uncon-sciously set up. The group encouraged her to explore her need to repeat the humiliation and betrayal she suffered vis-à-vis the airline by setting up such an excessive test of loyalty for the group that they were sure to fail her eventually.

At last Ms. A revealed a childhood memory[6] in which her best friend had fired a water pistol at her and told her afterwards that it was filled with poison. Ms. A remembered becoming extremely depressed and spending many anxiety-ridden hours preparing to die. The group and the leader then tried to help Ms. A make the connection between this memory and her fantasies about the group. Would the group betray her as she felt her childhood buddy had done? And continuing the thread of unconscious "set ups," now a theme in the group, they reinforced the interpretation that her demand of total loyalty from the group was unconsciously designed to lead to betrayal and thus recapitulate the betrayal by her friend.

Before the end of the training program, Ms. A was able to see more clearly the nature of her masochistic acting out as it had become delineated in her interaction in the group. She understood that this was not a one-time event; she often acted out a similar masochistic pattern, unconsciously setting up a betrayal that would subsequently justify acting out self-righteous rage. With the support of the group, she withdrew from the battle with the airline. Following the others' less pathological reactions to the same situation, she recanted her threats against the manager (albeit a bit grudgingly) and found herself another means of transportation home. The group afforded her the opportunity to observe, understand, and work toward altering a specific, significant piece of her overall character pathology.

Some Specific Contributions of Group Therapy to Analytic Treatment

In Case 1, the group as a treatment agent was able, often with more ease and efficacy than was the therapist, to help Ms. A question her own behavior and to introduce a dystonic element into an otherwise heavily rationalized, ego-syntonic behavior pattern. Group members were able, by their support, their questioning, their personal associations, and their associating in her stead, to help Ms. A through the process of exploring the unconscious meaning of her behavior and to identify some of the roots of that meaning. They were able to help her form the rudiments of a genuine working alliance that, it is fair to speculate, might never have begun had the therapist alone been responsible for accomplishing the job. Facing up to the underlying, avoided material is both

---

[6] The degree to which this "memory" itself was a fantasy or screen for more primitive material was not considered in this case because of the time-limited nature of the group. Had this been an ongoing group, the matter would have been pursued further, reinforcing and extending the gains made by the patient reported here.

frightening and painful and requires the best of the group, the therapist, and the patient to achieve. That the group was the primary vehicle
of intervention went a long way toward circumventing Ms. A's vulnerability to narcissistic damage in the exploration of her acting-out behavior. Many critical aspects of the therapy group played a role in this
positive outcome.

In this section some of the most important of these aspects are considered in more detail to further elucidate the role of the group in analytic
treatment.[7] Although the focus is on character pathology, it should be
remembered that these group factors are not dependent on diagnosis.
They simply become easier to identify when applied to more extreme or
more visible forms of pathology.

Foremost among the treatment requirements in dealing with character pathology are 1) in the intrapsychic domain, to make that which is
syntonic become dystonic (uncomfortable) to the patient, and 2) in the
interpersonal domain, to help the patient experience the transference as
a pathological phenomenon because it, too, tends to be quite ego syntonic. In both instances, the therapist in a dyad can be seriously hindered.
One general problem is that the syntonicity actually serves an important
defensive function. The very approach of the analyst in treatment, regardless of how delicate the approach may be, is often felt as dangerously
intrusive to the whole defensive structure that the patient has erected and
carefully maintained, often for most of a lifetime. Intended to operate
against the exposure of the most negatively experienced parts of the self,
this defensive structure tends to be protected at all costs. This is particularly true when the ego involved is very fragile. As the resistance begins
to relax, intense negative transference often makes its appearance, sometimes accompanied by such intense rage that the therapist is seriously
challenged countertransferentially.

Many aspects of the group, per se, and the group process as it unfolds
in that setting can be of assistance, to a large extent correcting for the
potential limitations of the dyadic modality. To stay with the example of
making that which is syntonic into a dystonic experience, the group has
several advantages. Group members can behave in many ways that are
specifically prohibited within the confines of acceptable behavior for the
analytic leader. Group members are not required to be neutral or objective. On the contrary, they are encouraged in the therapeutic contract to

---

[7] For a more complete discussion of the contribution of analytic group therapy to the
treatment of preoedipal character pathology, see Kauff (1991).

be spontaneous and uninhibited in their verbal responses to one another. Understandably, they are likely to be much more frank and confronting than the therapist could possibly be. Individually, they will say what they want, not limited by another member's demands or defenses. As a group they will not respond according to the patient's expectations, but will instead provide a new stage on which the old behaviors are played out. The patient will thus be faced with an unfamiliar, often negative, and surely unsettling response from his or her fellow group members to old, familiar (i.e., syntonic) behaviors that he or she had come to count on. To quote Alonso and Rutan (1984): "The member who brings syntonic character pathology into a group will soon find himself walking into brick walls of reality testing from the other members" (p. 1380). This phenomenon, typical of the group process, is often the first clue to a patient that he or she has been engaged in pathological behavior of which he or she was previously unaware.

To the extent that analytic data in the dyad come mainly from the patient's verbal reports as well as from his or her interaction with the therapist, the visibility of character pathology (which can be as subtle as it can be blatant) is often very minimal. Patients themselves do not view such pathology as problematic; it is "just me" behavior, both familiar and highly rationalized. Similarly, patients cannot report on the unconscious components (i.e., the dreaded fantasies, prohibited wishes, and unacceptable feelings that are being defended against). But group members do not have to depend on that which is reported. They do not need to be told; they can see how another member acts, reacts, and interacts in a richly stimulating yet controlled situation that is deliberately designed to encourage each member's most spontaneous behavior. As a result, they have an extensive view of each other's functioning, from the most pathological to the most adaptive.

Severe character pathology is often accompanied by a highly punitive superego, which increases the resistance against revealing more deeply buried, negative parts of the self. The therapist of the dyad has only his or her neutrality and objectivity, combined with the trust the patient is able to develop (oftentimes rather scant), to mitigate against such harsh superego prohibitions. The therapy group, in contrast, offers a unique opportunity for the patient to observe other people. When a heterogeneous group of individuals is brought together and encouraged to speak freely and behave in a spontaneous fashion, it is inevitable that at least one member will say or do precisely what another member vigorously defends against saying, doing, or feeling. When given the opportunity to observe that the anticipated drastic consequences do not occur, patients are often freed for the first time from the strangling constraints of their own defenses. They have been provided with a "bird in the mine" that the dyad can never offer. Until the patient finds it tolerable to deal with such expelled parts of the self (i.e., until the punitive superego is sufficiently neutralized), the group can allow the patient the relatively anxiety-free opportunity to expose or test the waters at his or her own pace. The patient actually gets a chance to anticipate a set of consequences different from those that he or she typically fears or expects, setting the stage, at least, for possible new behavior. In this sense, the group becomes a benign reality against which the overly punitive superego rarely survives in full force.

Related to the "bird in the mine" is the opportunity for group members to "mirror" one another in a very off-target way. In or out of therapy, people are generally able to see in others what they cannot or refuse to see in themselves, often with a speed and accuracy that surprises everyone concerned. In a therapy group, patients learn that when their own issues are being touched—including those of which they may not be aware—they are often unusually perceptive in detecting unconscious determinants of another's behavior. This experience is the beginning step toward acknowledging the presence in oneself of similar, previously rationalized or repressed problem areas.

As the rigid character structures start to relax, defended material often emerges in sometimes strenuous, negative transference. Such a transferential experience requires the support and empathy of the group because it can be both terrifying and painful to the patient involved. And although it is a necessary step in the course of treatment that such transferential material reach the level of outright expression in order to be subject to analytic interpretation, the therapist of the dyad frequently is handicapped in this function precisely because he or she must serve at once as the object and the interpreter of the transference (Racker 1968). In other words, the object of persecutory fantasies is hardly in a position to deny the reality of those fantasies; he or she is not even able, in many cases, to provide the support or empathy that must precede any effort at interpreting the more pungent transferential fantasies. The therapist of the dyad is even further hindered because his or her interventions are so often experienced as intrusive. In addition, because interpretations imply something unknown and therefore out of the patient's control, they are frequently experienced as a blow to the patient's omnipotent fantasies of self-sufficiency and can result in a major narcissistic wound in some instances (Glatzer 1969). Thus the therapist of the dyad can find his or her hands firmly tied behind his or her back just when he or she needs the greatest latitude in responding to the patient.

Members of a therapy group, on the other hand, are free to perform virtually all of the specific tasks that may be beyond the therapist's purview in such instances. To start with the most obvious difference, there is more than one other person present with the patient; thus there is the option for someone other than the therapist (the *transferentially negative object on most occasions*) to do the talking. To have a peer speak is usually far less threatening than to have an authority speak. Members of a therapy group are typically much better able to tolerate anything from simple comments to "plunging" interpretations when they are offered by another member than when the same ideas are offered by the therapist, regardless of how diplomatic his or her wording may be. Group members can and do speak as the therapist cannot. They are encouraged to confront and contradict other members' distortions. They are encouraged to interject reality when a fellow member's reality testing wavers or fails, as it does by definition in the transference process. They can literally say to one another, for example, "Dr. X never said that!" or "That may be how you perceived it, but you seem not to have realized what was really happening." And they are able to make such startling statements because of the horizontal trust that seems to develop inevitably in a well-functioning group, constituting for some patients the only working alliance they have yet achieved.

Group members can also pinch hit for another function: the capacity to associate. All patients lose this capacity on occasion, and the failure is often pervasive in patients who act out. Association is one of the critical tools of analytic technique because it facilitates access to material that has disappeared from (or sometimes never entered into) conscious awareness. Resistance easily interrupts this critical function, and the therapist in the dyad is constantly faced with the task of working through the resistance sufficiently to restore the associative process. Again, because they are not operating under the constraints that dictate proper analytic abstinence, group members can aid in the restoration of the associative process in at least two different ways: First, they can take over the associative process for the member, recalling what they have learned of the patient's history and what they have observed of his or her behavior over time. Using this information, they can literally associate for the member, saying things such as "That reminds me of what you said you felt as a child with your brother." Second, they can also associate to another member's material as if it were their own, thus using their thoughts and feelings as a substitute associative vehicle. In both cases, group members can retrieve unconscious material for a member who is unable to do so for himself or herself.

Patients typically become increasingly adept at associating for and with one another, a skill that greatly enhances the analytic process. Group members are able to perform this function largely because they are not under any prohibition against self-revelation. On the contrary, not only is self-revelation the very core of the working alliance in any treatment contract, but in group therapy it involves more than one patient and benefits more than just the patient revealing his or her associations at any moment. In addition, particularly for the more narcissistically vulnerable patient, the intimate sharing of thoughts, feelings, images, memories, and so forth that goes on during the process of mutual or reciprocal association has the secondary benefit of cushioning the narcissistic blow that interpretations from the therapist often seem to deal.

As the treatment progresses, and negative transference appears more readily, the therapist in the dyad may be subjected repeatedly, over a long period of time, to a barrage of negative affect. This is very difficult for most therapists to handle and is uncomfortable at best for virtually all therapists. In such cases, the therapy group can be enormously helpful, providing safety in numbers and serving as a haven for patient and therapist alike. The patient feels protected against imagined retaliation from the therapist for his or her "bad" behavior and also expects that the group will be able to help him or her control the worst of his or her real or imagined destructiveness. Similarly, the therapist feels protected by the group from the intense impact that negative transference and outbursts of rage can create. The presence of other group members grants the therapist time to recover from the impact and allows an opportunity to control any retaliatory countertransferential impulses that may have been provoked. In this sense, the group acts in a supervisory capacity, often interjecting reality for the therapist who is temporarily impaired. At the least the group's help gives the therapist an opportunity to shift gears and find a more salutary way of going forward.

Conclusions

The importance of detailing personality structure and functioning increases dramatically when the origins of psychopathology are considered to be less important than the individual's ability to successfully live his or her life. Such detailing requires as much creativity as is possible within the confines of the analytic situation. Analytic group treatment accelerates the process and enriches the scope of psychoanalytic treatment. It capitalizes both on the salutary aspects of the group, per se, and the group process generated among its members, frequently compensating for the inherent limitations in the dyadic modality. The analytic group adds a unique dimension to analytic inquiry, to the understanding of and the ultimate course of the story it aims to unfold.

References

Alonso A, Rutan JS: The impact of object relations theory on psychodynamic group therapy. Am J Psychiatry 141:1376–1380, 1984

Bion WR: Experience in Groups. New York, Basic Books, 1959

Durkin H: The Group in Depth. New York, International Universities Press, 1964

Durkin HE, Glatzer HT: Transference neurosis in group psychotherapy: the concept and the reality, in Group Therapy, 1973: An Overview. Edited by Wolberg LR, Schwartz EK. New York, Intercontinental Medical Book Corporation, 1973, pp 129–144

Freud A: The Ego and the Mechanisms of Defense. New York: International Universities Press, 1966

Freud S: The ego and the id (1923), in The Standard Edition of the Complete Psychological Works of Sigmund Freud, Vol 19. Translated and edited by Strachey J. London, Hogarth Press, 1961, pp 3–68

Foulkes SH, Anthony EJ: Group Psychotherapy: The Psychoanalytic Approach. Baltimore, MD, Penguin Books, 1965

Glatzer HT: Working through in analytic group psychotherapy. Int J Group Psychother 19:292–306, 1969

Glatzer HT: The working alliance in analytic group psychotherapy. Int J Group Psychother 28:147–161, 1978

Kauff PF: The interplay of countertransference, acting out, and the group process, in Acting-out, Acting-in, Acting Up: The Proceedings of the 5th Annual Conference of the Group Therapy Department, May 7, 1978. New York, Washington Square Institute for Psychotherapy and Mental Health, 1978, pp 7–33

Kauff PF: Diversity in analytic group psychotherapy: the relationship between theoretical concepts and technique. Int J Group Psychother 29:51–65, 1979

Kauff PF: The unique contributions of analytic group therapy to the treatment of pre-oedipal character pathology, in Psychoanalytic Group Theory and Therapy: Essays in Honor of Saul Scheidlinger. Edited by Tuttman S. New York, International Universities Press, 1991, pp 175–190

Klein M: Contributions to Psychoanalysis, 1921–1945. London, Hogarth Press, 1968

Racker H: Transference and Countertransference. New York, International Universities Press, 1968

See C: Golden Days. New York, Macmillan, 1986

Winnicott DW: The Maturational Process and the Facilitating Environment. New York, International Universities Press, 1965, pp 37–56

Wolf A, Schwartz EK: Psychoanalysis in Groups. New York, Grune & Stratton, 1962

Wolf A, Schwartz EK: Psychoanalysis in groups, in Comprehensive Group Psychotherapy. Edited by Kaplan H, Saddock B. Baltimore, MD, Williams & Wilkins, 1971, pp 241–291

CHAPTER 2

Group Analysis

Malcolm Pines, M.D.
Sylvia Hutchinson, B.Sc.

Introduction

The origins and development of group analysis lie in the pioneering work of S. H. Foulkes (1898–1976), a German psychoanalyst who came to the United Kingdom in 1933 (Pines 1983). What distinguishes group analysis from other approaches is its unique integration of psychoanalytic concepts within an open-systems, Gestalt framework that underpins both its theory and practice. Foulkes's exposure to the Gestalt ideas that flourished in Germany in the 1920s and 30s came mainly through the work of Goldstein, a neurobiologist whose emphasis on figure-ground relations and the determining effect of the total situation made a deep imprint on Foulkes's thinking. After psychoanalytic training in Vienna, Foulkes was appointed clinical director of the Frankfurt Sociological Institute, which was closely linked with the Frankfurt Psychoanalytic Institute. Together these institutes explored the possible integration of psychoanalytic theories of personality with sociological models that linked society to the person. These influences significantly shaped the development of group analysis in Britain and are clearly evident in Foulkes's writings (Foulkes 1948, 1964, 1975; Foulkes and Anthony 1965).

Gestalt, which conceptualizes our experience as being determined by the patterning or organization of its elements, permeates all aspects of group analysis. Gestalt postulates that what we see as "figure" is relative to "background" of other aspects of the whole and that the whole consisting of parts in relationship is different from the mere sum of the parts. Group analysis attempts to deepen our understanding by contextualizing experience and behavior as broadly and as deeply as possible (including the observer as part of the total field). In this holistic approach, Foulkes regarded the individual as an abstraction that acquires meaningful definition only in a social or relational context. The language of group analysis describes open, living communicative systems in dynamic equilibrium; these systems may be viewed from multiple perspectives. Each generates particular configurations and patternings that acquire meaning and validity in relation to a context.

Into this frame Foulkes incorporated his deep commitment to psychoanalysis, which he regarded as holding the key to the most profound insights and understanding of unconscious mental processes. Where he diverged, basically and explicitly, from classical psychoanalysis was in the importance ascribed to social influences. He rejected the Freudian notion that human social nature is a derivative of instinctual forces and instead ascribed primacy to it (Pines 1986).

In systemic terms, psychoanalytic and group-analytic models share the notion of a system in equilibrium, but they differ radically in the nature of the underlying paradigm. In energic terms, the Freudian tension-reduction model is a relatively closed system that operates according to mechanical principles to maintain a stable state of homeostatic equilibrium. The Foulkesian model, on the other hand, is based on a biological-organismic paradigm; it is an open system defined in terms of meaningful information, powered by social psychological forces. It is a system in

> . . . dynamic equilibrium. Dynamic means that it is never in a state of rest, has constantly to adjust actively to the ever-changing circumstances, milieu, conditions in which it lives. Such adaptation, however, does not take place mechanically following physical or chemical principles merely; there is always a creative element present, even in the simplest forms of adaptation. . . . Dynamic equilibrium therefore means the active and creative maintenance of a good balance. (Foulkes 1948, p. 1)

The incompatibility of Foulkes's basic paradigm with the Freudian model was not explicitly addressed in Foulkes's writing. Like that of Winnicott (Davis and Wallbridge 1981; James 1985), Foulkes' purely relational approach was not presented in opposition to Freudian theory. Perhaps if he had lived to write the promised theoretical companion volume to *Group-Analytic Psychotherapy—Principles and Practice* (1975), the contradictions would have forced further clarification. Instead, the evolution of group-analytic theory has seen the incorporation of psychoanalytic language consistent with the basic group-analytic blueprint of a relational matrix as primary. The language of structural and instinct theory has gradually disappeared. Psychodynamic concepts describing interactive processes (either intrapsychic or interpersonal) such as transference, projection, introjection, and projective identification are part of the basic grammar of group analysis.

The growth of group-analytic theory is singular in its capacity to absorb and integrate language and constructs from different theories consistent with its basic model. Paralleling its developmental model of growth as an open interactive system programmed to enhance its order, complexity, and coherence, the theory itself grows by what it can share with other theories. This constant cross-fertilization and reintegration enlarge and enrich our understanding.

Object relations theorists who emphasized the crucial role of the context both in development and the therapeutic situation (e.g., Winnicott [the holding environment] and Bion [containment]) provided models consistent with group analysis and a language that it can share (James 1985). Their notions of holding and containment are metaphors for the basic maternal functions that are essential for healthy growth. Winnicott and Bion focused, respectively, on the essential mothering function of providing a constant, stable, and "holding" enough environment and on the maternal capacity to transform painful affect by containment. It becomes evident during the course of this chapter that these constitute basic functions of the therapeutic group, underscoring the importance that Foulkes attributed to the conductor's capacity to create a culture in the group of safety, support, and tolerance (i.e., a "holding and containing" culture to enable therapeutic work to take place) (Zinkin 1989).

Contemporary developmental theorists studying the nature and development of early communication systems between mother and infant have a significant contribution to make to group analysis, particularly in its study of early communication systems in groups. Similarly, recent theories of self psychology offer a paradigm consistent in essence with group analysis (Pines 1985, 1987).

Comparison of Group Analysis With Tavistock and Other Group-as-a-Whole Models

There is frequent confusion about the group-analytic approach and the Tavistock group-as-a-whole approach. The source of this confusion may reside in their shared early history of psychoanalysts experimenting with group-dynamic approaches to the treatment of neurosis in wartime England. The work of Bion and, later, of Foulkes at the Northfield Military Neurosis Centre gave rise to two distinctly different models. Definition of the conductor role as adaptive and flexible clearly differentiates group analysis from the Tavistock approach, in which the task was narrowly defined as interpreting the basic assumption culture (Bion 1961) or the common group tension (Ezriel 1973). The frame in the latter instance is contracted to exclude all but a view of the dyadic relationship between the group as a whole and the analyst. The mobile perspective that characterizes group analysis, with its constant monitoring, contextualizing, and recontextualizing of all interactional components, including the conductor (i.e., therapy in the group, of the group, and by the group), contrasts sharply with the fixed-frame Tavistock model (i.e., therapy of the group, by the conductor).

The group-analytic conductor is mindful of the group-as-a-whole framework but is free to comment on and to interact with individual members. The validity of this freedom is both theoretical and practical. Changes in any one group member inevitably induce changes in other members of the group, who are participants in the group system. Changes in the one person facilitate the mobilization and activation of issues in the other members, which thus become available for therapeutic work (Pines 1989).

If the conductor restricts himself or herself solely to observations on the group as a whole, this will lead to a therapeutic situation where the conductor ceases to conduct (Brown 1985). To conduct is to identify themes, to recognize patterns, and to bring into play elements that contribute to the group process. To conduct is not only to make verbal interpretations. To conduct is to understand, reflect, and bring into play, enabling the "players" to recognize the process they are engaged in. Thus the conductor may sometimes closely engage with some member or members of the group to work with issues that they present such as resistance, depression, and isolation. The conductor's activity is a form of modeling that enhances the members' ability to participate therapeutically.

The conductor who restricts himself or herself to group-as-a-whole interpretations is invariably endowed with omniscience and omnipotence and is experienced as remote. The boundary between conductor and group member becomes clearly and strictly defined, and this is not to therapeutic advantage, although many have thought it to be so. For across this boundary the vital processes of mutuality, state sharing, and intersubjectivity do not develop. The therapist then reenacts the role of the distant giver who is not in tune with the needs and fears of the members. The group members have to adapt to the therapist either in compliance, submission, or rebellion, and the group becomes excessively leader centered. Each conductor has to find his or her own style, in which the therapist's role remains clearly defined but which nevertheless allows him or her to keep in close touch with the affective life of the group.

Some models, for instance that of Ezriel (1973), rely excessively on object relations theory to define group processes. The therapist relies on the activation of mutual projection and introjection cycles that result in a common group tension. The conductor believes that the interpretation will lead to resolution of the restrictive model. This model does not allow for the creativity of the group members, who constantly evolve new patterns of understanding and of relationship. In turn new experiences evolve that were unpredicted by the conductor and not necessarily understood at the time. The development and subsequent internalization of such new experiences comprise one of the processes of therapeutic change, which can be understood in terms of "corrective family group experience" (Grotjahn 1977) or of "transmuting internalization" (Kohut 1978).

Group-Analytic Therapy

Group-analytic therapy uses as its prime resource the group matrix—the network of interrelationships that evolve in a group. Its methodology guides practitioners in the creation and use of a dynamic group matrix to fulfill therapeutic aims. The standard group-analytic group has seven to nine members unknown to each other outside the group setting (the "stranger" group), meeting at regular intervals over time and bound by rules confining communication among members to the group setting. Members are encouraged to free-associate in the group in the absence of imposed task or structure. This basic structure allows for a shared observational field and a multidimensional frame (in which the shared history of the group interacts with the collective histories of individual members). This provides a backdrop against which ongoing communicative processes in the group may be articulated. The frame includes within it communications at many different levels, verbal and nonverbal, conscious and unconscious, and is constantly expanding as the interaction in the group over time adds to the total field (Pines 1984a, 1985).

Translating communication into meaningful language that can be shared and exchanged leads to the growth of an increasingly complex and coherent group matrix (Hutten 1983). Participation in this process, the constant interplay between embedding and differentiating the self from the group matrix, provides opportunities for restructuring psychic systems via processes of externalization and internalization. This in turn allows the individual to reintegrate aspects of the self that have been dislocated.

"Matrix" is the concept that refers to the developmental history of an analytic group, based on the communication network laid down by its participants over time. This communication network is the base on which a therapeutic group develops a form of psychological organization. It consists of shared experiences, evolving relationships, and growth in understanding. This shared history lays down the "dynamic group matrix" and evolving context against which transference patterns emerge, recur, and are experienced by all the group members who participate in their recognition, working through, and resolution (Roberts 1982).

The resolution of old patterns cannot be separated from the exploring of new ones (Pines 1990). The therapeutic power of the analytic group does not lie solely in the recognition, understanding, and working through of relationship issues that lead back to the past. The importance of doing so varies from person to person according to his or her own personality formations and the power of the neurotic interference in his or her psychic development. For some persons it is crucial to identify and to work with this neurotic interference because their problems lie in latent developmental potential that has not yet been released. But what nearly all group members are able to do is to engage in new ways of relating that will be sanctioned by the norms developed by the group. When these norms are facilitating, new ways are encouraged. When they are restrictive, old patterns will be reinforced (Whitaker 1985).

The working tools and constructs of group analysis guide the conductor in his or her task of observing and receiving communications on many different levels and in translating and organizing these data into communicable form. Foulkes (1990) defined *translation* as the essence of the therapeutic process. The theory provides a set of multifocal spectacles with which to view the matrix.

The group analyst attends both to the here-and-now patterns of interactions and communications, the ongoing dynamic *process,* and to the habitual, relatively stable, and continuous relationship patterns that occur over time and form the *structure* of the group. The *content* of communications is shaped by the process and structures through which they are transmitted (de Mare 1972; Foulkes 1964).

We can view the communicative process from various angles:

1. The level of current reality—directly observable by all participants.
2. The transference level (whole object level). Here the focus is on the manner in which different systems interact and link together—the transference of characteristic organizational features from one system to another, between intrapsychic systems of individual members, between members and the group as a whole, between members and the therapist, or various combinations of these.
3. The projective level (part-object level), which describes the movements and interchange of parts of members' intrapsychic systems (aspects of the self) and their relocation within the group network as a whole, and vice versa.
4. The primordial-collective unconscious level of communication (Foulkes 1964; Usandivaras 1986).

The following case example of a group session (as the 10th meeting) is used to illustrate a typical, multiperspective group-analytic view:

Case 1

The group began by commenting on how punctual the conductor was and how reliable she was in maintaining the time boundary. Then there was a tense silence, which Ms. A, giggling, tried to relieve by engaging Mr. B and telling him it was difficult to catch his gaze because he looked away. Mr. B told the group there was a neurological basis to his "shifty" look: he was only capable of discrete eye movements rather than steady object-tracking. He joked about dementing and said soon the group will have to hold his hand crossing the road.

While Mr. B was making light of his presentation of himself as a damaged and dependent object, Ms. C burst in. She described a "most terrible experience." She had just met two acquaintances nearby and had been caught out trying to cover up that she was a patient at hospital X. The group members readily shifted the focus away from Mr. B and onto Ms. C, sharing their anxieties about the social stigma attached to the label "psychiatric patient," and attempted to provide her with an alternative positive perspective of what it meant to be a member of a therapy group. Mr. D mischievously suggested that she should say it was something exotic like "rebirthing" or that it was mixed sexes and we all came here to strip.

A discussion followed of what kind of treatment group therapy was and what it meant to be having it. Did it mean being mad or dangerous? Mr. D talked of how it raised insurance costs. Mr. B countered with how, if you murder someone, treatment could be regarded as mitigating circumstances. The conductor pointed out how the balance between cost and benefit being described may reflect the balance between the painful demands of therapy and the holding and protection that it offered. The conductor's role in the group was discussed, and she was invested with omniscient and omnipotent powers—as the one who knows who they are and why they are here, and doesn't say.

Mr. D returned to the question of how members came to be in therapy, reminding us of Mr. E's account last week of the waking nightmare of dying and being annihilated that had precipitated him into treatment. The group, in an atmosphere of intense concentration and attention, resonated to the theme of recurrent anxiety dreams and nightmares. Mr. B disclosed his recurring anxiety dream of not turning up for, or failing, examinations. Mr. D shared with us his memories of an anxiety-ridden late childhood and recurrent nightmares of his pajamas turning to concrete—of being paralyzed and encased in concrete.

Mr. E encouraged others to talk. Ms. A told of an old recurring dream of being in a swimming pool with a shark or crocodile about to attack her mother and her feeling paralyzed. Ms. C said her dreams either were about unrequited love or were holocaust-type dreams where everyone, including her, is wiped out. Mr. D described a waking dream about a woman and stated his belief that this nightmare was the final trigger leading to his breakdown some years ago. He dreamed that she was the only person left who cared about him and he killed her. Mr. F, when asked, told us that he either did not dream or didn't remember his dreams.

Ms. C then elaborated on her chronic anxiety about destruction in the world and that harm will come to her mother. She revealed with some embarrassment that she used cleaning rituals to magically prevent something terrible from happening to her mother. Mr. E told of his walking to the group tonight and avoiding all the cracks but couldn't relate this to a particular anxiety. Mr. B chimed in that he counted car number plates and all was well if he didn't get the number 666!

The group then looked at the question of when a connection or link is meaningful and when it is coincidental. Ms. A told us that her ex-partner, with whom she had lived for many years, had returned and wanted to establish their relationship. Was the timing meaningful? She talked of her ambivalence—her longing for intimacy and fusion and her awareness that the relationship couldn't offer her what she wanted.

The conductor, having so far said little, now attempted to tease out a common theme in what had been presented—the anxiety about being in a dependent, helpless, or paralyzed state; the juxtaposition of images of mothering with those of annihilation and destruction; and the juxtaposition of images of closeness and fusion with separation and death. The conductor suggested that the emergence of these themes may be linked to her announcement at the end of the previous group of the oncoming break 4 weeks hence.

The group rounded on the conductor, unanimously rejecting this connection. She felt accepting of their refusal as she was aware that they had no experience yet of a break in the continuity of the group's life. She left it there as a link to be made available to use later. The issue of the break was then taken up, with Mr. D expressing surprise that there were any breaks and Ms. A and Ms. C denying the significance of them.

As the group drew to a close, Mr. F provided a voice for the denied feelings of dependence and need, expressing his frustration that the break was occurring at a time of maximum stress and anxiety for him in that he was getting married over Easter and feared a relapse into an acute anxiety state. After the group ended, Mr. F returned in a state of some agitation— he had mislaid his wallet.

In this group, reaching out to belong to each other and to find meaning in their common identity, group members took an active role in creating a facilitating environment for growth. All members participated in a free-floating discussion, sharing feelings about being a group member, sharing recurrent nightmares, and linking inner worlds of destruction and terror to the external reality that the internal worlds dominate.

The conductor's activities, leading the group in articulating common themes and linking the content to the context, were attempts to synthesize and integrate, to enrich meaning and enhance coherence. This is the view from the *current* level.

There were clear manifestations of transference in this group session, not (so much) between members but rather between the group as a whole and its relationship to the conductor and between one member, Mr. F, and his relationship to the group as a whole. The conductor accepted without challenge the group's transference onto her of omniscient and omnipotent qualities, holding for the group the strength and safety to contain experiences of helplessness, hopelessness, and despair. Mindful of the needs of the group, the conductor will step down from her pedestal in response to evidence of the group's increasing capacity to locate its own strength and wisdom in the group as a whole and its individual members. This movement has been described by Foulkes (1964) as a crescendo in the authority of the group and a decrescendo in the leader's authority.

Mr. F's direct expression of his dependence on the group and his frustration at the timing of the break was a manifestation of his *transference onto the group as a whole* the power to nurture and hold him safe and protect him from catastrophic anxiety. The group was idealized and protected him from his split-off and deeply repressed rage. He willingly positioned himself in the dependent role, and it took some time (well into his second year in the group) for him to allow into consciousness the anger and hate that go with the inevitable failure of the idealized parent.

Although projective processes were not clearly articulated in this group session, they were present in early form in the nonverbal communicative process. Mr. B, whose relationship to the group in the early stages was characterized by passivity and long periods of disengagement, presented a mirror surface to the group that was dark and empty, reflecting his isolation, hopelessness, and despair, and his fear of these overwhelming the group. Ms. A's attempts to engage Mr. B at the beginning of the group were part of a developing pattern (or structure) in which Ms. A took on the role of caring for Mr. B both inside and later outside the group-analytic field. For Ms. A, Mr. B acted as an electrical conductor to the pain that underlay feelings of helplessness and despair. When Mr. B risked bringing such feelings to the group, Ms. A would quietly weep. She could feel her feelings through Mr. B. It was only after much working through of depressive anxieties in the group at many levels that Ms. A was able to bring into the group her own despair and feelings of devitalization and her feelings of hopelessness at ever healing what had been broken and torn asunder.

Ms. C's deflection of attention away from Mr. B when she entered the group was also a pattern that repeated itself and reflected projective processes in the group. Her defensive distancing of Mr. B—her "not taking him seriously"—were linked to her fears of being, like him, isolated and depressed and of following his lonely path. Working through the reciprocal negative mirroring between Mr. B and Ms. C played an important part in their coming to terms with aspects of themselves that had previously been projected onto others (Pines 1984b; Zinkin 1983).

The search for underlying meaning and understanding always involves a recognition of, and an attempt to work with, transferential and projective systems. Many of the transferential distortions are corrected in the here-and-now ongoing interaction in the group; others may need articulating and analyzing, particularly when there is a "fit" between projective and introjective processes (projective identification). The importance of *mirroring* as a group-specific therapeutic factor was highlighted by Foulkes

(Foulkes and Anthony 1965). The *mirror phenomenon* is a higher-order dynamic concept based on complex processes of observing aspects of the self (both positively and negatively valued) in others and reclaiming projected parts of the self via identification processes.

Finally, Foulkes mentioned, but did not elaborate on, a fourth, more primitive view of the group: *the level of primordial images or collective unconscious* (see Usandivaras 1986). This view describes unconscious communication processes based on our shared identity as members of the human species sharing a certain genetic encoding and developmental programming. The collective-unconscious view is based on what Foulkes (1975) described as the "foundation matrix"—the basic culture that we all hold in common. In Case 1, the theme of separation and loss of the source of maternal security, triggered by the oncoming break, *resonated* in the group; it touched a deep chord in all members, who responded in different keys but to the same tune or shared structure. Participating in a resonating communicative matrix enhances a sense of belonging—of being embedded in the group matrix.

The Conductor: Tasks and Techniques

Having considered the key working constructs, we now take a closer look at the role and tasks of the conductor in group analysis.

The conductor's role in group analysis is conventionally described in terms of the dual function of the conductor as *dynamic administrator* and *analyst-interpreter.* The former term describes his or her executive functioning and is concerned with the *nontransferable* aspects of his or her role, in which the conductor is invested with the power and authority to make decisions affecting the creation, maintenance, and survival of the group. The latter term indicates that the conductor attempts to use the structure he or she has created and maintains to fulfill therapeutic aims. In this role the conductor's function is *transferable* to other group members, with the aim of the group itself becoming the agent of change (Hutchinson S: Styles in group analysis, unpublished paper, November 1986).

Conductor as Dynamic Administrator

Setting up a new group or maintaining the membership of a slow-open group (group-analytic groups tend to be either closed, fixed-term groups or, more typically, slow-open groups with a relatively stable membership) is a major part of the task of the dynamic administrator. The creative growth potential of a stranger group is laid down in the careful selection and preparation of patients for group analysis. Selection involves, in the first instance, an assessment of suitability for analytic psychotherapy (including motivation for change, capacity to use the analytic process, and so on). On the whole, most group analysts hold the view that patients suitable for psychotherapy can achieve therapeutic gains from either individual or group-analytic therapy, but that a group is the optimal setting for most such patients as it offers a richer, more stimulating context for therapeutic change (psychic inner restructuring) despite the reduced opportunities for methodical transference analysis.

The second crucial aspect of selection for group therapy is matching the patient, the nature of his or her problems, the degree of disturbance, and his or her current circumstances with the group and its composition, stage of development, holding and containing capacity, and culture.

The stranger group boundary, as defined by its fixed location in time and space, is both more and less flexible and accommodating than the individual boundary. For example, patients who are acutely depressed, distressed, or suicidal may need the flexibility of individual therapy with its possibility of increased frequency of sessions and its potential for greater direct and immediate control by the therapist over the analytic situation. Similarly, acutely psychotic patients who have lost or failed to establish a boundary between the self and other will need a more controlled and protected setting (groups in a special managed-care environment are possible).

On the other hand, some patients (e.g., borderline patients who may present the individual therapist with chronically negative transference responses that are difficult to endure) can be better accommodated in a well-selected and well-functioning group of neurotic patients. The transference effects are modulated by those patients who have capacities for understanding and responding that are not available to patients who are functioning at more primitive levels. In such groups of neurotic patients with one or two borderline patients, the basic parenting functions of holding and containment are combined with the developmental push to function at higher levels that characterizes good parenting (Loewald 1980; Pines 1978).

Once a group is set up and a relatively stable structure is established, the conductor's main task is to build a therapeutic culture in the group. This task includes

- Maintaining the boundaries
- Establishing therapeutic norms of tolerance and nonjudgmental acceptance
- Providing an atmosphere of safety, support, and containment; increasing participation and the range of expressiveness of members; and enhancing communication so that it becomes increasingly articulate and shareable

In his or her style of management and dynamic administration, the conductor brings to the group his or her internal authority relationships. The conductor presents the group with rules, exercises control, and enforces limits and may do so with varying degrees of firmness, consistency, and openness to challenge and questioning. The conductor's style will depend on how he or she carries the inherent contradiction between managerial function and the overall aim to facilitate the group becoming its own authority.

Styles vary according to whether they explicitly prescribe or implicitly model. If the conductor relies on prescriptive techniques (telling what and how to do) rather than modeling (showing by his or her own behavior what is appropriate and expected), he or she will bring to the fore issues of control and compliance in a way that does not easily allow for a "crescendo" in the authority of the group. Similarly, if the conductor uses social reinforcement to shape behavior rather than providing information and explanations about the purpose of rules and decisions, this will set the conductor in a fixed role that invites an adaptive response (e.g., submission and competition) rather than encouraging creative growth or self-initiated restructuring. Although prescriptions may sometimes be necessary and behavior shaping inevitable, their use was discouraged by Foulkes (1964, 1990), who warned against authoritarian-style leadership.

Conductor as Analyst-Interpreter

The interpreter-analyst role, on the other hand, is a complex one in which the tasks and functions are multifaceted, variable with respect to the stage of development of the group, and often paradoxical in their definition.

Foulkes (1964) urged the conductor to become a master of paradox by constantly directing him or her to function in the active and passive voice at one and the same time. The conductor "makes the group the instrument of its own therapy while he considers himself an instrument of the group" (Foulkes 1964, p. 57). The conductor is continuously concerned with directing the group to its own best benefit but he or she never does for the group what the group can do for itself.

The manner in which the conductor may address these therapeutic functions is infinitely variable; his or her effectiveness may depend on an appropriate balance between holding-containing activity and translating-analyzing activity.

In guiding the group toward establishing therapeutic norms, the conductor conveys his or her own characteristic way of saying yes and no simultaneously. He or she accepts all that is communicated while simultaneously resisting forces that block communication, change, and growth. The conductor's continuous assessment of the group's level of understanding and communication and its capacity to tolerate anxiety and other painful or threatening affects will determine how he or she holds the balance of these at any particular stage of its development.

How to accept what is communicated without colluding with or fostering defensive structures is the dilemma that constantly faces the conductor. Styles of noncollusive acceptance may vary; acceptance may be communicated nonverbally (by the quality of attention given) or verbally (by reflecting and clarifying in a way that conveys empathic understanding); failure to collude is communicated by attempts to translate communication and by facilitating the search for meaning (which will always involve a recognition of, and attempt to work with, transferential and projective systems).

On one hand, acceptance without structuring may lead to the development of a containing and safe group but one that does not promote growth and change. On the other hand, interpretations in the absence of adequate containing and acceptance may promote change at the cost of stability of membership, resulting in higher dropout rates.

Resistances in the form of blockages in the communication system are ubiquitous in groups. If a therapeutic culture has been established, the work of clarifying, analyzing, and translating the blockage is taken on by the group—accompanied by varying degrees of conductor participation, depending on the stage of development or particular circumstances impinging on the group at the time. Resistance may be expressed by acting out across the boundary (e.g., lateness, irregular attendance, and secret extra-group activity) and destabilizing the group, or it may be expressed by attempts to control the communicative process by imposing structures (e.g., turn taking), setting up antitherapeutic norms, resisting participation, or avoiding anxiety-laden issues.

The limits and potentialities of different styles of conducting manifest themselves most clearly in both the manner and the extent to which group resistances are worked through. It is here that the conductor's creative use of his or her own presence and skills has the most decisive impact on the developmental potential of the group.

A group-analytic view of resistance always involves the location of a resistant pattern within a framework (Sternberg 1982). A resistant structure controls and regulates change—it is set up in opposition to a real or imagined force that threatens the equilibrium or survival of the group. A conductor's relationship to an identified resistance varies according to the needs of the group. At the outset, the conductor will define his or her relationship to resistance as active or passive according to whether he or she directly intervenes to alter the resistance or allows the defensive structure to operate, intervening only in an indirect way by altering the context to facilitate the relinquishing of defenses. These different styles, broadly defined according to the directness with which the conductor interacts with the defense system, approximate the polarities occupied by the traditional versus the self psychological analytical approaches: the former emphasizing the "penetration-to-the-unconscious-via-the-overcoming-of-resistance model" (Kohut 1984, p. 113) and the latter emphasizing an "understanding of defence motivation in terms of activities undertaken in the service of psychological survival" (Kohut 1984, p. 115).

Let us examine these polarities more closely. A conductor may interact directly with a defensive structure in many different ways. He or she may describe and clarify and may engage in the analytic work of articulating the underlying conflict or threat that activates the resistance. He or she may hand over the analytic work of translation of the group. The manner in which the conductor does this may be more or less confrontational (Brown 1988) and challenging, or it may be empathic and providing of meaning and understanding. These metacommunicative messages are conveyed by the language used, the tone of voice, and the accompanying gestures.

Conductor Countertransference

Confrontation activity as an expression of conductor countertransference (i.e., the conductor's way of dealing with his or her own feelings and frustration, helplessness, and impotence in the face of resistance) is likely to harden resistant patterns or modify the form of their expression. This is especially true if 1) the conductor's confrontation activity simply reinforces transference projections (e.g., of the conductor as the demanding parent who can never be satisfied) or 2) they gratify attempts to locate such feelings in the conductor using mechanisms of projective identification. On the other hand, confrontation activity may shift defensive patterns if the countertransference is used to modify the transferential or projective aspects of the group's relationship to the conductor. For example, a group that collectively transfers onto the conductor the role of the anxious, fragile parent who needs protection from aggressive attacks may interpret the challenging behavior of the conductor as an expression of the conductor's capacity to sustain attacks. In such a case confrontation may shift resistance by failing to collude with the transference and by providing an alternative nonprotective model for relating (Skynner 1986).

In a similar vein, the effectiveness of interventions that reflect back and translate defensive structures in an empathic manner will depend on the degree to which they fit or gratify transferential or projective systems. If, for example, intensely envious feelings underlying resistance are expressed as a refusal to respond to a conductor's efforts to insert and attribute meaning, then the more he or she provides meaning or empathy, the more he or she fuels the envious attacks, thereby consolidating the resistance.

What we are suggesting above is that conductor styles that are either consistently confrontational or consistently providing and empathic will limit the group's potential development. As such, they may constitute countertransference impediments to the work. Skynner's work (1986) provides an elegant model for how the conductor may use his or her own presence to shift defensive systems. Flexibility of role and creativity of function in the conductor will enhance possibilities for the development of complex and creative group cultures.

Conclusions: The Expanding Frame

The group-analytic movement has rapidly grown and consolidated its professional identity. This is reflected in the expanding international network of the Group Analytic Society (founded by Foulkes in the early 1950s as a forum for the exchange of ideas about group analysis), in the vitality of its journal *Group Analysis,* and in the proliferation of training courses in the United Kingdom and Europe. The Institute of Group

Analysis, London, established in 1971, is responsible for training and professional qualification in group-analytic psychotherapy.

The scope of this chapter allows only a brief sketch of the wider application of group-analytic principles. These principles have been successfully applied to large-group therapy, family therapy and couples groups, and adolescent and children's groups. The eclectic but coherent multi-disciplinary features of group analysis are finding ever-widening application and form a very interesting and powerful sector in the field of group therapy.

References

Bion WR: Experience in Group and Other Papers. London, Tavistock, 1961

Brown D: Bion and Foulkes: Basic assumptions and beyond, in Bion and Group Psychotherapy. Edited by Pines M. London, Routledge & Kegan Paul, 1985, pp 192–219

Brown D: Confrontation in the group-analytic matrix: towards a classification. Group 12:191–197, 1988

Davis M, Wallbridge D: Boundary and Space: An Introduction to the Work of DW Winnicott. London, Karnac Books, 1981

de Mare PB: Perspectives in Group Psychotherapy. London, Allen & Unwin, 1972

Ezriel H: Psychoanalytic group therapy, in Group Therapy: An Overview. Edited by Wolberg LR, Schwartz EK. New York, International Medical Books, 1973, pp 183–210

Foulkes E (ed): Selected Papers of S. H. Foulkes: Psychoanalysis and Group Analysis. London, Karnac Books, 1990

Foulkes SH: Introduction to Group-Analytic Psychotherapy. London, Heinemann, 1948

Foulkes SH: Therapeutic Group Analysis. London, Allen & Unwin, 1964

Foulkes SH: Group-Analytic Psychotherapy: Methods and Principles. London, Gordon & Breach, 1975

Foulkes SH, Anthony EJ: Group Psychotherapy: The Psycho-Analytic Approach, 2nd Edition. London, Pelican Books, 1965

Grotjahn M: The Art and Technique of Analytic Group Therapy. New York, Jason Aronson, 1977

Hutten EH: Meaning and information in the group process, in The Evolution of Group Analysis. Edited by Pines M. London, Routledge & Kegan Paul, 1983, pp 151–166

James C: Bion's containing and Winnicott's holding in the context of the group matrix. Int J Group Psychother 34:201–214, 1985

Kohut H: The Search for the Self, Vols 1 and 2. Edited by Ornstein P. New York, International Universities Press, 1978

Kohut H: How Does Analysis Cure? Chicago, IL, University of Chicago Press, 1984

Loewald HW: Papers on Psychoanalysis. New Haven, CT, Yale University Press, 1980

Pines M: Group-analytic psychotherapy of the borderline patient. Group Analysis 11:115–126, 1978

Pines M (ed): The Evolution of Group Analysis. London, Routledge & Kegan Paul, 1983

Pines M: The frame of reference of group-analytic psychotherapy, in Spheres of Group Analysis. Edited by Lear TE. London, Group-Analytic Society Publications, 1984a, pp 20–28

Pines M: Mirroring in group analysis as a developmental and therapeutic process, in Spheres of Group Analysis. Edited by Lear TE. London, Group-Analytic Society Publications, 1984b, pp 118–136

Pines M: Psychic development of the group analytic situation. Group 9:24–37, 1985

Pines M: Psychoanalysis, psychodrama and group therapy: step-children of Vienna. Group Analysis 19:101–112, 1986

Pines M: Mirroring and child development: psychodynamic and psychological interpretations, in Self and Identity: Perspectives Across the Lifespan. Edited by Honess T, Yardley K. London, Routledge & Kegan Paul, 1987, pp 19–37

Pines M: The group-as-a-whole approach in Foulkesian group analytic psychotherapy. Group 13:212–217, 1989

Pines M: Group analysis and the corrective emotional experience: is it relevant? Psychoanalytic Enquiry 10:389–409, 1990

Roberts JP: Foulkes' concept of the matrix. Group Analysis 15:111–126, 1982

Sternberg T: Defence mechanisms and the working through of resistances in group therapy. Group Analysis 15:261–277, 1982

Skynner ACR: What is effective in group psychotherapy? Group Analysis 19:5–24, 1986

Usandivaras RJ: Foulkes' primordial level in clinical practice. Group Analysis 19:113–124, 1986

Whitaker DS: Using Groups to Help People. London, Routledge & Kegan Paul, 1985

Zinkin L: Malignant mirroring. Group Analysis 16:113–126, 1983

Zinkin L: The group as container and contained. Group Analysis 22:227–234, 1989

Endnotes

1. *Group Analysis: The Journal of Group Analytic Psychotherapy,* edited by Malcolm Pines and published quarterly on behalf of the Group-Analytic Society (London) by SAGE Publications, Ltd., frequently has special sections devoted to such topics as Jungian analysis and group analysis, group analysis with children and adolescents, group therapy with affective disorders, studies of shame, and others.

2. *The International Library of Group Psychotherapy and Group Process,* edited by Malcolm Pines and Earl Hopper and published by Routledge & Kegan Paul, has several volumes in the series written from a group-analytic perspective.

CHAPTER 3

Self Psychological Contributions to the Theory and Practice of Group Psychotherapy

Margaret N. Baker, Ph.D.
Howard S. Baker, M.D.

Introduction

In a 1984 review, "The Cutting Edge in Psychiatry," Strauss et al. surveyed leading American psychiatrists for their views on the most important developments in the field in the last decade. The contributions of self psychology joined advances in psychobiology and diagnosis as particularly valued contributions. For those interested in group therapy, the theory initially advanced by Kohut (1971, 1977, 1978, 1984) is particularly useful in two ways. It helps integrate interpersonal and intrapsychic dimensions of human behavior, and it clarifies the therapeutic process in ways that can yield effective intervention. Although Kohut did not work directly with groups, one of his supervisees, Dr. Sheldon Meyers, has. He presented a paper applying the principles of self psychology to group process at the Twelfth Annual Conference on the Psychology of the Self (Meyers 1989). Bacal (1985a), Harwood (1983), Lofgren (1984), Schwartzman (1984), Weinstein (1987), and Whitman and Stone (1977) also made important contributions to our understanding of group process from a self psychological perspective.

The purpose of this chapter is to elaborate how self psychology elucidates group process and treatment. A brief elaboration of salient aspects of self psychological theory precedes an explanation of ways that it can clarify and enrich group work. (For a more complete overviews of the theory and treatment process, see Baker and Baker 1987 and Wolf 1988.) Case examples are used to illustrate dynamic emphases in a self psychological approach. Data obtained in both individual and group sessions are presented to show how patients experience the salutary effects of the group. Throughout the chapter, it is assumed that the reader has only a minimal understanding of self psychology. Therefore, occasional detours to clarify its concepts are necessary throughout.

A Review of Self Psychological Theory

The concepts of the *self* and of *selfobject* are the cornerstones of self psychology. According to Kohut (1971), preserving the experience of the self as vital, cohesive, and integrated is the principal motivating force and need in human behavior. This need is supraordinate to all other needs, drives, and wishes. It was the realization of selfobjects and selfobject transferences, however, that Kohut (1984) believed was his most powerful contribution to understanding the human condition. A selfobject is another person, thing, or life event that we experience as if it were a functioning part of our endopsychic life. Intrapsychic representation of the other person or thing serves to facilitate our emotional development and sustain our well-being. Selfobjects are intimately involved in regulating self-esteem, calming and soothing the self, and channeling and containing affects and drives. Selfobject needs may not be met because of real relationship failures or because of transferential distortions and needs. Consistent failure to meet selfobject needs leads to developmental arrests and resultant defensive reactions, and "good enough" availability of self-selfobject relationships facilitates healthy growth and development throughout the life cycle (Baker and Baker 1987).

Self psychology defines three basic lines of selfobject development: mirroring, idealizing, and twinship. The relationship of an actor with his or her audience illustrates how others may be used as mirroring selfobjects. The actor relies on the applause of the audience to maintain self-esteem. He or she looks to the audience to function as a mirror. The reflection they provide partially determines the actor's experience of self-worth. Applause consolidates the feeling of worth and vigor, whereas indifference may precipitate terrible anxiety and calamitous loss of self-esteem. For the developing infant, the response of parents is analogous to the audience response.

Of course, the actor is not entirely dependent on the audience. The more endopsychic capacity that he or she has to regulate his or her self-esteem, the less critical the audience response is to self-esteem maintenance. The development of these self-regulatory capacities requires a consistent selfobject environment. Thus children who are repeatedly disappointed and/or traumatized are less able to establish these internal capabilities than are those raised in more health-giving environments. As adults, they remain encumbered with developmental arrests in self-sustaining capacities. A person's need for selfobject experience, then, is a function of

- The strength and flexibility of internal capacities to maintain self-esteem
- The availability (both past and present) of a varied network of self-selfobject relationships
- "Atypical" biological vulnerabilities (dyslexia or another physical limitation, for example)
- External stress

Idealizing self-selfobject relations help us regulate affect, tensions, and drives. For example, when a patient is frantically anxious and a therapist quietly communicates his or her understanding of this affective state, the patient may be able to use this interaction to consolidate himself or herself. The therapist's sustaining force then provides a selfobject experience that consolidates the patient, enabling him or her to calm down and return to productive work.

Twinship self-selfobject relationships focus around a sense of human likeness to others and being a valued and important member of a group, such as a family, professional, or leisure activity group. From this association a person feels included, accepted, and affirmed; this is particularly true when we know we are essential and useful to the maintenance of the other members and to the group as a whole.

Self psychology differentiates selfobject needs from object needs. An object is an autonomous being, an independent center of initiative. Objects are valued, loved, or hated for who they are. In contrast, selfobjects are valued for the internal functions and the emotional stability they provide. They are experienced as destructive and catastrophically disappointing when they fail to meet that need. In other words, the selfobject need being met is more important than who meets it.

Self psychologists often refer to intrapsychic structures that facilitate the vital self-sustaining functions of self-esteem and affect regulation. What does intrapsychic structure mean? It is, first, the pattern or way an individual organizes information. What actually happens to a person and what he or she understands to have happened are not always synonymous. For example, a patient constructs his or her therapist's foot jiggling to mean that he or she is boring and not worth the therapist's concentration. This construction of meaning constitutes an important aspect of transference and colors all human interactions, leading one to more or less enjoyable and useful perceptions of what is happening.

To return to our analogy, the therapist may merely have thought that his or her foot itched. But did it? Did it itch then because the therapist was actually bored? The answers to the question may not matter. What always matters is that the patient grasps that the therapist understands that the patient felt injured and why he or she felt that way. An absolute requirement for effective therapy is that the patient experience that he or she is empathically understood by another.[1] Without this vital first step, correcting distortions of reality usually leaves the patient feeling diminished. With that understanding, correcting those transferences often becomes unnecessary because the patient comes to realize the uselessness of the perceptual pattern. Empathic understanding establishes and maintains a therapeutic bond. This bond provides the holding environment that consolidates a patient's self-cohesion, providing a stable platform on which to begin to reorganize and resolve transference patterns.

When there is a disruption in the self-selfobject relationship, one can schematize the resultant sequence of pathological behavior as three steps. An important self-selfobject relationship is disrupted (step 1). This precipitates a loss of self-cohesion (step 2), which leads to symptomatic affect, behavior, or defenses (step 3). Either the affect dissipates or intrapsychic defenses and/or symptomatic behaviors are called into play. These are understood to be the patient's best (although often misguided or short-sighted) effort to restore self-cohesion or to repair the disrupted relationship. Krueger (1989) pointed out that many therapeutic efforts prior to self psychology have failed to consider the initial links in the

---

[1] Empathy is often misunderstood as "being nice" to someone or knowing "what I would feel if I were in your place." What self psychologists mean is to grasp both cognitively and emotionally what another experiences from his or her own unique perspective. What one does with this information may be kind and helpful or cruel and misguided.

symptomatic chain. When understood from a self psychological perspective, then, symptomatic affects are direct expressions of the anguish of loss of self-cohesion because of a selfobject loss, and so-called ego defenses and psychiatric symptoms are efforts to restore a depleted or fragmented self. Thus substance abuse might be understood as an effort to revitalize a depleted self after an argument with a loved one, rather than as a covert gratification or compromise formation necessitated by libidinal or ego conflicts.

Returning to the foot-jiggling therapist, when the therapist's empathic stance is maintained, the patient may come to the conclusion that he or she was interpreting the data according to his or her own peculiar patterns. A second possibility is that the jiggling foot was not the problem. A few minutes earlier the patient felt dropped from the experience of being understood. The therapist didn't seem enthusiastic about a recent success. A quiet frustration of a mirroring need was denied; and the patient slowly lost self-esteem, attaching the insult to the jiggling foot. Dealing with the foot won't help. Tracking down the actual precipitant (no matter how trivial it may seem) and understanding it (in this case an unrecognized mirroring need) are required.

What makes a person feel understood varies. In one instance, the therapist may nod approvingly and say nothing. At another juncture the therapist may make an interpretation or gratify a mirroring need. In self-psychology, Kohut (1984) described how "optimal frustration" is necessary to alter internal organizing patterns. A patient experiences a need that is not overwhelming or depleting. The need is not met; it is interpreted. When sustained by a sufficient selfobject transference, the interpretation—rather than the gratification of the need—both enables and requires that the patient alter his or her pattern of organization. The interpretation undergoes what Kohut (1971) called a *transmuting internalization*. This awkward term was intended to convey that some element of the therapist-patient relationship will be internalized, combined with other elements of the patient's personality, and formed into a healthier intrapsychic pattern (or structure).

Kohut (1984) remained constant in his original opinion that some frustration was necessary for growth. Although they are aware that frustration is part of any relationship, Bacal (1985b) and Terman (1988) turned to current developmental research and noted that growth seems to proceed best under the condition of "optimal responsiveness." This led them to question the concept of therapeutic abstinence. As a function of empathic immersion in the patient's experience, a therapist should seek to maintain the selfobject bond with the patient (whether called by that or some other name). This may mean that sometimes a therapist confines himself or herself to interpretation and at other times gratifies a mirroring or idealizing need—or the therapist may just listen. The goal is to provide a therapeutic environment in which the patient feels safe and trusting and thus is able to disclose his or her innermost thoughts and feelings. A therapist may feel compelled to remain detached, to withhold a response, or to insist on an interpretation when it is apparent from the patient's distress that the therapist's behavior is aggravating to the patient. In some cases, the therapist may be adhering too rigidly to an abstinent stance, not realizing that his or her posture is affecting the intersubjective field between patient and therapist. At the present time, self psychology is in considerable flux in trying to understand the optimal balance between frustration and responsiveness.

There is complete agreement, however, that the way a person constructs reality can create that reality. A patient's rage at our inattentive foot will initially seem puzzling if we don't understand the patient's perspective. If the patient persists in his or her rageful attacks on our indifference, we may well become angry. At this point an interpretation of the patient's transference distortion will be helpful—to us. We will be reassured that we are good therapists and that only the reemergence of feelings of neglect that began in childhood can explain the patient's misconceptions of us. We will, in other words, organize information about the patient in a way that preserves our self-esteem and our belief that we are good therapists. Unfortunately, as we do this, we treat our own countertransference needs rather than respond with appropriate empathy to the patient's needs. This will further rupture the relationship and confirm, rather than alter, the patient's way of understanding the interaction. The possibility of the patient reorganizing his or her perceptions is precluded, and further transference-countertransference impasses may occur (see Stolorow et al. 1987).

By providing an external source of self-esteem or affect regulation, the self-selfobject relationship provides a "splint": a function that is simply not internally available to the patient at crucial times. The intrapsychic construction of this relationship grants stability and comprehensibility to the entire way that the patient understands what is happening to him or her and who he or she is. Because someone else provides essential functions (optimal responsiveness) that the patient cannot provide for himself or herself, the patient can risk new thoughts, feelings, or behavior without an internal collapse. Empathic understanding is not synonymous with "being nice"—agreement with or placating the patient. It is communicating that we understand the patient's experience. The most bizarre affects and ideas can be understood in a way that is free of judgment and evaluation.

Intrapsychic structure is ineffective when perceptual transference patterns create a distorted, crippling picture of the self. There may also be lack of structuring in certain areas. For example, an anorectic patient may have no intrapsychic organization of her body image (rather than a severely distorted one). Consequently, she insistently needs other people's evaluation of her (whether that mirror is a reflective surface or the opinion of a boyfriend, a friend, or her mother). The last mirroring experience determines what she transiently believes until the next mirroring experience.

In summary, an intrapsychic structure that is the conduit for the transference may be distorted or partially or totally absent. A sustaining selfobject surround is the fundamental requirement to reorganize or to form intrapsychic structure belatedly. It may be necessary to help the patient establish patterns where none had previously existed, create new interactions between perceptual patterns, and generate new skills and talents.

Proponents of self psychology maintain that these goals are best achieved within an empathic selfobject surround, one that can function to provide missing sectors of the patient's personality. The task of reorganization is inherently threatening. The process disassembles old patterns, making mechanisms that had contained anxiety and consolidated self-esteem less functional. Ongoing external help in accomplishing those tasks is, therefore, necessary. The selfobject surround must step in and meet and/or interpret those intrapsychic needs interpersonally (optimal responsiveness) until the patient has reestablished new and more effective information-processing modes within his or her own psyche. As old structure is reformulated, an external "splint" is temporarily vital. The process of examining the establishment, disruptions, and repairs of these self-selfobject relationships, moreover, facilitates the reorganizational and developmental processes. The process that was thwarted in childhood is given a second chance. A belated process offers opportunities to understand and compensate for developmental arrests and deviations.

A difficult problem in creating meaningful reorganizations and change is helping the patient return to less mature levels of development with the goal of unearthing archaic affects. Patients often see what they want to change but are frustrated when they can't. They may even recognize the origins of this problem and how they want to change. What keeps them "stuck" is the part of them that is still laboring like a two-year-old or a six-month-old in the old arena of their original caregivers. They were traumatized or left with psychological deficiencies that are unconsciously still organizing their experience. Treatment must help them return (not in time but in psychic configuration) to this old stamping ground, to "peel off" false self-accommodations and defenses in order to reexperience their authentic needs (in self psychology their mirroring, idealizing, and twinship needs) in the safety of the self-selfobject bond with the therapist. This ever-deepening and trusting relationship with an optimally responsive therapist creates the opportunity for this descent into the emotional past.

Self Psychology and Group Therapy

A self psychological perspective may be readily applied to group therapy. In the following discussion, we focus on specific ways that self psychology can enhance understanding of the group process:

1. The group offers a multitude of opportunities to examine self-selfobject relationships.
2. The group provides a selfobject surround that holds the members so that they may reorganize their perceptions and develop more effective psychic organization.
3. The group simulates a family group and stimulates the development of sibling rivalry and parental transferences.
4. The inevitable disruptions and repairs in the relationships among group members and with the leader offer opportunities to understand the vicissitudes of the patient's intrapsychic response to these cycles. Habitual defenses and coping mechanisms are thus clarified.
5. When opposing "functioning realities" are observed to create disruptions between two group members, those who are not involved are provided with an opportunity to understand that someone can empathically grasp and understand divergent "realities," even when they genuinely conflict.
6. For members who are in concurrent individual therapy, still further opportunities are available to examine and reorganize their responses to alterations in self-selfobject relationships.
7. Helping other members grow grants a sense of competence and consolidates self-esteem.

8. New interactions that do not recapitulate past traumas actually happen, and when they are perceived, patients are afforded the possibility to reorganize perceptions. Interactions can be understood in ways that are currently appropriate rather than in ways that were determined by old injuries.
9. New ways to establish and use mature self-selfobject relationships can be established.
10. The group as a whole becomes the source of self-selfobject experiences for the members and leader.

Case Examples

The main thrust of a self psychologically oriented group is to facilitate the development and examination of self-selfobject relationships among the members and with the leader. The leader encourages group members to examine their moment-to-moment responses to each other. What was their affective and cognitive reaction to what was said? What was the impact of their particular response on the interaction? What was the experience of uninvolved members during specific dyadic interactions? When members get fluent with this means of examining their reactions and interactions, the leader then helps them clarify what function other members hold for the maintenance of their self-cohesion and vigor. How do interactions affect self-esteem? How are others used to soothe upset, relieve boredom, and otherwise contain and modulate both positive and negative feelings? This leads to a growing acceptance of and dependence on each other as important and vital to effective functioning. As the vicissitudes of these interactions are examined in depth, the patients begin to establish more effective, independent self-sustaining structures.

A group's process is strongly influenced by the theoretical orientation and countertransference of the leader. The most fundamental concept that orients a self psychological group is the self-selfobject experience. The intervention of choice is whatever intervention facilitates the members' ability to clarify what they need from others, how to ask for it, and what they experience when they do and don't get some level of optimal responsiveness. Consequently, what happens in sessions varies widely, although the therapist should keep the interaction as spontaneous as possible.

For instance, one usually reticent patient said he needed help understanding his relationship with his lover of many years. Discussing an "outside" situation violated the norm of talking principally about what happens in the group here and now. The therapist's empathic immersion in the group process led her to conclude that it was more salient that this particular member was taking a huge risk by exposing aspects of his relationship and asking for something for himself. His trust and reliance on the group was strengthened when they understood and responded to his dilemma. Had she intervened and said, "I wonder what is going on in the group that [the patient] is asking to talk about an outside issue," she would have interrupted his initiative and robbed the other members of their experience of efficacy in helping a usually quiet member. (She might well have brought the detour to outside material to the group's attention, but only later and if it still appeared salient). She also could have addressed his defiant rule-breaking and worried that devoting the whole group to his issue ignored the other members and created individual therapy in a group setting. This was not done, because the most fundamental guideline is to do what is appropriate and necessary to enhance the ability of the group members to empathically understand and respond to each other. The deeper the trust that all members have that they will be heard, understood, and responded to, the greater the level of involvement, disclosure, and working through.

Operating from a self psychological perspective imposes no particular limitations on patient selection. A balance of men and women with a maximum of eight in a group is optimal. A balance of active and passive members helps ensure ongoing group movement. Members should be within the same general level of functioning. It is best if all group members are (or have been) in individual therapy, although not necessarily with the group therapist. The latter, however, may cause some problems for both the therapist and the group members because the therapist won't know the patient as well. The patient may then feel at a disadvantage and envious of his or her other group siblings who have a stronger selfobject tie to the therapist. However, these issues can be worked out by taking it out in the group and maintaining contact with the group member's individual therapist.

Intense use is made of the relationships among members. The selfobject relationship with the therapist functions in the background. Persons for whom group therapy is contraindicated include

- Persons who are skeptical about group therapy and have to be prodded to join
- Overtly suicidal patients unless they are in an inpatient setting

- Persons who are highly defensive and are so narcissistically vulnerable they would have an "allergic reaction" to the group process
- People who have a meaningful relationship with each other outside the group (or whose spouses and friends are significantly involved with group members)

How Do Self Psychology Groups Work?

The "how" of this growth process is illustrated by providing specific case examples of the 10 elements of the therapeutic process listed above. All of the material is drawn from three, long-term, ongoing therapy groups led by the first author (M.B.).

1. Group process offers members repeated opportunities to examine the habitual, repetitive ways that others are used to meet selfobject needs. The therapist also has a chance to observe and clarify the patient's transference dynamics in relation to himself or herself and other members, as the following case example illustrates:

Case 1

Mr. A, a 47-year-old professional man, had joined a group as his 17-year-long, dysfunctional marriage was dissolving. He had been extremely isolated both as a child and in his marriage. His basic pattern was to try to be good and respond to others' needs by promising the sky. He would then do more or less what he thought they wanted; but he would always alter it slightly, leaving them more disappointed by the unfulfilled promise than satisfied by his efforts. Frustrated because no one appreciated him, he would withdraw into sadoerotic fantasies.

When Mr. A entered the group, he was anxious and tangential. He was superficially supportive of others and made no overt demands for attention for himself. Others liked his "filling air time" at first. His rambling got everyone off track and created distance among the members. They tired of this, but they could not confront such a "nice guy trying so hard." I stepped in and helped him try to articulate his anxiety and what he wanted from the group. At the same time, I asked him what impact he thought he was making on the group. He was fully aware he was alienating people, but he had no idea how not to do this.

Mr. A's case illustrates a disruption in his relationship to the group. We all worked together to help him ask for what he needed for himself. When he could articulate this (it took a long time) and when he saw most group members wanting to respond in some way to his needs (even if it was "I don't think I can give you what you want although I understand your need"), he was deeply touched. He could begin to accept how much he needed other people and how they could function for him. To experience this, he went through weeks of paralyzing fear and attempts to withdraw. But with each successive effort he came to trust the group members as reliable sources of understanding and support.

2. By providing a selfobject surround for the members, the group itself gratifies intrapsychic needs.   These needs are initially met extrapsychically, using the group experience to further understand and deepen selfobject bonds within the group and provide "real" experience. This real experience and gratification of narcissistic needs bolster hope of change and can give courage to work more intensely in both group and individual therapy, as the following case illustrates:

Case 2

Mr. B, a 34-year-old narcissistically vulnerable man, entered the group full of impatience, arrogance, and a need for constant attention and reassurance. He would express his need for attention by being falsely responsive to others and unctuously thankful for any direct recognition he received. The group members couldn't stand him at first. They would try to ignore him. When that failed, they tried to confront him. When they did, he would become instantly hostile and attack others and threaten to leave the group. Some of the members would have been delighted, and, at times, so would have I. After sessions of going through this pattern and at the suggestion of the other members that he might do better if he asked directly for what he wanted for himself, he was very slowly able to be more direct. At the same time, he was working in individual therapy on these issues. What emerged in both group and individual sessions was his terror of being ridiculed and abandoned. His mother had constantly criticized him and competed with him. The only contact he had with her was a negative struggle of wills. If he ever let down his defenses, she would lecture him unmercifully about his faults—including that his complexion was bad, his nose was odd looking, he didn't dress right, and he had no friends. The only early memory he had was taking his feces and wiping them all over the bathroom.

As Mr. B came to trust the other group members, he was able to begin to experience that they were not out to get him. As they were able to function for him by understanding his feelings (no suggestions or interpretations, only understanding), he was able to experience himself not as a greedy, defective monster as his mother had convinced him he was, but as a person both craving affection and worthy of being responded to and cared about. (When under pressure, he can lapse into his old self-perceptions, but his new sense of self is building with each positive encounter with both me and the group.)

3. The group setting stimulates sibling rivalry.   Self psychology encourages the development of an intense and archaic self-selfobject relationship with the therapist. The more archaic this transference is, the greater the affect charge the therapist will have to the patient. Given this intensity, patients can experience other group members as threats, not the source of selfobject experience. The therapist then has a difficult situation to manage. Each patient-therapist–self-selfobject bond has its own unique character. Patients have different vulnerabilities and some variation in developmental level and degree of therapeutic regression in individual therapy. The therapist's countertransference to each patient varies.

When sibling rivalry issues arise directly in the group, the therapist communicates his or her understanding of the patient's subjective experience. Exploration continues in both the group and individual therapy. When the therapist is confronted in the group (as when one patient says, "You [the therapist] are always more attentive to him [or her] than to me"), the best policy is to be nondefensive, honest, and willing to examine the contents of the confrontation in both group and individual therapy. The following case example illustrates that even seemingly trivial group interactions can trigger "psychic earthquakes":

Case 3

Ms. C was an attractive, confident woman. Mr. D was tall and roundish and has a depressed and solemn demeanor. When Ms. C came into the room she greeted me with a big smile and lively small talk. Mr. D came in as if he would have preferred to be invisible. He ignored everyone until group started. I enjoyed Ms. C's upbeat presence and felt saddened by Mr. D's distancing himself from the group. If I ignored Ms. C to protect Mr. D, I would have cut Ms. C off from a natural exchange. Ms. C's presence in the group intensified Mr. D's competitiveness and withdrawal, yet he was not able to articulate this in the group. In individual therapy he began to work with renewed fervor. Here I was able to immerse myself fully in his experience. As he got beyond some of his rage, he would have the opportunity to confront Ms. C in the group.

4.   Habitual defenses and coping mechanisms are clarified and processed.   Disruptions in relationships between group members or between a group member and the leader inevitably occur. These disruptions often lead directly to intrapsychic experiences of loss of self-cohesion, which are affectively felt as fragmentation, depletion, and/or depression. Fragmentation, in turn, precipitates a symptomatic effort to restore self-cohesion. Disruptions and consequences can be examined in the group setting, as the following case example illustrates:

Case 3

> Ms. E, a 34-year-old woman, had been in group and individual therapy with me for 3 years. We had reached an impasse. She wanted to come only once every 2 weeks and be told how to structure her schedule so as to accomplish her goals. I had tried to work this way with her and only found myself experiencing a disappointment with her, not unlike what she felt with me. When I suggested that she come more often and work on underlying problems, she refused. I felt hopeless and frustrated. I was asked to do something I couldn't do given the situational constraints and my countertransference reactions. I suggested that we not continue with individual therapy. We had worked through many issues. Maybe it was time to try someone else who might feel more comfortable with how she now wanted to work. She was both furious and relieved. As she started with a new therapist, her rage at me in the group became paralyzing. She would sit in the group red faced and silent. No one could function. I extended myself with no result.
>
> After three excruciating sessions like this, the other group members rallied and said unless Ms. E worked this out with me, they wanted her to leave the group. She exploded and accused me of abandoning her, giving up, and letting her fail. I accepted her storm. I acknowledged that I had become part of the problem. My own feelings prevented me from being as helpful to her as she needed someone to be. She was able to resolve her resentments enough to continue in the group and make steady and sustained progress with the new therapist.

5.   Group process may facilitate the appreciation that there is often more than one way to construct the "functional reality" of a situation. Before their very eyes, group members frequently see others reaching a perception about themselves or their relationships that is clearly at variance with conclusions that seem obvious to everyone else. These people have created a functional reality that is unlike the more consensual reality shared by the rest of the group. It is often possible to observe how the functional reality leads to behavior that begets its own confirmation (i.e., the self-fulfilling prophecy). The members may even come to realize that many events lend themselves to more than one construction of reality. When this happens in interactions between people, and when one person listens with care and does not insist on the correctness of his or her own reality, the impasse is often resolved. Both people may shift their understanding of what happened. Not only do the involved participants benefit, uninvolved observers may come to realize two useful principles: 1) people—themselves included—regularly construe the intent of others in ways that are comprehensible but not useful or intended and 2) relinquishing a rigid insistence on habitual patterns of perception can lead to resolution of differences, as the following case example illustrates:

Case 5

Mr. F, a 42-year-old divorced man, was seen in individual and group therapy. He complained that people did not respect him or like him, and he believed that this was because he was a completely boring person. He was able to help others readily. When he talked about himself in the group, he felt that people rapidly lost interest. He was not nearly as weak as he believed himself to be. When I gave him feedback about how I experienced him in the group, he was shocked that he came across at all. On further exploration and association, he came up with an image of himself as a bland, invisible, wraithlike youth. No matter what kind of feedback he got, it did not register. He was not able to change until he internally experienced the full impact of this self-perception in individual therapy.

Other members of the group were regularly astounded that Mr. F could see himself in a way that seemed so out of touch with how they saw him. As his internal image came to correspond with a more consensually accepted reality, several members began to wonder whether they, too, were locked into deceptive patterns of observing themselves and their relationships.

6.   For members in concurrent individual therapy, still further opportunities are available to self-selfobject relations in the group.   This is illustrated by the following case example:

Case 6

Ms. G had made progress understanding her fears about work success and relating intimately to others. However, she found it very difficult to implement what she came to know about herself. Instead, she would continue to isolate herself and procrastinate finding a regular job. No amount of time or interpretation altered her sitting on the edge of change.

After a few sessions in the group, Ms. G had become assertive in wanting to give advice to others and looking to them for support. Although the other members liked her, they told her she could be very controlling and distancing. In particular, she had a way of relating that was very cognitive and reasoned, but not very emotional.

During one group, Ms. G was feeling awful and went into a lengthy explanation about it. The group pressed her to share how she was feeling. In doing so, all were able to say how much closer they felt to her. She felt some enduring relief. Her perception of herself as a closed-off, impenetrable person who was easily overwhelmed at the slightest demand began to change through repeated interactions of this sort. She started to make productive career moves and to reach out to more appropriately responsive people.

7. Helping others to grow grants a sense of confidence and self-esteem. The awareness that one has facilitated the personal growth of someone else provides a mirroring function that reveals the self as caring and capable. The "we-ness" of the group experience also lends a feeling of identification with others who also try to help. The knowledge the members have that they and the leader have had a hand in this growth draws a parallel between the self and someone who is seen as powerful and effective. In self psychological parlance, this is both a twinship and an efficacy experience, and it gives people a needed sense of community, collegiality, and effectiveness, as illustrated in the following case example:

Case 7

Ms. H, a 32-year-old borderline woman, had attended the group erratically for over 6 months. She projected onto the members an attitude that they disliked her intensely and could give her nothing. Throughout this time, despite herculean efforts on the part of many group members, she was unable to experience much support or caring for her. When the subject of her attendance came up, she fully anticipated an angry, rejecting response. Instead, the members understood that there were genuine and unavoidable problems imposed by her job commitments. They genuinely valued her because she was so perceptive about others. They wanted her to continue despite her intermittent attendance. The accepting feedback she experienced when she was fully anticipating being banished improved her attendance markedly. The group members shone with pride that their responses to her had made a significant difference.

Ms. H gained enhanced self-esteem when she realized that she had a helpful impact on people in the group. The group members, in turn, gained assurance when they saw that their support and caring had consolidated Ms. H in a way that improved her behavior.

8. Interactions that do not repeat old traumas serve as potential self-selfobject experiences.   A person may behave in certain ways and either consciously or unconsciously anticipate certain consequences. When group members react differently or when they act as anticipated but with a desire to understand "just what happened" in the group, the person may use the experience to help him or her reorganize perceptions of himself or herself and others, as the following case example illustrates:

Case 8

Mr. I, a 30-year-old married man, had been in the group for 2 years. He had earned the reputation of being like a venetian blind: he would dart out to say something and then halt and retreat in mid-sentence as he was overcome with terror that his comment would be taken over, stolen from him, or used in another equally painful way. His fear was so intense that he could do or offer very little that might actually garner encouragement and support. When supportive responses were available, he could not appreciate them, because they would precipitate fears of and longing for compliant, passive merger with the other person.

After a breakthrough in individual therapy, Mr. I began to roll the blinds up and out of the way. He would make direct comments and then visibly cringe, waiting for some entrapment or rapelike exploitation of his contribution. With increasing frequency, he would beam from ear to ear when he realized that he had found affirmation. He was not engulfed as he was by his parents. He had gotten healthy responses before, but he could not recognize them. His blinders were off. Although caution persisted, he found that support was available.

9. Both within the group and in their outside lives, group members gain confidence that they can have relationships with others that will meet selfobject needs.   The life experiences our patients have seem to grant them a paucity of life-affirming encounters. As the following case example illustrates, when patients discover and experience new patterns in the group, they begin see new opportunities both in and out of the group:

Case 9

Ms. J had had a series of inappropriate relationships with very imaginative but weak men. She herself was very artistic and creative. She was proud of her difference and at the same time began to see how it isolated her. She had always thought of herself as different and had a hard time thinking that anyone "normal" would think well of her. As she settled into the group and got affirmation and praise for her liveliness and difference from those she viewed as normal, she was able to end an unproductive relationship. She began to build confidence that she would eventually find a genuinely appropriate partner. The impact of six other people liking her and valuing her was crucial to her ability to sustain herself through the breakup.

10.   The group as a whole becomes a meaningful self-selfobject experience.   This final case example illustrates how the concept and experience of the group gestalt can consolidate a member's sense of self:

Case 10

Ms. K, a 42-year-old narcissistically vulnerable sociopathic woman, had a propensity for being victimized, having suffered assaults and rape. She was detached in the group, preferring to tell stories about devastating events and then pulling back or becoming defensive if anyone responded directly. However, when she was away from the group, thoughts of it were a source of comfort to her. She would describe how she would think of people in the group and the group process. She wanted them all with her so much that she would feel disappointed because they weren't really there. Experiencing imagined contact with the whole group gave her a vicarious selfobject experience she was often too frightened to experience directly in the group.

Conclusions

Whether in childhood, later in the life cycle, or belatedly in therapy, psychological development proceeds best (and in some cases only) in a milieu of optimal self-selfobject relationships. Furthermore, Kohut (1984) stressed that self-selfobject relationship needs persist in varied form throughout the life span. He even concludes that an appropriate and important goal for successful analysis is improving the analysand's abilities to establish and maintain successful ongoing self-selfobject relationships. All psychopathology and emotional health are understood best, therefore, in the context of the individual's empathic, partially empathic, or unempathic surround.

Although conflict and drives are clearly involved in psychopathology, developmental arrests are understood as more centrally based on a "dread to repeat" (Ornstein 1974) previous traumatic experiences. The consequent withdrawal from healthy relationships conflicts with the need and wish to reinstitute development. Group therapy is ideally suited to explore the vicissitudes of both object and selfobject relationships, and it can facilitate the development of a vigorous, resilient, and cohesive self.

References

Baker H, Baker M: Heinz Kohut's self psychology: an overview. Am J Psychiatry 144:1–9, 1987

Bacal H: Object-relations in the group from the perspective of self psychology. Int J Group Psychother 35:483–501, 1985a

Bacal H: Optimal responsiveness and the therapeutic process, in Progress in Self Psychology, Vol 1. Edited by Goldberg A. New York, Guilford, 1985b, pp 202–226

Harwood IH: The application of self psychology concepts to group process and group therapy. Int J Group Psychother 33:469–487, 1983

Kohut H: The Analysis of the Self. New York, International Universities Press, 1971

Kohut H: The Restoration of the Self. New York, International Universities Press, 1977

Kohut H: The Search for the Self, Vols 1 and 2. Edited by Ornstein P. New York, International Universities Press, 1978

Kohut H: How Does Analysis Cure? Chicago, IL, University of Chicago Press, 1984

Krueger D: Body Self and Psychological Self. New York, Brunner/Mazel, 1989

Lofgren LB: The self in a small group: a comparison of the theories of Bion and Kohut, in Kohut's Legacy. Edited by Goldberg A, Stepansky P. Hillsdale, NJ, Analytic Press, 1984, pp 203–214

Meyers S: Group therapy and the disorders of the self: theoretical and clinical considerations. Paper presented at the Twelfth Annual Conference on the Psychology of the Self, San Francisco, CA, October 1989

Ornstein A: The dread to repeat and the new beginning. Annual of Psychoanalysis, Vol 2. New York, International Universitites Press, 1974, pp 231–248

Schwartzman G: The use of the group as selfobject. Int J Group Psychother 34:229–241, 1984

Stolorow R, Brandschaft B, Atwood G: Psychoanalytic Treatment: An Intersubjective Approach. Hillsdale, NJ, Analytic Press, 1987

Strauss GD, Yager J, Strauss GE: The cutting edge in psychiatry. Am J Psychiatry 141:38–43, 1984

Terman D: Optimal frustration: structuralization and the therapeutic process, in Learning from Kohut: Progress in Self Psychology, Vol 4. Edited by Goldberg A. Hillsdale, NJ, Analytic Press, 1988, pp 113–125

Weinstein D: Self psychology and group therapy. Group 11:144–154, 1987

Whitman RM, Stone W: Contributions of the psychology of the self to group process and group therapy. Int J Group Psychother 27:343–359, 1977

Wolf E: Treating the Self. New York, Guilford, 1988

PART II

Groups in Hospital and Medical Settings

CHAPTER 4

Group Psychotherapy for Chronically Mentally Ill Patients

Walter N. Stone, M.D.

Introduction

Group psychotherapy, combined with the administration of medications when indicated, is an optimal cost-effective therapeutic approach to fulfilling many of the sociopsychotherapeutic needs of severely ill patients. Indeed, several reports have demonstrated the effectiveness of group intervention using therapists with limited experience and training, such as medical students (O'Brien et al. 1972), psychiatric residents (Alden et al. 1979), and minimally trained nurses (Malm 1982). Nevertheless, many of the initial hopes that this treatment approach would be widely applied and effectively utilizedwith this population have not been realized.[1]

The quality of these individuals' lives is positively linked to the formation of satisfactory interpersonal relations. Healing relationships offer the best way to influence and assist patients in their quest for more meaningful lives. In this chapter, I provide an overview of the patient population and an adumbrated review of dynamic theories of individual and group processes that are relevant to working with chronically mentally ill patients within the context of the impact of interpersonal influence on

---

[1] It is beyond the scope of this chapter to discuss the neglect of the chronically mentally ill patient, but group treatments are only one element in the widespread difficulty in engaging and maintaining patients and therapists alike in the treatment endeavor. Lamb (1979) poignantly enumerated many of the causes.

mental illness. I review the elements necessary to establish group treatment and describe one treatment model that has evolved at the Central Psychiatric Clinic, the outpatient service of the Department of Psychiatry at the University of Cincinnati. Case examples are used to illustrate some of the treatment strategies and techniques.

Patient Population

Bachrach (1988) characterized the chronically ill patient by examining the three D's: diagnosis, disability, and duration. The diagnostic spectrum represented in this patient population is considerable. Historically, schizophrenic patients have received the most attention, which is well deserved because of the chronic and disabling nature of their illness (Breier et al. 1991; McGlashan 1984). Many patients with affective disorders recover only partially with medications (E. Frank et al. 1991), whereas others with debilitating personality disorders respond minimally to medication. More recently, widespread substance abuse has been found in this population, thereby adding another dimension to the clinical diagnosis (Ananth et al. 1989).

Duration of illness is harder to define, but it generally is measured in years if it does not date to early childhood. A recent study (Walker and Lewine 1990) found that experienced and inexperienced therapists who were shown family home movies of two siblings, one of whom was later to be diagnosed with schizophrenia, could identify the child in each family who would become ill beyond what would be expected due to chance. The movies covered the period from birth to 8 years of age, and judgments were based on motoric and affective characteristics.

The disability associated with chronicity is variable, but it is measured against a societal standard that individuals successfully assume a functional role. Such a standard may be ideal, but for many patients is unattainable. Broad-based deficits in social skills including social anxiety, self-deprecation, unassertiveness, or, conversely, overassertive or aggressive behavior contribute to social dysfunction (Curran et al. 1980). Nonverbal aspects of impairment may be present in personal hygiene, facial expressions, responsiveness, or a variety of gestures or postures (Morrison and Bellack 1987). Thus chronically ill patients suffer multiple deficits, and treatment goals must be designed to respect the various disabilities without evoking undue therapeutic pessimism.

Theory

Successful psychotherapy with chronically mentally ill patients requires a sophisticated understanding of social, group, and individual dynamic processes. In most instances the goals of treatment are supportive, and exploratory strategies aimed at helping patients gain insight into their unconscious drives and conflicts are to be eschewed.

Social Forces

Before any therapy can be effective, concrete survival issues must be addressed. First, and then concurrently, these patients must be helped to obtain adequate and stable housing, food, clothing, transportation, and basic medical care. Governmental support is usually an essential part of the safety net on which many chronically ill patients depend. Their therapists must be fully informed about current public laws and policies regarding food stamps, housing, and so on. (Of course, patients generally are more informed than their caretakers about the ins and outs of the system, and not only do they provide support and information for one another, but they educate their therapists.) In essence, these most severely ill of psychiatric patients naturally require multidimensional interventions.

Interpersonal Dynamics

Chronically ill individuals require a comprehensive evaluation of their biopsychosocial needs. The diagnostic efforts should not be focused merely on eliciting psychopathology, but also should include a careful assessment of each patient's strengths, particularly in the sector of interpersonal relationships. Intrapsychic conflicts and developmental deficits primarily become manifest in interpersonal transactions. In group therapy the drive derivatives, internal object relations, or selfobject needs are visible as problems in basic trust, dependence and independence, closeness and distance, boundary and self-esteem maintenance, and narcissistic vulnerability.

The dynamics of interpersonal relationships in recovery from psychotic illness were described by Breier and Strauss (1984) using a two-stage model. In the initial convalescent stage, patients reported that their recovery was facilitated by ventilation, reality testing, social approval and integration, material support, problem solving, and constancy. In the second rebuilding stage, material motivation, reciprocal relating, and symptom monitoring were deemed more important. These stages were not conceptualized as discrete, but as overlapping with considerable individual variation.

The place of affect in these dynamics is reflected in the emerging literature on family therapy of schizophrenia and the concept of expressed emotion. Studies have shown that patients whose families make a preponderance of critical and hostile statements or are overly involved are prone to exacerbation of their illness (Brown et al. 1972; Falloon et al. 1984). Group processes may mirror family dynamics in that direct expression of hostility may be countertherapeutic (Kanas 1986). Patients seem able to discuss disappointment, loneliness, depression, and loss without the intrapsychic disruption they experience with discussion of anger or hostility.

Group Dynamics

For the purposes of this discussion, the model emphasizing the similarity of group development to childhood attachment and separation and individuation processes is used. Patients entering a group form a dependent attachment to the therapist (mother). Gradually they disengage from the therapist and begin to form peer relationships. However, there appears to be a "pregroup" phase in which meaningful emotional relationships are not apparent. This phase can be conceptualized as one of patient self-absorption and self-protection. Movement out of the pregroup phase is similar to the severely traumatized child's willingness to trust strangers or mother. Through a series of unconscious and preconscious tests and direct observations of the therapist's consistency, patients are willing to risk new attachments (Stone and Gustafson 1982). However, the step may be tenuous because the therapist is perceived ambivalently and is said to represent both the nurturing and the devouring mother (Scheidlinger 1974). These polarities correspond with the individual's wish for closeness and fears of loss of self secondary to boundary instability.

The developmental step from the maternal-therapist attachment to involvement with peers is similar to young children engaging in parallel play in which the children seem to be engaged in the same activity but do not genuinely interact.

The succeeding step is similar to the development of interactive play. It is this stage that signals the formation of a cohesive group in which members are most amenable to peer influences. However, at all stages, members influence each other to varying degrees.

A fictive illustration of how the developmental process may proceed might go like this: A formerly silent member (pregroup phase) tentatively tests the group ambience by presenting a problem of not having received the expected ration of food stamps. At first, the therapist is seen as the only helpful resource (dependent phase). Eventually, others may respond by talking about their individual problems with various bureaucracies. They ignore the first member and use the situation to express their own troubles (parallel-play phase). Finally, they may ask questions or use their experiences to help the distressed member or encourage attempting novel solutions (cohesive phase). The interaction enhances the patient's feelings that others can be trusted and the group may be helpful, thereby furthering cohesion. These processes fit very nicely with Breier and Strauss's findings (1984) of the value of problem solving, reality testing, and social integration in the convalescent stage of recovery.

In most groups of chronically ill patients, these developmental sequences are distorted by inconsistencies in attendance. Chronically ill patients do not attend on the same regular basis as individuals in higher-functioning groups. Instead, some patients attend regularly, forming a core group, and others participate on an irregular basis, forming a peripheral subgroup (de Bosset 1982). Over an extended period both core and noncore subgroup members gain a feeling of belonging (McIntosh et al. 1991). Evidence for this process is patients' recall of important life events of both core and peripheral members, as well as the names of members' children or spouses—details that the therapist may not recall. A dramatic example of this bonding occurred when a woman returned to a meeting unannounced.[2] She had discontinued her group therapy about 8 months previously after only 4 months of membership. In that period her long-standing delusion that chipmunks would enter her bedroom and bite her while she was asleep had disappeared (antipsychotic medications had not been altered). She had stopped attending after choosing to live with her elderly mother in a retirement village. Although

---

[2] Patients are not encouraged to return for a visit, but on occasion, as in this instance, a patient returns and enters the meeting. The therapist greets the ex-patient warmly and attempts to understand why the person may have come on this particular day. Sometimes it is a signal of decompensation; other times it is primarily to inform the old members of how well someone is doing. In either instance, it represents an important message about the bonding that has taken place in the group.

she was not a core member, two others accurately recalled the date of her last visit as the week before Easter. They asked about her move and about her mother as if she was an intimate friend. The therapist had been unaware of and was quite surprised by the positive affect toward this patient. The strength and the importance of the member-to-member interpersonal bonds can easily be underestimated by a therapist whose own object world is a comparatively rich one.

Attending to the biopsychosocial needs of these patients in a group is a complex challenge that requires careful and specific therapeutic techniques. Treatment boundaries extend beyond the group room, as therapists may need to have contact with family members, other community agencies, or hospital personnel. Patients are to be informed in advance and concurrently of the indications for and content of these meetings.

Organizing the Group

Administrative Considerations

In initiating an outpatient program for treating chronically mentally ill patients, the therapist(s) must establish an alliance with the clinic administration. Administrators need to be involved with the project to ensure satisfactory patient referrals, adequate treatment space, secretarial support, and so on. On the surface many clinics seem to harbor an abundance of chronically ill patients, but appropriate referrals may be slow unless there are good connections with intake workers, who have the responsibility for assigning patients. Often efforts to begin these groups founder on the basis of lack of patient flow.

Therapists' personal needs also demand attention (Stone 1991). They have increased time demands related to the number of patients seen in the group. Among the additional tasks are paper work requirements (i.e., regular treatment summaries and correspondence with other agencies), need for contact with families, and interaction with staff of emergency services and, inevitably, with staff of inpatient facilities. These extra demands may seem daunting. In many settings therapists receive "bonus" credit for leading groups. Such an arrangement not only reflects the reality of the work and boosts morale, but it is a clear statement of administrative support for the enterprise and a recognition of the unique value of group therapy in the treatment of chronically mentally ill patients.

Therapists thrive when they have continuing opportunities to review and learn from their work. The barriers to therapists' effectiveness include not only traditional countertransferences, but, as described by Friedman (1988), interferences with therapists' ability to fulfill their treatment plan, satisfy their curiosity, or consistently establish meaningful emotional contact with their patients. Therapists are best able to maintain their balance and therapeutic commitment when administrators also demonstrate their commitment by arranging for supervision, employing an outside consultant, or providing monies to attend relevant conferences.

Group Structure

The following discussion is a description of the group format used in our clinic. Groups are diagnostically heterogeneous. Over an extended treatment period diagnoses do not seem to matter with respect to patients' functioning in a group.

The group census ranges from 12 to 15 patients, which ensures that 5 to 8 patients will be present at any given meeting (McGee 1983). Sessions are held weekly for 60 to 75 minutes. The final 15-minute segment of each meeting is used to review and, if necessary, adjust medications. Members are free to remain or leave during this time. When the clinician leading the group is not a physician, the psychiatrist prescribing medications joins the group during this final segment. The group's therapists provide pertinent clinical information for the psychiatrist, and, of course, they are privy to any decisions made regarding medications.

Most groups have coleaders. In our setting the optimal arrangement has been for one therapist to be a permanent staff member who provides continuity of care and one to be a psychiatric resident who may remain with the group for 1 or 2 years. Singly led groups are provided with a designated alternate therapist who meets with the patients in the absence of the regular leader.

As many problems as possible are managed within the group. However, some patients referred from other therapists continue their individual sessions with an ultimate goal of containing all regularly scheduled treatment within the group. During periods of crises, however, individual appointments may be necessary and are best handled by the group leaders.

Patient Selection

The chronically ill patients selected for group therapy represent a cross-section of the population that requires aftercare treatment services.

They generally are of lower socioeconomic status, are dependent for basic necessities on their family and/or public funds, and have few aspirations of becoming gainfully employed.

Almost all patients can be accepted into the diagnostically heterogeneous groups. There are few absolute contraindications, but a number of relatively important reasons exist to exclude or delay entry of a particular patient. Acutely psychotic, severely depressed, or significantly organically impaired patients are not accepted until the more florid symptoms are under control. Individuals who have the capacity to use more intensive treatment in the service of increasing the level of function should be offered such treatment when possible. Unfortunately, many patients are quickly diagnosed as having chronic illness and are assigned to treatments that limit their potential for growth.

Patient Preparation and the Group Contract

As with any responsible group endeavor, patients are interviewed by the therapists before entering the group. This statement seems simplistic, but in some settings the status of groups for chronically ill patients is such that patients are "dumped" into groups without prior contact with the therapist(s). This practice undermines the patients' acceptance of and collaboration in their treatment.

The individual session(s) serves diagnostic needs and provides an opportunity to begin a relationship between patient and therapist and to establish a therapeutic contract (Rutan and Stone 1984). In contrast to higher-functioning patients, chronically ill patients often are unable to articulate their therapeutic goals, which has been suggested as a primary condition for joining a group. Rather than reject such individuals, therapists might spend several sessions helping to identify one or two general goals such as learning to talk with others, feeling less alone, or having a place to talk about making it in the community. These goals seem sufficient (McIntosh et al. 1991). The single limited wish to have a place to receive medication is insufficient to motivate a patient to remain in a group.

Other elements of the traditional group contract are modified for this patient population. As noted above, chronically mentally ill patients have difficulty complying with the requirement to attend all scheduled meetings. An alternative to this portion of the contract is discussed below as the flexibly bound group model. It is sufficient to note that therapists are ill advised to enter into a contract that they are unwilling to abide by. If patients, because of their psychopathology, are unable to keep their portion of the agreement, the therapist must either modify the arrangement or end up ignoring certain of its elements. This latter response does not provide a model of consistency with which the patients may identify and in which they can feel safely held.

Limiting extra-group contacts among members is difficult and perhaps not desirable. With the impaired capacity for forming satisfactory interpersonal relationships, outside meetings among members might represent important treatment progress. For instance, members may ride the bus to and from the clinic together. Indeed, one phobic woman, who had been brought to the clinic by her family members, risked coming to her group alone because she knew that another member would meet her at the bus stop. Certainly there are dangers of destructive subgrouping, but the agreement to talk about contacts among members outside the group is frequently interpreted by patients as a prohibition. Consequently, patients may inhibit such contacts or not reveal them if they do take place.

Like patients who enter into the traditional contract, chronically ill members are instructed to talk about the important events and problems in their lives and to comment on what others have said. Patients are *not* instructed to discuss their internal responses to one another. This condition is eliminated from the contract because such commentary is linked with increased negative or hostile affect, which is very difficult for patients to manage. Eventually there will be opportunities to directly examine intermember transactions, but this should be delayed until the members feel sufficiently safe. Moreover, patients are firmly told that they are to try to express themselves with words, not action.

Generally, therapists are not directly responsible for patients' fees. In most public clinic settings, fees are set and monitored by billing offices. Nevertheless, clinicians should include in their discussion of the contract the requirement that patients collaborate with the financial manager, which would include compliance with requests to complete forms or provide documentation of income.[3]

Finally, as in all group treatment contracts, the members need to be told that what takes place in the meetings is to remain confidential. An

---

[3] In an unpublished Ph.D. thesis, Englander (1989) found a significant and positive relationship between a group contract that attended to fees and the development of group cohesion. This finding held for patients in groups in the public sector as well as in private settings.

optimal way to present this point is to state that if members discuss their group experiences outside, no member should be identified by name or in a manner that would allow someone else to know who they were talking about.

Flexibly Bound Group Model

The concept of the flexibly bound group follows from our experiences with patients' difficulty in adhering to their agreement to be present at each scheduled meeting (McIntosh et al. 1991). The flexible-boundaried group contract is modified to provide patients with more flexibility and autonomy and yet maintain the boundaries of group membership. In this model, patients are asked to come weekly for four sessions. Then, in the presence of the others, they are given an option of attending once weekly to once monthly. The patients thereby have increased control over closeness and distance and a feeling of autonomy in this sector of their treatment. Some patients will opt to come weekly, whereas others will choose to come less frequently. The model enables the group to incorporate members who would be excluded from treatment under the more customary contract and provides a viable alternative for patients who otherwise would not engage in traditional group therapy.

Treatment Goals

The initial treatment goal for most chronically ill patients is psychological stabilization and prevention of social deterioration. A substantial portion of the patients, however, have the potential for developing more satisfactory interpersonal relationships and an improved capacity to manage their everyday affairs. The group provides an opportunity to work toward these goals.

Treatment is conducted within a psychodynamic framework. Ultimately, through improved interpersonal relationships and enhanced problem solving, patients will achieve more stable and flexible internal psychological structures. These are not achieved through the acquisition of genetic insight, but within a supportive environment, through acquisition of adaptive strategies and development of self-understanding of current interactions.

Using psychodynamic principles, the therapist searches for themes that emerge in each meeting. These themes are embedded in and modified by the stage of group development. Knowledge of the stages assists the therapist in choosing where or how to intervene. Moreover, the therapist also uses group development to foster interpersonal influence among members, and to that end he or she attempts to maintain and promote a sense of safety and group cohesion. However, the nature of a particular intervention depends on the therapist's skill and sensitivity.

Leadership Functions

The leader of a therapy group of chronically ill patients must perform six primary functions:

1. Identifying themes
2. Managing boundaries
3. Bonding members
4. Managing affect
5. Promoting problem solving
6. Handling metaphors

Identifying Themes

Finding the central theme is not always an easy task, and often there are several important themes during a single meeting. Many of the themes involve patients' anxieties about establishing and maintaining personal boundaries. Discussions of family members, bureaucrats (i.e., the welfare or public support personnel), or less intimate acquaintances all may contain messages about patients' fear of intrusion, control, or danger to their person. Metaphors for boundaries are contained in discussions of the value of peepholes in apartment doors, the pushiness of drug dealers, and children being accosted in the streets or being asked for protection money at school. An additional expression of the patients' boundary problems is evident in their fears of emotional contagion and their anxieties about listening to others describe symptoms. The patients fear that they may develop similar problems.

Themes of isolation, loneliness, and aloneness are frequent. Discussions of separations, loss, death, and changing neighborhoods all have the potential for conveying the patients' concerns about being alone, losing support, and feeling isolated.[4] A theme of loneliness and loss emerged in the following fragment of interaction in a flexibly bound group that had been meeting for almost 8 years:

Case 1

At the meeting to be described, five of the six patients present had participated on a regular "intermittent" basis for more than 6 years. All but one, Ms. A, were diagnosed as having chronic schizophrenia. Ms. B began by saying that she had been very upset the preceding week and had driven to the emergency room twice, but then did not register because she feared that she would have to go into the hospital and she did not want to leave her two young children. Mr. C, a rather withdrawn man, surprisingly asked several questions that clarified the extent of Ms. B's depression. The therapist observed that Ms. B had been separated from her husband only 10 days and was now living in her new apartment. Ms. A nodded her head, and the therapist asked her what she was thinking. Ms. A, recalling the preceding week's meeting, told Ms. B that she shouldn't let her husband come and see the kids whenever he wanted. She continued that if they got back together, he would walk all over her, which is what happened to Ms. A when her own husband had left. Mr. C commented that Mr. D had gotten sick when his brother had died (a piece of information unknown to the therapist). Mr. D responded that his mother had died when he was born, and an aunt and then an older sister who had cared for him died. He said he had three mothers who left him (he did not mention his brother). Mr. E then recalled how upset he had been when his mother had died, and how it had been useful to talk about this in the group.

In this instance the themes focused on death, loss, and loneliness. The associations were emotionally cohesive and reflected the involvement these patients had with one another.

Managing Boundaries

The primary vehicle for managing the group and creating a safe environment is the group contract. In a pilot study (W. W. Stone, D. McIntosh, M. Grace, unpublished data, January 1989) comparing patients in a flexibly bound group with those in a traditional group (i.e., a group in which patients agree to attend all scheduled meetings), members of the flexible group were accepting of those who attended as scheduled and felt that it was not necessary that everyone be present at every meeting. Therapists should encourage discussion of missing members to convey a concern for them. Often those present object to such discussions because "it's like talking behind someone's back." The therapist needs to convey a concern similar to that of a parent for a missing family member (Grotjahn 1982).

Patients alter the traditional group boundaries in their outside contacts. In addition to those contacts described above, the therapist needs to decide whether to inform the group about a patient's reason for missing a meeting. If a member is ill, either physically or psychologically, the therapist has to consider whether to reveal that information, and if members wish to contact or visit the ill person, whether information should be provided to enable that to take place. In supportive treatment, providing such information creates the opportunity for members to have outside contact and indicates the therapist's concern, but it may run the risk of creating insular subgroups.

Patients properly use one another for support. In many instances they readily exchange last names and phone numbers and call each other. Outside contacts may be an important way of entering and sustaining membership in the group. J. D. Frank (1957), in describing the positive impact of such meetings, observed that some individuals may take greater risks if they have an ally among their peers. In this context, therapists may explore outside contacts as a positive adaptation, rather than as a resistance.

Envy, competitiveness, or feelings of exclusion are common responses of members who are excluded from the extragroup contacts. The therapeutic management of these affects is difficult. Resentments may remain within consciousness but are not verbalized. One strategy is to focus on the hurt underneath the more aggressive, angry feelings. The therapist's judgment in how or when to intervene is complicated by the recognition that outside contacts may be supportive of an individual and counterproductive for the group.

Bonding Members

When chronically ill patients enter a group, their most salient issues are safety, boundary management, and trust. How they manage particular elements of the joining process is variable. Members provide one another with models for identification that help newcomers become integrated into the treatment process. For instance, a member who is afraid to join verbally may observe another person seeking and receiving support from the therapist. Another who is overly dependent on the therapist may observe others successfully interacting with peers. Therapists can support such steps with nods of approval or through verbal recognition.

A less frequently appreciated method of linking is through the discussion of somatic complaints. Patients often will remark about their physical illnesses and the treatment they receive.[4] These individuals experience their families or friends as unable or unwilling to listen to complaints about their physical illnesses, and they find it confirming to be respectfully listened to by the group. The therapist's task is to determine the meaning of such discussions. Is it a resistance to talking about emotional states, or is it a message about the care they are receiving (i.e., a transference)? In the entry phase of the group, rather than interpreting the content of the discussion, the therapist may draw attention to similarities of the patients' concerns. This strategy promotes bonding and allows them to proceed.

Managing Affect

Many chronically ill individuals have deficits in identifying and tolerating affects. These deficiencies coincide with the developmental level of self and object representations and libidinal organization (Krystal 1975; Schmale 1964). Therapists serve a valuable therapeutic function by identifying and labeling specific feeling states such as shame, joy, pleasure, or guilt.

Affects are often readily identifiable in group themes (Stone 1990). Anxieties about loss of self or being intruded on are not uncommon. Emotional contagion, particularly around fears of decompensation and loss of control in the presence of an overtly psychotic member, requires active intervention on the therapist's part. At times a patient has to be removed during the middle of a session, both to protect the individual and the group as a whole. The therapist then should explore the members' responses to this event. It is not unusual for the patients to respond with somatic complaints. This can be understood as a

---

[4] It is important to recall that there are significant medical illnesses among chronically mentally ill patients. They often receive inadequate care, characterized by having to wait for extended periods in crowded public facilities. There is a real basis for their complaints, because it is clear that the quality of medical attention is unevenly distributed in the population. A significant proportion of chronically ill psychiatric patients have medical problems that contribute to their overall disability (Roca et al. 1987).

resomatization of feelings under the regressive pressures of affect stimulation (Krystal 1974).

A considerable data base has emerged supporting the clinical finding
that unrestrained exploration of anger in schizophrenic patients is counterproductive (Kanas 1985). It is our experience that these findings hold
for other chronically ill patients as well. Usually, anger or rage is a response to narcissistic injury. Therapeutic interventions directed at the
underlying feelings of hurt, abandonment, and loneliness generally are
more readily integrated by the patients than efforts to "get anger out"
(Stone and Whitman 1977). Optimally, patients learn to become more
self-assertive in the face of injury and to gain control over their rage. This
is a developmental step that is difficult to achieve in the light of the
patients' extensive experiences of withdrawal, somatization, or destructive outbursts.

Promoting Problem Solving

Consistent with treatment goals, the therapist encourages problem solving. This involves a two-step process. After identification of a theme, the
therapist encourages patients to elaborate on its relevance to themselves. Tactically, clinicians may address individuals and then identify the
common issue (Horwitz 1977). They should be prepared to actively engage the patients, even if the data supporting a theme are incomplete.
Silence promotes regression and increases patients' self-absorption. If
the therapist is successful in promoting interaction, the interpersonal influences in the recovery from chronic illness are enhanced.

The therapist then engages patients in exploring coping strategies.
This element in the treatment approach reinforces the sense of competence and self-esteem through addressing a common task, gaining new
ideas, and providing an opportunity to be of assistance to others. Patients
are experienced in solving a variety of problems in living that are perplex-
ing to the therapist. For instance, when family members are unavailable
to help with grocery shopping, members may know of cab companies
whose drivers will carry groceries into an apartment. Frequently, conflicts
arise around dealing with bureaucracies of the welfare system or other
public agencies. Patients bring to the group an impressive series of stories
of both successful and unsuccessful experiences in dealing with the inevitable frustrations in negotiating with the "system" to fulfill their needs.

The problem-solving element should not be pursued too rapidly. Patients need sufficient time to feel understood and to share their difficul-

ties before embarking on problem solving. Sharing enhances a sense of belonging and provides a base that enables patients to take new risks. The model of the flexibly bound group dictates a lessened continuity between sessions. Nevertheless, themes are carried forward from one session to the next by members of the core group, and therapists can judge the level of group involvement with a particular issue and time their inquiries into problem-solving responses accordingly.

Handling Metaphors

The therapist identifies many themes as metaphors that communicate the status of the group development or of the group or individual transferences. Considerable therapeutic work can be accomplished in the metaphor, without threatening nascent and precarious patient-to-patient or patient-to-therapist bonding (Katz 1983). Many boundary alterations, such as entry of new members or patient or therapist absences, can be directly addressed. For instance, safety issues are often discussed when new members enter the group, and those can be directly linked to the presence of the newcomer. The therapist's interventions should be framed in a manner that indicates that the patients' responses are understandable and are not peculiar to them as "sick" individuals. Over a period of time chronically ill patients gain genuine insight into their patterns of response to such real-life group events.

Many metaphors are statements about the therapist and the patients' wish for the therapist to provide greater safety, more nurturing, or magical cures. These metaphors are compatible with the level of individual and group development. When the therapist directly addresses these metaphors as wishes, group fragmentation or regression often occurs. Patients are better able to problem solve in the displaced derivative. This strategy conveys to the paients that the therapist has understood the common message, respects their vulnerabilities, and attends to problem solving.

For instance, in one group after the therapist's absence, one of the schizophrenic members reported a dream in which her father adopted a younger sister "who was just like me until she became violent and blew up a building [similar to the one in which the group met] because she had become angry with her father." The patient had no thoughts about the dream. The therapist asked what the others thought, and the response was a series of associations to mistreatment by parents or authority figures. The therapist wondered how they could let parents know that they had been hurt. This led to a lively discussion of their helplessness as children and several members' animated illustrations of their successes in standing up to mistreatment. The angry feelings directed at the therapist were not explored. The dream was used to explore adaptive solutions, rather than rage at the therapist.

The following case example illustrates many of the elements present in working with chronically mentally ill patients in groups:

Case 2

The group, which had been meeting for over 2 years, was led by a nurse and a psychiatric resident. This particular session occurred 2 months after a change of residents. The nurse cotherapist was absent, as had been previously announced. Three core group members were present, Ms. F, Mr. G, and Ms. H. A fourth member, Ms. I, ordinarily attended biweekly, but at the suggestion of the nurse-therapist had returned in 1 week to continue discussing her feelings of rage at her mother, who Ms. I felt had mistreated and ignored her.

Ms. I opened the discussion by stating that she couldn't recall what had happened the preceding week and why she had been asked to come. Ms. H immediately began to talk, saying that she wasn't at the meeting the preceding week because her mother had died. Her mother had been ill with cancer for an extended period, and Ms. H felt relieved because her mother's suffering was over. Mr. G said that he wanted to bring in his collection of memorabilia from World War II airplanes to show the doctor.

The resident, rather than directly responding to Mr. G, asked Ms. H to talk more about her feelings about her mother's death. Ms. H repeated that her mother had been ill a long time and it was a relief when she died. Ms. I, without actually making the linkage from the prior week, said that she had been upset because her individual therapist had left the clinic and she was worried about what her new therapist might be like. She recalled that as a child she had been locked in closets by her father and she had become fearful of closed and locked doors. The therapist commented how important it was for people to be able to find somebody they could trust and who would reliably be there for them. The therapist continued that they all seemed to have suffered important losses. Ms. I responded by telling a story about how her mother really had never been available to her. As a little girl she was sexually molested in the park in the presence of her mother, who ignored what was happening. Ms. I continued that she told her mother that if she didn't help get rid of this boy she would have a screaming fit and embarrass her.

At that point Ms. F, who had been present the preceding week, entered. With pressured speech, she described coming from visiting her friend in the intensive-care unit. She was quite pleased with herself for being able to help in a crisis. She continued, asking the therapist if her son had called. The therapist indicated that indeed he had, and he had been concerned that his mother (Ms. F) was hyperactive and was becoming sick again. Ms. F responded that essentially she didn't want to be bothered with her son and that he really wasn't reliable. She exemplified his unreliability, recalling that when she had been ill, she had asked him to scrub all the floors in her apartment and he said he didn't want to do it. The remainder of the session was a further discussion of how children weren't available or reliable and how parents were not reliable either.

Case 2 illustrates a number of elements present in working with groups composed of chronically mentally ill patients. The central theme of loss and the various ways of protecting oneself against the affects associated with loss are readily identifiable. Mr. G tried to cope by making linkages to the therapist. Ms. F's solution was to care for others, and she also avoided affects by coming late. Additionally, Ms. F's decompensation may have been linked with the theme of loss. Ms. I complied with the therapist's request, but forgot why she was returning. It should not be surprising that Ms. I could not recall the problem of her anger, which is a particularly threatening topic. In this context, because of the intensity of the losses experienced by others, it was difficult to help Ms. H grieve. Ms. H herself had considerable resistance, but the presence of others may have enabled her to proceed with the grief work more effectively because it was a shared experience.

This case also brings into focus several technical issues for the therapist. Should the therapist assist Ms. I in recalling the reason for coming to the group this week? How should she respond to Ms. F's question regarding her son's call? How can she evaluate the extent of Ms. F's decompensation? How might she respond to Mr. G in a way that will move the process forward and yet not injure him or the others? It is not unusual for therapists to feel somewhat disorganized and off balance in the face of these questions. Indeed, as might be anticipated, the problems do not stop at the close of the session. The therapist reported that she was awakened at 3 A.M. by a call from the emergency room where Ms. F had gone after having stopped a motorist in the middle of the street to say that she was upset. This situation also illustrates the responsibility associated with caring for those chronically ill patients who intermittently decompensate and require extra group contact for the best continuity of care.

Summary

The major emphases of this chapter have been the review of the individual and group dynamics that are salient to conducting group psychotherapy with chronically mentally ill patients. The group contract was described, with the modification that after attending four sessions patients could determine the frequency with which they would attend treatment. This modification, labeled the *flexibly bound group,* enables patients to feel more empowered in deciding about their therapy.

Treatment strategies that emphasize building bonds and interactions among patients were described. Typical themes that may be addressed are related to reality factors associated with everyday survival issues, fears of psychological decompensation, and underlying feelings of loneliness. After elaboration of a theme, the therapist engages the members in sharing their coping strategies. Technical considerations that address the management of affects (in particular, anger) in the context of the underlying helplessness and deprivation were explored.

References

Alden AR, Weddington WW Jr, Jacobson C, et al: Group aftercare for chronic schizophrenia. J Clin Psychiatry 40:249–252, 1979

Ananth J, Vandewater S, Kamal M, et al: Missed diagnosis of substance abuse in psychiatric patients. Hosp Community Psychiatry 40:297–299, 1989

Bachrach LL: Defining mental chronic mental illness: a concept paper. Hosp Community Psychiatry 39:383–388, 1988

Breier A, Strauss JS: The role of social relationships in the recovery from psychotic disorders. Am J Psychiatry 141:949–955, 1984

Breier A, Schreiber JL, Dyer J, et al: National Institute of Mental Health longitudinal study of chronic schizophrenia: prognosis and predictors of outcome. Arch Gen Psychiatry 48:239–246, 1991

Brown GW, Birely JLT, Wing JF: Influence of family life on the course of schizophrenic disorders: a replication. Br J Psychiatry 121:241–258, 1972

Curran JP, Miller TW III, Zwick WR, et al: The socially inadequate patient: incidence rate, demographic and clinical features, and hospital and post hospital functioning. J Consult Clin Psychol 48:375–382, 1980

de Bosset F: Core group: a psychotherapeutic model in an outpatient clinic. Can J Psychiatry 27:123–126, 1982

Englander TR: The facilitating environment, cohesion, and the contract in group psychotherapy. Unpublished Ph.D. dissertation, Fielding Institute, Santa Barbara, CA, 1989

Falloon IRJ, Boyd JL, McGill CW: Family Care of Schizophrenia. New York, Guilford, 1984

Frank E, Kupfer DJ, Perel JM, et al: Three-year outcomes for maintenance therapist in recurrent depression. Arch Gen Psychiatry 47:1093–1099, 1990

Frank JD: Some determinants, manifestations, and effects of cohesiveness in therapy group. Int J Group Psychother 7:53–63, 1957

Friedman L: The Anatomy of Psychotherapy. Hillsdale, NJ, Analytic Press, 1988

Grotjahn M: Talking behind a patient's back. Group Analysis 15:163–164, 1982

Horwitz L: A group-centered approach to group psychotherapy. Int J Group Psychother 27:423–439, 1977

Kanas N: Inpatient and outpatient group therapy for schizophrenic patients. Am J Psychother 39:431–439, 1985

Kanas N: Group therapy with schizophrenics: a review of controlled studies. Int J Group Psychother 36:339–351, 1986

Katz GA: The non-interpretation of metaphors in psychiatric hospital groups. Int J Group Psychother 33:56–68, 1983

Krystal H: The genetic development of affect and affect regression, in The Annual of Psychoanalysis, Vol 2. New York, International Universities Press, 1974, pp 98–126

Krystal H: Affect tolerance, in The Annual of Psychoanalysis, Vol 3. New York, International Universities Press, 1975, pp 179–219

Lamb HR: Roots of neglect of the long-term mentally ill. Psychiatry 42:201–207, 1079

Malm U: The influence of group therapy on schizophrenia. Acta Psychiatr Scand Suppl 297:1–65, 1982

McGee TF: Long-term group psychotherapy with post-hospital patients, in Group and Family Therapy 1982. Edited by Wolberg L, Aronson ML. New York, Brunner/Mazel, 1983, pp 93–106

McGlashan TH: The Chestnut Lodge follow-up study, II: long-term outcome of schizophrenia and affective disorder. Arch Gen Psychiatry 41:586–601, 1984

McIntosh D, Stone WN, Grace M: The loosely bound group: format, technique, and patients' perceptions. Int J Group Psychother 41:49–64, 1991

Morrison RL, Bellack AS: Social functioning of schizophrenic patients: clinical and research issues. Schizophr Bull 13:715–725, 1987

O'Brien CP, Hamm KB, Ray BA, et al: Group vs individual psychotherapy with schizophrenics. Arch Gen Psychiatry 27:474–478, 1972

Roca RP, Breakey WR, Fischer PJ: Medical care of chronic psychiatric outpatients. Hosp Community Psychiatry 38:741–745, 1987

Rutan JS, Stone WN: Psychodynamic Group Psychotherapy. New York, Macmillan, 1984

Scheidlinger S: On the concept of the "mother-group." Int J Group Psychother
    24:417–428, 1974

Schmale AN: A genetic view of affects. Psychoanal Study Child 19:287–310, 1964

Stone WN: On affects in group psychotherapy, in The Difficult Patient in Group.
    Edited by Roth BE, Stone WN, Kibel HD. Madison, CT, International Univer-
    sities Press, 1990, pp 191–208

Stone WN: Treatment of the chronically mentally ill: an opportunity for the
    group therapist. Int J Group Psychother 41:11–22, 1991

Stone WN, Gustafson JP: Technique in group psychotherapy of narcissistic and
    borderline patients. Int J Group Psychother 32:29–47, 1982

Stone WN, Whitman RM: Contribution of psychology of the self to group process
    and group therapy. Int J Group Psychother 27:343–359, 1977

Walker E, Lewine RJ: Prediction of adult-onset schizophrenia from childhood
    home movies of patients. Am J Psychiatry 147:1052–1056, 1990

CHAPTER 5

Inpatient Group Psychotherapy

Howard D. Kibel, M.D.

Introduction

On admission to a psychiatric unit, patients are in a state of decompensation. The attendant loss of independent function and decision-making capabilities is demoralizing (Rutchick 1986). On the unit, patients are required to surrender part of their usual autonomy. They must conform to the regulations of the unit and submit, in part, to the decisions of the treatment team regarding treatment and discharge planning. They find themselves drawn to the staff, yet somehow pitted against them. In a dynamic sense, ambivalence and resistance are an inherent part of the treatment and form an intrinsic part of the hospital treatment alliance with clinicians and other members of the treatment team (Kibel 1987a).

The psychiatric unit is like a large group in which all these factors are played out. The small psychotherapy group, which meets briefly and intermittently, functions much like a subgroup of the larger unit. Indeed, its dynamics have been found to symbolically reflect those of the milieu within which the group resides (Klein and Kugel 1981). The small therapy group can be considered as a biopsy of the unit (Levine 1980) because it reveals the overall dynamic forces of the unit as expressed in the patient subculture. Alternately, it serves as an interface between the intrapsychic experience of each member and the shared conflicts that are activated within the system at large (Kibel 1987b).

This perspective on the psychotherapy group defines its position in a functional way, one that complements the general goals of inpatient treatment. This stance has evolved over time. Although most practitioners today would agree with this viewpoint, there is diversity in its application.

Historical Overview

The first use of group psychotherapy with inpatients is credited to Edward W. Lazell (1921). At the end of World War I, Lazell, a psychoanalytically oriented psychiatrist, established lecture classes for war veterans at St. Elizabeths Hospital in Washington, D.C. Advantages of the group method, he reported, included socialization, reduction of fear of the psychiatrist, and minimal social contact for the inaccessibly regressed. He observed that even the latter retained the information of his lectures and that afterwards patients shared this information and compared symptoms. Ten years later, L. Cody Marsh (1931), who was influenced by Lazell, employed a similar approach at Worcester State Hospital in Massachusetts. However, he added ward discussion groups to the lecture format. These groups averaged fewer than 20 patients and included what today would be called group exercises to promote rehabilitation and reeducation. Marsh (1935) was committed to the then-innovative notion that patients could be supportive of each other.

Louis Wender (1936) was the first to apply psychoanalytic concepts to the small inpatient group. Wender worked in a private mental hospital with nonpsychotic patients. He took pains to distinguish his group method from the educational and directive techniques of his time by describing relationships within the group in terms of transference and contending that these were symbolic of the family of origin. Understanding them, he believed, could shed light on the dynamics of behavior, lower resistance, provide an opportunity to rework some unresolved family conflicts, and facilitate partial reorganization of the personality (Kibel 1989).

During World War II, group therapy was practiced in a number of military hospitals. One such hospital was Northfield Military Hospital in England. There Bion, Foulkes, and Main began working with groups and developing approaches that were later applied to outpatients (Rice and Rutan 1987). Of these, Foulkes (1965) did the most to describe applications to inpatient treatment. He noted the healing qualities of the group as a whole and came to view the hospital itself as a large therapeutic group of which the small therapy groups were only a part. He appreciated the complex interrelationship between the group and the psychiatric unit. The former influenced the latter, so that the work in the small group helped the unit develop a therapeutic milieu. By the same token, group life was profoundly influenced by the larger community.

After World War II, there were several years in which hospital group work flourished. Elvin Semrad and colleagues (Mann and Semrad 1948; Standish and Semrad 1951) at the Boston State Hospital described a method in which the therapist abandoned the usual authoritarian role in favor of facilitating group interaction, recognition and acceptance of patients' underlying emotions, and tolerance for their psychotic productions. They emphasized the experiential aspect of the patient-therapist relationship by attempting to understand what the patient was trying to say and verbalize it in terms of what he or she felt. They did little in the way of interpreting, but directed their efforts toward improving relatedness.

Concurrently, Powdermaker and Frank (1953) did similar work with Veterans Administration patients at Perry Point, Maryland. They also noted how the experience of being in a group was beneficial in itself. In a subsequent summary, Frank (1963) emphasized the importance of group cohesiveness as support, the need for role models in the group for behavior modification, and the use of group interactions to help each patient get a more accurate picture of himself or herself in relation to others. Like Semrad, Frank believed that improved communication within the group spills over to and benefits the social structure of the hospital.

This enthusiasm for inpatient group psychotherapy soon waned. Frank (1963), among others, had hoped that a traditional psychoanalytic group would help patients gain insight into symptoms and their causes. Yet rather than producing ego mastery, the focus on feelings heightened anxiety in a way that seemed to impede therapy. Consequently, Frank's writings and those of others began to reflect the preference for task groups, social skills training, and decreased emphasis on verbal psychotherapy. Part of the problem was that inpatient groups were initially modeled after outpatient treatments. But the conditions for treatment are markedly different. The average length of stay on an inpatient unit is less than 1 month, patient turnover is rapid, the population is heterogeneous, and motivation is questionable (Marcovitz and Smith 1986). In addition, there are many confounding variables created by the milieu within which the group resides (Klein 1977). By creating ambiguity, the nondirective method only aggravated these patients' confusion.

Nonpsychodynamic Approaches

Some therapists introduced nonverbal exercises into groups (Cory and Page 1978), and others used psychodrama and related experiential techniques (Farrell 1976). Still others used didactic approaches (Druck

1978) or educational techniques (Maxmen 1978). Certain workers advised use of a graded group program geared to the patient's level of functioning (Betcher et al. 1982; Griffin-Shelley and Trachtenberg 1985). With some of these plans (Leopold 1976; Youcha 1976), patients progressed from the highly structured and supportive group for regressed psychotic individuals to one in which directive techniques were used to promote interpersonal skills and finally to one composed both of outpatients and inpatients who were nearing discharge. However, in other schemata (Yalom 1983), inpatients were divided into populations according to their level of functioning (high or low), and different methods were applied to each.

In contrast to these level-based approaches, some authors excluded those patients who were actively psychotic and disorganized (Marcovitz and Smith 1983; Maxmen 1984) or simply developed a method that was suited to better-functioning, motivated patients, that is, a therapy that had an interpersonal focus (Brabender 1985). Kanas (1985) developed a method designed for homogeneous groups of schizophrenic patients that is supportive and discussion oriented (Kanas and Barr 1983). In this method, patients are encouraged to talk about the problems they have interacting with others. Sharing emotions and symptoms is promoted. There is an attempt to improve reality testing and to help patients cope with disorganizing experiences. Advice is given about practical matters. Expression of anger is discouraged, however, because it is seen as poorly tolerated, anxiety promoting, and potentially disruptive.

Common to most inpatient methods are the use of support and structure, active interpersonal engagement by the therapist, problem spotting, and problem solving. These are typified by the methods of Yalom (1983), described below, and Maxmen (1978). The latter's often-quoted educative model has as its goal the rapid reduction of the problematic behavior that led to hospitalization. Patients are encouraged to identify their maladaptive behavior and to detect and avert those situations that could lead to a recurrence of symptoms. The leader's role is to train patients to work therapeutically with each other (Marcovitz and Smith 1986). Through this experience it is hoped that patients will be more accepting of professional help in the future.

Yalom (1983) developed a structured method for here-and-now, interpersonal learning. Actually, there are two such methods, one for patients functioning at a higher level and one for patients functioning at a lower level. The former is better known and more widely used. The lower-level group for more impaired patients employs systematic verbal tasks that consist of a series of prescribed, graded, sentence-completion exercises. The higher-level group works with an agenda created by the patients to modify maladaptive behavior. In this regard, Yalom's method is focused and pragmatic, like many others mentioned above. Patients are encouraged to play out their self-identified, interpersonal problems within the here and now of the group session. Yalom restricted the focus to interactions within the therapy group itself. He eschewed any consideration of genetic, current life, or milieu issues.

Yalom's method has several characteristics. It is structured and stylized, leader directed, and behaviorally oriented. As such, it is adynamic. Because it is pragmatic and freely teachable, it is made for ready application.

Psychodynamic Approaches

There are a few approaches that claim to be psychodynamic. Battegay (1965) worked supportively, but exploratively, with inpatients, whereas Rice and Rutan (1987) advocated consideration of group transferences, resistances, and genetic factors. But these authors elaborated general principles of treatment and did not develop a specific methodology. In isolation stand reports such as those by Malawista and Malawista (1988) and Cutler (1978), who employed psychoanalytic techniques but did not make a convincing argument for their wide use.

Evidence for the effectiveness of one method over another is lacking. Models that stimulate intense affect have been shown to be of no value (Pattison et al. 1967), and those that uncritically transpose outpatient, expressive techniques can be frankly detrimental (Beutler et al. 1984). Despite earlier negative reviews of controlled studies, recent ones generally support the notion that group therapy is effective for inpatients (Kanas 1985). The question remains: which method is best? In the following section, I discuss recommendations for a dynamic method that integrates the small therapy group into the overall treatment on the unit (Kibel 1981, 1987a, 1987b).

Conditions of Practice

The establishment and conduct of inpatient group psychotherapy require careful attention to the role of the group in the overall treatment program, including its structure and its goals. Practice may vary from one psychiatric unit to another depending on its patient population, length of stay and rate of patient turnover, staffing patterns, availability of therapists to lead the group, and logistics. The parameters of group treatment discussed below should be modified in accordance with the needs of a particular setting.

Forming the Group

For a group program to be successful on a psychiatric unit, it must have solid administrative and staff support. When inaugurating the program, the group therapy coordinator or group leaders must actively seek alliances with key members of the medical and nursing staffs, educating them about the practice and benefits of group therapy. It is also important to show staff how group therapy will benefit them directly by making patients more receptive to milieu treatment. Often it is advantageous to involve the staff directly in the program, such as having key nursing personnel join the program as cotherapists or having staff observe sessions on a systematic basis. On one unit the staff (that is, physician administrators, primary therapists, social workers, and nursing personnel) regularly sat in an observers' circle during group sessions. These sessions were followed by treatment rounds in which patients' behavior in the group became the basis for discussing their functioning in the milieu. The group process itself was not discussed in these rounds (Oldham 1982).

Whether to use cotherapists or one therapist is a multifaceted question with outpatient group psychotherapy. However, with inpatients cotherapy is best. Any disadvantages are outweighed by the support cotherapists can give one another. Such support is needed more with inpatient treatment because the countertransference pressures here are so great.

Once the group program is in place, the group therapists must establish and occasionally redefine arrangements with the unit's staff and its administrators. This has been called the "outside" contract (Rice and Rutan 1981) to differentiate it from the "inside" one (i.e., the usual treatment contract with the patients). The outside contract is designed to maintain the group's boundaries so that it can function in a viable way and includes several elements:

1. The goals of group therapy must be consonant with those of the overall treatment system. The staff must be made to feel that the group therapists are supporting their work. Lack of congruence invariably produces conflict with other staff.

2. Group therapy should have a defined role and be viewed as a primary mode of treatment within a multimodal system and not be subordinate to other treatments.
3. Staff should expect patients to participate in group therapy just as they are expected to cooperate with other treatment prescriptions, such as taking medicine, attending activities, meeting with the social worker, and so on.
4. Assignment to group therapy should be made by the treatment team shortly after admission.
5. The time and place of group therapy must be respected. Other treatments and diagnostic procedures should not be scheduled at that time. When scheduling conflicts are unavoidable, the group therapist should be included in the planning so that he or she can relay the information to the patients in the group and explain what happened. Failure to do so lets the patients know that the staff and group therapists are working at cross purposes, which puts the patients in a bind that will defeat the aims of treatment.
6. Therapists must communicate relevant information from group sessions. Sequestering the group with a rationalization of a need for confidentiality only fosters staff distrust of psychotherapeutic treatments. Communication is simplified when the group therapist is a member of the treatment team or observers are used.
7. Therapists must keep informed of relevant events on the unit, because they will have an impact on the group treatment. Consequent reactions by patients are to be worked out there.

It should be noted that this contract contains elements that spell out the therapists' and the staff's obligations. It stresses their interdependence and will work to their mutual benefit.

Patient Selection

Outpatient selection criteria do not apply to inpatient groups. The very patients who are excluded from outpatient groups are the ones who populate the inpatient units. Therefore, criteria for inclusion need to be quite broad. When the method of treatment is designed to complement the overall hospital treatment program, virtually all patients can benefit from group therapy. The exceptions would be limited to patients who are too confused or too disruptive to participate. More specifically, it is advisable to exclude the following types of patients (Rutchick 1986):

1. Patients with cognitive impairment, such as that seen in patients with marked organic brain syndromes
2. Patients with severe regressions that impede communication of even the simplest of needs
3. Patients who are unable to tolerate even modest external stimulation
4. Patients with tenuous impulse control that threatens the group's safety
5. Patients who exhibit extreme self-injuriousness that requires close, constant observation lest they mutilate themselves
6. Patients who cause the therapist to feel unduly anxious for realistic reasons as opposed to countertransference problems

In applying these criteria the therapist must recognize that his or her attitude toward one patient affects the entire group. Thus intolerance of bizarreness in one patient (e.g., by excluding him or her) can be experienced by the others as a rejection of their psychotic potential. This is antitherapeutic. On the other hand, it is necessary that the group be a safe place where patients need not fear others and where they can say what they wish without concern that it will precipitate aggressive or self-destructive behavior.

Group Composition

Some psychiatric units employ a serial hierarchy of groups, each geared to a particular level of patient functioning (Leopold 1976; Rice and Rutan 1987; Youcha 1976). However, in most settings this approach is not practical because there are an insufficient number of therapists available. Usually, the choice is between the establishment of either two-level groups or team groups.

With a level-based group approach, patients are segregated according to their level of functioning, with better-functioning patients in one group and more regressed patients in the other. Level of functioning may be determined by the Global Assessment of Functioning Scale (American Psychiatric Association 1987), a clinical assessment of patients' current state, or an assessment of the level of patients' internal personality organization. On admission, patients can be divided into two groups, depending on their presenting clinical "state": 1) those who seem to have a predominantly psychotic illness and 2) those who suffer from severe character pathology or affective illness, including manic-depressive patients who readily recompensate (Rutchick 1986). Patients can also be sorted according to an enduring "trait," such as borderline personality organization versus psychotic personality organization (Kernberg 1977).

Team groups require less fine clinical tuning. Patients in team groups are clustered along lines that parallel the administrative structures of the unit. Group therapists are part of specific treatment teams. There are definite advantages to a team approach: 1) communication within the staff is facilitated so that treatment is well coordinated and 2) the assignment of therapists clearly conveys to the patients that the group is an integral part of the treatment system.

In some settings an additional group is provided. This group is for those few patients who meet some of the exclusionary criteria and are not yet ready to join the standard psychotherapy group. They may be included in a separate, very small, intake group (Leopold 1976) that meets daily for abbreviated sessions.

Patient Preparation

In most treatment settings patients have virtually no preparation before entering the group. They may not even have been evaluated by the group therapist, but rather by other clinicians on the team. They are given minimal information before entry beyond the facts of time and place. On some units, they attend the next scheduled session. This is typical for those with a very short length of stay (e.g., 7–10 days). However, on units with longer lengths of stay, even if only 2–4 weeks, it is best for the patient to wait out the next session and join the group thereafter. This short delay allows the new patient to get used to the unit and the other patients to acclimate to him or her.

The "inside" contract (Rice and Rutan 1981) is best kept simple and confined to bare essentials. On some units, it is presented to each patient before entry. But on most units, its major elements are included in an opening, orienting statement at each meeting. The elements include

1. Structural boundaries of the group, namely, the time of the meeting, its length, frequency of sessions, and its location.
2. Explanation of the flow of information (i.e., the informational boundaries) between the milieu and the group. This means that
   a. Members (both patients and therapists) are to discuss outstanding events on the unit, and patients are to include significant information regarding their treatment.
   b. Participants will not discuss information revealed by other group members with patients who are not in the group.

c. Members will bring outside, group-related discussions back to the sessions.
d. Therapists will share information on a selective basis with other members of the treatment team.

Not every part of this contract is spelled out. For example, items *a* and *d* simply become part of the unit's culture of treatment. Likewise, expected norms for behavior on the unit implicitly apply to the group.

Whenever there are new members, the opening statement of that session should include an explanation of the group's purpose, namely, to discuss and clarify any concerns patients have relevant to their problems, their treatment, or their experience on the unit. This statement is usually followed by a go-round of introductions. Although many therapists ask new patients to state why they have come to the hospital, I advise against it. Revealing symptoms associated with decompensation is embarrassing and serves as a narcissistic wound. Usually, no such initiation statement is necessary. On certain units, acculturation can be facilitated by asking the newcomer to state what it was like for him or her to enter the hospital. This open-ended approach gives patients some latitude with their answer.

Structural Elements

It is best if the group meets on or adjacent to the unit so that patients with limited hospital privileges and status are able to attend—preferably a quiet, comfortable place apart from the usual activity of the unit. The size of the group may vary. With fewer than 5 members, interchange is limited. With more than 12 members, even with cotherapists, communication becomes unwieldy. In practice, 7 to 9 members is optimal.

The length of sessions can vary from 45 to 75 minutes. The upper limit is more suited to better-functioning patients. Less than 45 minutes allows little time for orientation, introductions, discussion of topics, and closure. In practice, 45 to 60 minutes is optimal. The frequency of sessions can vary from two to four per week. In general, the shorter the length of stay, the more frequent the sessions.

Method and Technique

There is no consensus in the literature as to the method for inpatient group psychotherapy. Some authors advocate what amounts to a leader-centered approach in which the therapist sets the agenda for the session and orchestrates every move (Yalom 1983). A laissez-faire approach is not advocated by anyone. All agree that it can have deleterious effects (Beutler et al. 1984), because patients lack the ability to tolerate the anxiety engendered by an unstructured group. All agree that the leader needs to be active, moderately directive, accepting, noncritical and, in general, very supportive. Some encourage a focus on maladaptive symptoms and use gentle confrontations to effect change. They might view the group as an arena for social skills training. But others (such as myself) encourage a focus on milieu issues and their effect on patients and rarely confront individuals. Thus the goals for these different approaches will affect technique. The choices are many because the group, and especially the group in context, has a myriad of dynamic possibilities. The following discussion, although attempting to encompass a variety of practices, does reflect my biases.

Goals for Treatment

The goal for treatment should be to help patients understand their experience in the milieu or, at least, to make it more benign. Other benefits will accrue. These include improved relatedness, enhanced appreciation of reality, bolstering of self-esteem, management of aggression, and improvement in the hospital treatment alliance.

Patients' relations with others are usually characterized by manipulation, projection, or projective identification in which they manage to induce in others the noxious, unwanted, and punitive attitudes and/or responses that they find in themselves. In the group, many of these interactions happen but in a more controlled and toned-down way. For this benefit to occur, the therapist must set the tone by reacting to patients in an accepting, noncritical manner, while promoting intermember relationships.

Benign group interactions permit the therapist to assist patients with their sense of reality. Patients struggle with bizarre fantasies that are projected onto others and form the basis of anticipated responses. This is somewhat true with peers, but it is especially true with authority. Therefore, clarifying milieu events, particularly in ways that expose actual staff responses while dispelling distorted ones, improves reality testing. Typically, patients fear that most authorities have malevolent tendencies. These persecutory fantasies ultimately are focused on the therapist. By tolerating them, not responding in kind, and even accepting them while clarifying the reality context, the therapist improves reality testing and helps patients manage their aggression. The following case example shows how a therapist sanctioned group members' anger and by doing so facilitated discussion:

Case 1

> An example occurred on one unit during a period of administrative disor-ganization that happened near the time that the therapists (psychiatric residents) were scheduled to leave the unit. At one session, after acknowl-edged errors by the staff had fouled up passes for several patients, group members were particularly unforthcoming. The therapist tried to get them to talk, but it was like "pulling teeth." The few comments patients made showed that they viewed the nurses as critical and callous, almost malicious. The therapist said that he could understand how, given these errors, the presence of changes on the unit, and the pending rotation, patients would feel frustrated, of course with him too, and not want to talk. The therapist said that the least he could do was to work to prevent any recurrence of such errors. After this statement the patients were more forthcoming and the pace of discussion quickened.

In Case 1, the therapist could be said to have "detoxified" (Kibel 1987b) and "contained" (Bion 1962) these patients' aggression. He ac-cepted their feelings as manageable and demonstrated that he would not retaliate. Reality testing was improved when he failed to respond as antic-ipated.

Reality testing is "the ability to evaluate the external world objectively and to differentiate adequately between it and the internal world" (Stone 1988). It should be differentiated from judgment, which reflects choice. Many therapists make the mistake of confronting patients, basically chal-lenging them on their opinions, under the guise of so-called reality test-ing. This is usually a response to countertransference pressure.

With therapeutic, member-to-member interaction comes enhanced self-esteem. Feelings of hopelessness and powerlessness are countered as patients interact with one another and gain a sense of mastery, particu-larly over their own responses to environmental events. The world is no longer a confusing and frightening place. Moreover, patients learn that their reactions to events are understandable by normal standards of human responsiveness. Statements by the therapist that clarify and ex-plain this process promote empathic linkages among the patients. More importantly, ego mastery is promoted when patients learn that their chaotic reactions are capable of being understood. The following case example shows how therapists' acceptance of patients' aggression—clarifying its nature and explaining how the environment and/or milieu upset them—served to calm the patients down:

Case 2

This group session took place on a unit with an average length of stay of 4 weeks. It occurred just 1 week before the vacation of one of the cotherapists. The session was shaped against the background of three recent events. First, 5 days previously, an unattended razor had been discovered on the unit. Second, 3 days previously, Mr. A had tied some cord around his neck while at the hospital gymnasium. When this was discussed at the next community meeting, it was dramatized in that it was said that he had fashioned a noose for his neck. Finally, 2 days previously, a borderline patient did not return from an authorized pass. Notably, this patient had been initially admitted after she had scratched her abdomen with a razor blade. These events were reflected by an atmosphere on the unit of uneasiness and impending doom.

The session began with a standard orientation statement from one therapist. At that point, Mr. A spoke up and identified himself by another patient's name. He claimed that everyone in the group had the same name. His statements were characteristic of the early phase of this session, which was disjointed and chaotic. One patient talked about another's insomnia. A regressed patient said that he wanted a job. Another babbled about medication and physical fitness. Mr. A said he envied those patients who have liberal hospital privileges because such freedom permitted them to exercise on their own whenever they pleased. Another patient reported that he believed the staff restricted his privileges out of fear that he would "pop pills." He complained that they were prejudiced against those who have used marijuana. The regressed man began to talk about cars and girlfriends, but his speech quickly degenerated into unintelligible ramblings. Mr. A next cataloged a series of complaints about the unit, ranging from the unavailability of marijuana to the unproductivity of most of the treatments available. When describing his frustration with these, he mumbled, "That's why I did it."

Up to this point, the session had sounded like bedlam. The references to physical fitness and exercise were meaningful to the therapists because they related to the incident at the gymnasium. The references to marijuana were less clear. The therapists were unable to organize the discussion until it crystallized into a barrage of complaints about the treatment program. They showed acceptance of the patients' anger by postulating that their dissatisfaction must have caused them to feel frustrated with the staff. The patients agreed and more complaints followed. At one point, Mr. A characterized the atmosphere on the unit as one of a "war between the patients and the staff." The therapists further commented that the recent events could have easily caused the members to feel as if they were in an unsafe environment, attended to by uncertain staff and therapists. The impending vacation of one may have added to this sense of instability.

These interventions helped to calm the group members. Conditions became favorable for an orderly discussion of the recent untoward events. This discussion was developed by the patients, but was orchestrated by the therapists. At one point, one therapist remarked that when events get out of control, as they had recently on this unit, patients feel frightened, become disillusioned and frustrated with their therapists, and may even wonder whether illicit drugs have played a role. The patients agreed and reported that some others were dissatisfied with their therapists and wondered if these patients were "pot heads." (The following week it was learned that some marijuana had been on the unit before all these events.) Near the close of this session, one therapist explained that when a unit feels unsafe patients get frightened and that the difficulty they had had at the beginning of this session reflected such anxiety. This was understandable, he said, because anyone in such a situation would become quite anxious. By the end of the session, the patients were much calmer, their conversation was both organized and relevant, and they were more related to each other.

Techniques of Intervention

Appreciation of the rationale for treatment and its goals is more important than the study of technique. From understanding flows the method. Only general guidelines can be stated here. Like all forms of psychotherapy, application of treatment principles is an art. As noted, the therapist of an inpatient group needs to be active, supportive, and noncritical. First, he or she should use interventions that mobilize the patients, interest them, and promote member-to-member interaction. Second, he or she ought to ensure that relevant milieu issues are introduced so that the group discussion will be immediately meaningful to the patients. These two strategies are related.

Support can be provided in subtle as well as in overt ways. Examples of the former can include offering one patient a chair or another a tissue, inviting some to join the circle, attending to each one's physical comfort, and sitting next to a disturbed patient who needs additional attention.

The therapist needs to attend to his or her own behavior. He or she should apologize for his or her mistakes (e.g., lateness) and then make up the lost time. Patients should be told well in advance of any structural or schedule changes, including missed sessions due to holidays, vacations, and so on.

Patients respond well to praise, but only if it is genuine and not gratuitous. This praise may include a word of appreciation to an anxious patient who sat through an entire session or to another for trying to promote the therapeutic process. Likewise, it is well to show interest in what patients say, no matter how negative or bizarre it may seem. Even a complaint about medication can reflect feelings, for example, fear of authority. One should never label patients' comments or questions as "inappropriate." The word conveys denigration. Interest in a patient's jumbled thoughts shows respect for the psychotic potential in others. When members need to be cut off or topics deferred, this should be done tactfully. The focus ought to be on people, not on their symptoms.

Overall, support is given when the therapist provides structure. This includes starting each session on time, ending without cutting patients off, welcoming newcomers, orienting them, and carrying out the provisions of the treatment contract as previously outlined. It is the therapist's job to engage the retiring members, for example, by asking silent ones for their observations or merely checking in with them by asking how they are managing. When problems in the process arise, the therapist must handle them if the patients are unable. In this regard, silences must not last too long. The therapist should feel free to introduce topics, especially those related to life on the unit, if these are not forthcoming from the membership. The active therapist is one who quietly orchestrates the flow of the session without imposing his or her preconceived ideas.

Group interaction is promoted when the therapist gently deflects attention and interest away from himself or herself and toward the patients. This can be done by inviting opinions and observations on particular issues. Likewise, it helps to present topics in which all have an investment. It is important to ask questions in a manner that allows for a concrete focus rather than an abstract response. Thus patients respond better when asked "what happened?" rather than "how did you react?" Because these patients have difficulty "owning" their own responses because of their paranoid stance, unit events may first be discussed in terms of how others were affected before patients are asked to describe the events' impact on them. Noting their ability to be forthcoming and their success in helping one another is a way to give implicit praise.

When impasses occur or structural difficulties are encountered, the therapist can ask members for help. This shows respect. Yet it is the therapist who must manage intermember conflict and diminish scapegoating. A useful device here is to explain or interpret the process. Interpretations have a way of correcting this behavior by explaining that its sources lie beyond conscious intention. They can also serve as gentle admonition. Invariably, an interpretation tends to move action, thought, and affect from the realm of the ego-syntonic to the ego-dystonic.

The therapist can weave group cohesion in several ways. Experiences of one patient can be generalized to the others. Similarities among members can be noted. Sometimes the therapist can respond to one patient by using the words or phraseology of another. Likewise, references to previous sessions help give the members a sense of continuity. Lastly, showing members how they respond to particular events is the most powerful group-bonding technique.

The most fascinating part of group psychotherapy is discerning meaning from metaphors. With inpatient work the task of making so-called interpretations is more complicated than with other kinds of groups. First, when the content reflects a concern of the membership, the therapist needs to do more than merely translate its meaning. He or she must relate it to the event to which the patients are reacting. In fact, discussion of the event is often more important than exploration of its effect. The aim is to improve the hospital treatment alliance, not to gain insight. Second, the process of translating metaphors should be indirect. Strict interpretation of group themes can be narcissistically wounding to patients because it unduly implies that the metaphoric content has little face value. It is much better to decode the material by drawing analogies to the precipitating event or even to raise the latter as a parallel issue. For example, if the stimulus is an explosive outburst by an acutely manic patient and the metaphoric content is about angry parents, the therapist might say that feeling helpless and frustrated in the face of an unpredictable, impulsive parent must be analogous to what the patients experienced when the index patient lost control of himself. Again, if a smooth transition from one topic to another is not possible, the therapist can merely raise the milieu issue in a timely fashion.

It is important that explanations of patients' reactions to events contain several elements, as previously indicated. Their reactions must be identified as understandable and bearing semblance to those of other people in like situations. The therapist should empathically describe the patients' aggressive reactions in gentle terms, for example, to say that they might be frustrated (instead of angry). The therapist must acknowledge that these reactions are also directed toward the treatment team, including himself or herself. For example, in the instance of the manic patient who lost control, the therapist could empathize with the patients' "frustration" that the staff could not contain that individual and state that he expected that they would be frustrated with him too because he is part of the treatment team. These interventions help to work out problems in the alliance through the transference in the group.

Conclusions

This chapter is far from inclusive. Further descriptions of technique are not possible here. (For an excellent review of techniques, see Rice and Rutan 1987.) Likewise, countertransference is an exhaustive subject that is beyond the scope of this chapter. Inpatients virtually thrive on inducing noxious reactions in others so as to convince themselves that the problems are "out there," not inside themselves. (For discussions of this issue, see Brabender 1987 and Hannah 1984).

By the same token, supervision is required for junior therapists, and peer supervision or regular, outside consultation is needed for more experienced therapists. This recommendation underlines an important aspect of inpatient work; it is arduous. But it is extremely rewarding.

References

American Psychiatric Association: Diagnostic and Statistical Manual of Mental Disorders, 3rd Edition, Revised. Washington, DC, American Psychiatric Association, 1987

Battegay R: Psychotherapy of schizophrenics in small groups. Int J Group Psychother 15:316–320, 1965

Betcher RW, Rice CA, Weir DM: The regressed inpatient group in a graded group treatment program. Am J Psychother 36:229–239, 1982

Beutler LE, Frank M, Schieber SC, et al: Comparative effects of group psychotherapies in a short-term inpatient setting: an experience with deteriorating effects. Psychiatry 47:66–76, 1984

Bion WR: Learning from Experience. New York, Basic Books, 1962

Brabender VM: Time-limited inpatient group therapy: a developmental model. Int J Group Psychother 35:373–390, 1985

Brabender VM: Vicissitudes of countertransference in inpatient group psycho-therapy. Int J Group Psychother 37:549–567, 1987

Cory TL, Page D: Group techniques for effecting change in the more disturbed patient. Group 2:149–155, 1978

Cutler MO: Symbolism and imagery in a group of chronic schizophrenics. Int J Group Psychother 28:73–80, 1978

Druck AB: The role of didactic group psychotherapy in short-term psychiatric settings. Group 2:98–109, 1978

Farrell D: The use of active experiential group techniques with hospitalized pa-tients, in Group Therapy 1976. Edited by Wolberg LR, Aronson ML. New York, Stratton Intercontinental Medical Book Corp., 1976, pp 44–51

Foulkes SH: Therapeutic Group Analysis. New York, International Universities Press, 1965

Frank JD: Group therapy in the mental hospital, in Group Psychotherapy and Group Function. Edited by Rosenbaum M, Berger M. New York, Basic Books, 1963, pp 453–468

Griffin-Shelley E, Trachtenberg J: Group psychotherapy with short-term in-pa-tients. Small Group Behavior 13:97–104, 1985

Hannah S: Countertransference in inpatient group psychotherapy: implications for technique. Int J Group Psychother 34:257–272, 1984

Kanas N: Inpatient and outpatient group therapy for schizophrenic patients. Am J Psychother 39:431–439, 1985

Kanas N, Barr MA: Homogeneous group therapy for acutely psychotic schizo-phrenic inpatients. Hosp Community Psychiatry, 34:257–259, 1983

Kernberg OF: The structural diagnosis of borderline personality organization, in Borderline Personality Disorders. Edited by Hartocollis P. New York, Interna-tional Universities Press, 1977, pp 87–121

Kibel HD: A conceptual model for short-term inpatient group psychotherapy. Am J Psychiatry 138:74–80, 1981

Kibel HD: Contributions of the group psychotherapist to education on the psy-chiatric unit: teaching through group dynamics. Int J Group Psychother 37:3–29, 1987a

Kibel HD: Inpatient group psychotherapy: where treatment philosophies con-verge, in The Yearbook of Psychoanalysis and Psychotherapy. Edited by Langs R. New York, Gardner Press, 1987b, pp 94–116

Kibel HD: A historical memoir on group psychotherapy, in Group Psychodynam-ics: New Paradigms and New Perspectives. Edited by Halperin DA. Chicago, IL, Year Book Medical, 1989, pp 3–28

Klein RH: Inpatient group psychotherapy: practical considerations and special problems. Int J Group Psychother 27:201–214, 1977

Klein RH, Kugel B: Inpatient group psychotherapy: reflections through a glass darkly. Int J Group Psychother 31:311–328, 1981

Lazell EW: The group treatment of dementia praecox. Psychoanal Rev 8:168–179, 1921

Leopold HS: Selective group approaches with psychotic patients in hospital settings. Am J Psychother 30:95–102, 1976

Levine HB: Milieu biopsy: the place of the therapy group on the inpatient ward. Int J Group Psychother 30:77–93, 1980

Malawista KL, Malawista PL: Modified group-as-a-whole psychotherapy with chronic psychotic patients. Bull Menninger Clin 52:114–125, 1988

Mann J, Semrad EV: The use of group therapy in psychoses. Journal of Social Casework 29:176–181, 1948

Marcovitz RJ, Smith JE: An approach to time-limited dynamic inpatient group therapy. Small Group Behavior 14:369–376, 1983

Marcovitz RJ, Smith JE: Short-term group therapy: a review of the literature. International Journal of Short-Term Psychotherapy 1:49–57, 1986

Marsh LC: Group treatment by the psychological equivalent of the revival. Ment Hyg 15:328–349, 1931

Marsh LC: Group therapy in the psychiatric clinic. J Nerv Ment Dis 82:381–392, 1935

Maxmen JS: An educative model for inpatient group therapy. Int J Group Psychother 28:321–338, 1978

Maxmen JS: Helping patients survive theories: the practice of an educative model. Int J Group Psychother 34:355–368, 1984

Oldham JM: The use of silent observers as an adjunct to short-term group psychotherapy. Int J Group Psychother 32:469–480, 1982

Pattison EM, Brissenden E, Wohl T: Assessing special effects of inpatient group psychotherapy. Int J Group Psychother 17:283–297, 1967

Powdermaker FB, Frank JD: Group Psychotherapy: Studies in Methodology of Research and Therapy. Cambridge, MA, Harvard University Press, 1953

Rice CA, Rutan JS: Boundary maintenance in inpatient therapy groups. Int J Group Psychother 31:297–309, 1981

Rice CA, Rutan JS: Inpatient Group Psychotherapy: A Psychodynamic Perspective. New York, Macmillan, 1987

Rutchick IE: Group Psychotherapy, in Inpatient Psychiatry, 2nd Edition. Edited by Sederer LI. Baltimore, MD, Williams & Wilkins, 1986, pp 263–279

Standish CT, Semrad EV: Group psychotherapy with psychotics. Journal of Psychiatric Social Work 20:143–150, 1951

Stone EM: American Psychiatric Glossary, 6th Edition. Washington, DC, American Psychiatric Press, 1988

Wender L: The dynamics of group psychotherapy and its application. J Nerv Ment Dis 84:54–60, 1936

Yalom ID: Inpatient Group Psychotherapy. New York, Basic Books, 1983

Youcha IZ: Short-term in-patient group: formation and beginnings. Group Process 7:119–137, 1976

CHAPTER 6

The Community Meeting

Cecil A. Rice, Ph.D.

Introduction

The *community meeting*—sometimes called a *ward meeting*—is the most pivotal treatment of the psychiatric hospital. (Except when clarity demands otherwise, I will use the term "hospital" to refer to a psychiatric hospital or a psychiatric unit that is part of a general hospital.) It is the meeting in which the hospital culture, values, and practices are passed on from one patient generation to the next. It is the meeting at which all the other treatments and the many other meetings, both casual and professional, converge. It is also the meeting in which the intrapsychic worlds of numerous individuals, patients and staff alike, come together and play themselves out in a network of interactions that give voice to the primitive, unconscious, and irrational inner worlds of the participants as well as to their mature, conscious, and rational worlds. These interactions sometimes result in melodramatic meetings and at other times in meetings punctuated by empty, dreadful, or seemingly meaningless silences. Most meetings fluctuate somewhere between these extremes.

Despite the many difficulties in leading and participating in a community meeting, a well-run meeting can be a very effective container and articulator of the needs and desires of its members. The optimal expression of those desires in the community meeting, accompanied by occasional commentary, significantly reduces the potential for their being repetitiously acted out on the floors and grounds of the hospital, thus

I want to thank Burns Woodward, M.D., and Marianne McGrath, L.C.S.W., of Westwood Lodge psychiatric hospital, Westwood, Massachusetts, for their careful review of this chapter and for their helpful comments.

avoiding additional trauma to individual members and to the hospital community. In brief, the community meeting can be the treatment that holds together and informs all the other treatments and activities in the hospital, both individual and communal.

In this chapter, I seek to provide readers with some understanding of the community meeting and to suggest ways in which staff may both participate in and lead it effectively. I address the following areas: the history of the community meeting, the relationship of the community meeting to the hospital, the dynamics of the community meeting, and finally, leading the community meeting.

A Brief History of the Community Meeting

Communities have been vehicles for healing since before recorded history. Ellenberger (1970) noted, "Primitive healing is almost always a public and a collective procedure" (p. 39). The primitive healer, who was often the central figure of his or her tribe, usually worked with patients' families and other members of the tribe to relieve them of their physical and psychic pain by using rituals that resemble modern psychodrama. Examples of these community rituals were found among the Zuni (Stevenson 1901–1902), Navaho (Pfister 1932), and Huron Indians (Raguenau 1897) and among the Amhara of Ethiopia (Almond 1974), among others. In more recent times, especially in the first half of the nineteenth century during the era of Moral Treatment, healing in psychiatric hospitals often included the active participation of patients and staff alike (Rice and Rutan 1987). And for centuries, religious groups of many persuasions and cultural heritages have made extensive use of the community to shape and control the behaviors and values of their members and to provide succor in times of stress.

Since the beginning of the twentieth century, the histories of group therapy and community meetings have been closely entwined. Many of the group therapies of the early 1900s were more akin to community meetings as we know them than to modern group therapy. Marsh (Rice and Rutan 1987), one of the early founders of the group therapy movement, used a variety of group approaches. One method was to lecture patients about the nature of their illnesses in groups with as many as 100 members. Staff also participated in those large groups. Around the same time, Lazell (Rice and Rutan 1987) used a similar model.

There is little doubt that the community meeting received a major impetus after World War II with the rise of the Therapeutic Community movement. Founders of the movement (such as Maxwell Jones [1953]; its putative father, Main [1946], who coined the phrase; and Foulkes [1977], who also claimed paternity) made large meetings of the entire staff-patient community an essential part of their approach. Since that time, community meetings have become an integral part of most psychiatric hospitals in Western societies.

Relationship of the Community Meeting to the Hospital

For inpatients, being hospitalized in a special environment where they are separated from their normal everyday activities is the primary mode of treatment. All other modes of treatment, while necessary and even essential, are derivative. Further, as Jones (1953) and others (e.g., Foulkes 1977; Kindts and Verhaest 1980) have made clear, the nature of that special environment determines the effectiveness of all treatments that take place within the hospital.

The import of the hospital environment is often taken for granted until something goes wrong. A helpful analogy is the early history of the general hospital. It is well known that patients admitted to a general hospital used to contract additional illnesses, sometimes worse than the illness for which they had been hospitalized, because the equipment, beds, sheets, food, and air were contaminated. In a similar manner, the atmosphere of the psychiatric hospital can be contaminated by unresolved stresses and conflicts and by negligent, cold, or hostile attitudes among the staff. That contamination can quickly lead to exacerbations of patients' illnesses. The rapid turnover of patients means that tensions between and among staff and patients need to be addressed more immediately than in longer-term units, where resolutions can be allowed to evolve more slowly. Paradoxically, the brevity of each patient's stay tempts us to allow difficulties to be resolved by waiting for troublesome patients (and staff) to move on.

Arguably, the community meeting contributes more to the climate of the hospital, for good or ill, than most other daily events in the hospital. Clearly, the community meeting is not the only contributor, but as stated in the introduction, its centrality makes its direct and indirect influence on the hospital atmosphere very telling.

In systems terms (von Bertalanffy 1968), the community meeting is the largest subsystem of the hospital and contains most of the other subsystems of the hospital within it. Within the community meeting are the subsystems of the individual members, including the subsystems of their pathological structures and pathology-free structures, and the individual, group, and occupational and medication therapy subsystems, among many others. There are also representatives of the hospital system itself, such as the medical and clinical directors and the heads of various departments. Hence during a community meeting the boundaries between and among the hospital and its various systems and subsystems are at their most permeable, leaving each system receptive to information from all the other systems, including the community meeting itself. In brief, whatever transpires within the community meeting becomes a part of the hospital and its many subsystems.

The converse is also true. Whatever is taking place in the hospital at large or in its various subsystems has an immediate effect on the community meeting. For instance, the unresolved conflict in a recent group therapy session or in the coffee shop will be carried into the community meeting and affect the meeting and its subsystems. In addition, the manner by which that conflict is addressed in the community meeting will not only determine its effect on the meeting but will also determine how it penetrates the other subsystems and how it reenters the group in question, or the patients' meal time.

In summary, the transfer of information and experience between the community meeting and its subsystems and the hospital system takes place on a continuous feedback loop. Thus interventions of the therapist-leaders[1] in charge of the community meeting play an important role in determining whether that feedback loop results in an atmosphere conducive to healing. Interventions that enable the concerns of the community meeting members to be optimally articulated and contained will, as a rule, create a safer and more helpful environment both in the hospital at large and within the other treatment modes. By contrast, ineffective leadership of the community meeting can result in an acute regression of patients and staff that will limit the effectiveness of all other treatments and contaminate the hospital atmosphere.

In the section on leadership of the community meeting I address more

---

[1] Throughout I refer to the leader or leaders of the community meeting as "therapist-leaders" or simply "therapists" because I view the community meeting as a form of therapy and not simply a management meeting.

specifically the role of therapists' interventions. It is sufficient at this point to emphasize the centrality of the community meeting and its influence, for good or ill, on the hospital at large and on the other treatments.

Dynamics of the Community Meeting

Elsewhere (Rice and Rutan 1987) I use the metaphors of the town meeting and the family meeting to describe the dynamics of the community meeting. Here, I am adding a third metaphor, namely, the community meeting as theater. These metaphors approximate the political, interpersonal, and intrapsychic aspects of the community meeting. In Bion's terms (1959), they may also be viewed as a gradual movement from the task group to the basic assumption group. For the sake of clarity I address each metaphor separately; however, in practice these features of the community meeting are closely interrelated, transforming and being transformed by each other.

Community Meeting as Town Meeting

The community meeting is like a town meeting in that it is concerned with aspects of community management and addresses and performs numerous tasks essential to the running of the community. It is the art of the possible in a hospital setting. For our purposes, the dynamics of this political dimension of the community may be viewed as largely secondary process in nature, logical, and akin to Bion's work group (1959). Clearly, there are other powerful unconscious forces in operation, which I address in the third metaphor.

At this level of organization the community meeting is concerned with such management tasks as 1) *information exchange*[2] (Almond 1974); 2) the discussion of hospital policies, changes, and procedures as they relate to the patients and their treatment; and 3) the general management of everyday events.

Information exchange can include an endless variety of things. Among the more common are announcements of meal schedules, changes in menus, new additions to the staff, staff vacations, and the addition of new buildings or the repair of existing buildings, advice on ex-

---

[2] The term was first used by Winer and Lewis (1984) to describe the reciprocal sharing of information between patients and staff in the community meeting.

posure to the sun while on medication, explanations of on- or off-grounds privileges, and so on. Patient information to the staff may include concerns such as drug dealing on the floor, suicide threats, discharge plans, the benefits of medication and various treatments (as well as difficulties with same), and problems with washing machines and dryers.

Discussion also may be generated by events external to the community meeting and by experiences of staff and patients within the hospital that raise questions about hospital policies and procedures. For instance, during a rather quiet community meeting, a thoughtful, middle-aged man raised the following issue with the staff and the therapist-leader of the community meeting:

> "Last weekend while on pass I saw the movie *One Flew Over the Cuckoo's Nest.* I was horrified at that movie, so I want to know what the policies of this hospital are regarding shock treatment and restraints."

The meeting was no longer quiet. Others had seen the movie and demanded to know the hospital's policies. A lively discussion ensued.

This request can be understood on a variety of levels. Clearly, whatever else it may imply, it is a question addressed to the policy of the hospital and it can and should be addressed at that level.

Management of everyday events draws the community meeting's attention to those numerous small and large happenings that take place in any hospital. These happenings may arise in response to a crisis or may simply be the mundane tasks necessary to the smooth running of any community. Common examples include the following: Who will take the minutes of the community meeting? Can we get a group of staff and patients together to go to the movies this weekend? Let us agree that when people answer the patients' telephone they do not give out the name of the hospital. Can we ask the chef to make sure the milk is fresh in the morning and not sour as it has been recently?

Management of everyday events also includes the management of information exchange in the hospital at large. For instance, who speaks to the chef about the sour milk—the patients or the staff or both? Patients concerned about the payment of their fees may be directed to discuss the situation with their therapists and the business office, as well as discussing it in the community meeting.

Some aspects of the management of everyday events fall into a gray area between the community meeting as town meeting and the community meeting as family meeting.

Community Meeting as Family Meeting

The community meeting is like a family meeting in that it addresses the pleasures, conflicts, attractions, dislikes, loves, fears, and angers that arise among and between people who live, work, eat, and sleep under the same roof. At this level of organization, the community meeting is concerned with interpersonal aspects of the community more intimate than those addressed in the previous section.

The community meeting, for instance, plays a significant role in enabling new patients and staff to bond with the family community. It is during community meetings that new patients and staff are first introduced by name to the whole community. During these introductions, patients and staff may also share a little about themselves to facilitate the bonding. New patients, for instance, may simply acknowledge the welcome, or they may add a comment about where they come from, with whom they share a room, or whom they have met since coming to the hospital. New staff may also simply acknowledge the welcome or they may describe their particular functions in the hospital. Other members of the community may respond to these introductions in ways that range from limited to expansive. Whatever the response, the initial process of bonding has taken place.

From this tentative beginning, as Kirsch et al. (1981) noted, patients and staff alike begin to develop a membership identity. They begin to see and experience themselves as members of the family-community.

At the other end, the community meeting performs the important function of enabling members to say goodbye to their family-community. Bonding and terminating are intimately related. For some patients the fear of loss is so great that bonding is precluded so that losses may be avoided. For others bonding is readily accepted, whereas ending is denied and tenaciously resisted, or the original bonding is denied to make the ending bearable. For still others the fear of losing a sense of self in relationships or in large groups is so great that attachments can be acknowledged only when endings are taking place. Thus in facilitating the "hellos" and "goodbyes" the community meeting not only strengthens the family-community but also provides patients with an opportunity to address issues that are often intimately related to why they came to the hospital in the first place.

Between the hellos and goodbyes, the community meeting addresses an endless variety of other interpersonal and family issues, such as two patients fighting over the use of space in their bedroom, an argument between a patient and a staff person, a patient stealing from another patient, a patient playing the piano loudly while others are trying to watch television, a rumor of an intimate relationship between a patient and a staff person, the development of a tight group that excludes other patients, or a "strange" patient who frightens others.

At this level of organization, the community meeting provides an opportunity for direct talk among the individuals involved, the optimal expression of feelings and concerns, a related reduction in anxiety and paranoia, and a cessation of the offending behavior. Clinical experience suggests that this also results in greater safety throughout the hospital.

Community Meeting as Theater

Theater is frequently the window into the soul of humankind. Like the myth, theater can be viewed as the dream of the community in which human archetypes find expression in acceptable and disguised form. As Bergman (1987) so persuasively argued, many of Shakespeare's plays, like the Greek myths, address complex and distressing aspects of love in acceptable forms, providing catharsis and possible resolution for the audience. He noted also that the audience project their conscious and unconscious conflicts around love and sex onto the actors and identify with them as they play out and demonstrate the numerous themes of love and sex.

The community meeting is like theater in that the patients project onto the meeting and its leadership and staff a variety of unconscious and preconscious concerns and conflicts and identify with the therapists' and staff's responses to them, real or imagined. Indeed, the force of those projections can be so powerful that, to paraphrase Bion (1959), therapist-leaders and staff may feel like actors in an impromptu play scripted by the patients. Those projections often contain a variety of object and part-object representations and their associated sexual and aggressive drive derivatives; these can be of fantastic proportions that imbue staff and therapists with immense powers to heal or destroy. The meeting, therapist-leaders, and staff become endowed with charismatic power (Almond 1974; Rice and Rutan 1981).

For example, in one community meeting, there was a lively and heated debate about the impact of modifications of the hospital structure and related policies on the patients and their treatment. Finally, a very irate man turned to the community meeting leader (a hired member of staff) and said, "Doctor, if you own this hospital I do not see why you cannot just go out there and change these policies and stop those builders from interfering with us." This illustration not only portrays the power of patient projections, but also makes clear that the community meeting as theater profoundly affects the community meeting as town and family meeting. The irate man was concerned about matters related to hospital policies and politics and deserved to be addressed at that level. But his statement also revealed his flattering and distorted perception of the therapist and the nature of his expectations and disappointment in him.

From this perspective, the earlier example about the response to the movie *One Flew Over the Cuckoo's Nest* takes on a new and richer meaning. In a political sense, the patients had a right to know the hospital's policy about shock treatment and restraints. However, the illustration must also be understood in terms of the helplessness and fears patients may feel toward the staff and the corresponding projection onto them of their own frightening and destructive desires.

Community meeting size also significantly affects the nature of the members' projections and the resultant dynamics of the meeting. The size of most community meetings is such that it is difficult or impossible for members to maintain face-to-face contact. Under these circumstances, members' projections tend to become increasingly fantastic and disorganized because the lack of eye-to-eye contact deprives them of the "otherness" of members whose verbal and nonverbal behavior can give feedback that may correct or modify those projections. In the words of Buber (1958), the lack of eye-to-eye contact tends to reduce a "thou" to an "it," with a resultant decrease in the containment of projections. This is especially true if the meeting is run in an unstructured manner. Such an increase in the fantastic nature of the members' projections can also prove threatening to their sense of identity (Kernberg 1980; Turquet 1975).

There are several solutions to this dynamic problem. The most common one is an increase of projections onto, and of identification with, the therapist-leaders and staff of the community meeting (Greene et al. 1980). This helps to contain the projections and to solidify each member's identity. The idealization and charismatic elevation of the therapists and the staff are then increased, creating what Bion (1959) called a dependency assumption group; Rice and Rutan (1987) referred to this as the dependency culture of the hospital. The converse of this idealization is also true. The elevated staff can readily be demeaned if, as is inevitable, they fail in the charismatic role, at which point they may become recipients of primitive aggressive and destructive projections.

Another solution, especially when the first one fails, is to choose a patient as leader. Kernberg (1980) noted that certain narcissistic patients are particularly able to provide organization for the community meeting, often better than members of staff. He suggested that "the lack of deep conviction regarding his own values makes it easy for the narcissistic personality to swim with the currents of the group" (Kernberg 1980, p. 250). He added that the narcissistic patient's desire for center stage and his or her capacity to manipulate others make him or her a great leveler of the group's tensions. Such a patient can become a leader of the community meeting, sometimes in a destructive manner against the staff as a whole, a particular staff member, or a particular patient.

Another solution is for the community meeting to break into small groups or for members to form special one-to-one bonds within the meeting. Thus the members can identify with their small group or pair and project unpleasant and primitive concerns onto others outside the small group. In brief, the community meeting can regress from a dependency group to a series of what Turquet (1974) and others (McMillan 1981; Morrison et al. 1985) have called oneness assumption groups, in which splitting is the primary defense. Not uncommonly, those projected concerns are turned into actions that can be damaging to individual patients and staff. They are certainly disruptive to the community meeting and to the hospital as a whole and frequently lead to increases in iatrogenic anxiety and regression that seriously limit the effectiveness of treatment.

Although my focus has been almost exclusively on the projections of the patients, it is important to note that staff members may have the same projections as the patients, thus adding to the complexity of the community meeting dynamics. Other things being equal, however, it is expected that the staff will have better mastery of their like projections, feel less overwhelmed by them, and be less prone to act them out than the patients. Staff, however, may have more difficulty dealing with the demands of patients' projections on them and with the reciprocal projections they may stimulate. The charismatic elevation of staff members, for instance, along with their own desires to heal, may result in overwhelming frustration with the limited responses of the patients and sometimes lead, to their own embarrassment, to angry and sadistic behavior.

Leading the Community Meeting

For a community meeting to run effectively, it is essential that its boundaries be optimally maintained. They should be open and permeable enough to allow for information to enter from and, having been processed, to return to other parts of the hospital. The boundaries should also be open and permeable enough to allow for adequate communication among the participants.

The boundaries must be firm enough to clearly distinguish the community meeting from other functions in the hospital. They should also be firm enough to allow for clear distinctions between and among the members and between patients and staff.

Well-maintained boundaries also play an important role in reducing the iatrogenic anxiety, regression, and splitting noted earlier. In doing so, the boundaries prevent the community meeting and the hospital from becoming, in terms of an earlier metaphor, a contaminating environment.

There are a variety of boundaries around and within the community meeting. As noted above, these include the boundary between the community meeting and the rest of the hospital and the boundary between the patients and the staff. These boundaries are especially influenced by and dependent on two aspects of community meeting leadership: contracts and meeting structure.

Community Meeting Contracts

The community meeting contract is among three sets of parties: hospital administration, staff, and patients.

Agreements with the administration.   No community meeting can function effectively without the active support of the administration. Hence, it is important that the administration openly agree to support the community meeting therapists and staff in their work. Such agreements should include three features:

1. The administration acknowledges the importance and centrality of the community meeting.
2. The administration agrees that no other treatments, patient, or staff activities will take place during the community meeting time. Clearly, exceptions are made for emergencies, coverage for patients unable to attend the meeting, and so on.
3. The administration expects all treatment staff (e.g., nursing staff and other floor staff, administrators of patient care, psychiatrists, psychologists, social workers, occupational therapists, and other clinicians)

on duty at the time of the meeting to attend. Again, exceptions for emergencies and the like can be made.

Agreements with the staff. The agreements with the staff are consistent with and reiterate those made with the administration:

1. The staff agree to attend all community meetings when they are on duty.
2. The staff agree to participate.
3. The staff agree to arrive on time and stay for the full session.

Agreements with patients. The agreements with patients are similar to those with the staff and are consistent with the agreements made with the administration. The staff must, on occasion, make clinical judgments regarding the extent to which any given patient can understand and live up to those expectations and how much it will help the patient to do so.

1. Patients agree to attend all meetings unless it is clearly detrimental for them to do so or detrimental or dangerous to the other members of the meeting.
2. The remainder of the agreements are the same as those for the staff.

Structure of the Community Meeting

The structure of the community meeting should facilitate the achievement of the meeting's goals, which are to aptly voice and optimally address the issues of politics, family, and theater within the meeting. Thus the structure of the meeting should not be so rigid as to preclude the opportunity to address the affective and unconscious communications of the members, nor so loose that the passions of the theater remove all order and the possibility of critical review.

Within these parameters the structure of a community meeting can vary considerably. The following is an example of a fairly common structure of a community meeting.

The beginning phase: welcome and announcements. The beginning phase of the community meeting is usually quite well structured and facilitates the settling in of the members. In this phase, after a punctual beginning, therapists invite the members to introduce themselves. This is often done in a fairly rote manner by going around the room. This activity helps draw new members in and gives all members an opportunity to put names to faces. Clearly, this process can be overdone, especially in those hospitals where the population is very stable. However, this is an increasingly rare phenomenon, because rapid turnover of hospital populations is much more common. And in these latter circumstances, or in situations where patients' memory traces have been severely compromised by years of illness, the naming of others can be very helpful and act at least as an initial acknowledgment of their existence, if not as an initial step toward tentative bonding.

During this introductory process it is also helpful to state very briefly and in everyday language the goals of the community meeting. For instance, therapists might say, "This is a meeting where we can talk about what it is like to live and work together in the hospital, try to resolve our differences, and understand what we do and say."

This introduction is often followed by announcements by both staff and patients. The therapist-leaders will usually make general announcements about hospital events. Staff members may also have important announcements to make, such as vacation plans, modifications in treatment schedules, and resignations. Patients may also have announcements to make and should be given the opportunity to do so. These may include their discharge plans, room changes, and privileges.

A transition phase: discussion of announcements. The next part of the community meeting is transitional in nature and usually involves responses and dialogue about the announcements, often encouraged by the leader(s) and the staff. This discussion can be very helpful because it allows patients to voice any uncertainties, feelings, or concerns they may have about the various announcements.

From this transition the meeting usually moves into the middle phase, in which the major discussion of the meeting takes place.

The middle phase. The middle phase may simply be a continuation of the second (transition) phase. The issues and concerns raised by the announcements and related data may be sufficient to warrant at least one meeting, and sometimes more, to discuss them thoroughly. Not uncommonly, however, announcements may be routine and patients may have other things to discuss.

Thus after the announcements therapists may invite an open discussion of other concerns. This discussion can sometimes be effectively seeded when the therapists mention having heard in conversations with staff and patients a number of things that are bothering members of the community.

The ending phase.   The last phase of the community meeting is the ending. As the meeting began on time, so it should end on time. In conjunction, these two acts help to clearly define the space-time of the community meeting and distinguish it from other events in the hospital. Clinical observation indicates that clear beginnings and endings also help contain and reduce the anxiety of the members.

The last phase also gives the members an opportunity to say goodbye to those who are leaving and to wrap up the meeting. Therapists should allow sufficient time for this process to unfold.

Although therapists should indeed allow adequate time for these phases and their content and, when necessary, help introduce them, it is also important to recognize that this structure follows the natural development of the meeting. All groups have beginning, middle, and ending phases. This is especially true when the beginning and ending times are clear (Mann 1973). Thus the timing of the introduction of the various phases does not imply an arbitrary procedure, but rather means that therapists must carefully listen to and follow the movement of the meeting and introduce each phase as much as possible in harmony with the meeting's own development. I address this issue more fully below.

Listening, Intervening, and Interpreting

Listening, intervening, and interpreting are closely related functions of community meeting therapists. Therapists' interventions and interpretations are dependent on how they listen to and hear the communications, both verbal and nonverbal, of the members. Interpretations are a particular kind of intervention that seek to bring understanding to issues of theater. Also, listening itself can be an intervention.

Listening is one of the most important and often most difficult tasks of community meeting therapists. The amount of data that therapists receive before and during a community meeting is extensive. Before a meeting therapists will hear from other members of the treatment team about the varied events that have happened on the floor, what patients are saying and doing, which staff are missing, what crises have taken place, and numerous other details. Patients will also approach therapists before the meeting to inform them about the community, sometimes in a clear manner, often by innuendo or humor or in a confused metaphor. From these sources therapists will also have gotten some initial clues concerning the mood of the patients and staff. Once in the meeting, therapists hear a great deal more information, much of which may be hard to follow. On some occasions information may be communicated silently and nonverbally. In addition, there are the personal physical and intrapsychic communications of the therapists themselves, such as the degree of physical comfort or discomfort they experience, their feelings and moods, and their endless variety of fleeting thoughts and fantasies.

Given this volume of information, how can therapists and staff[3] listen effectively during a community meeting, let alone make effective interventions? It is not surprising that some therapists prefer to decide in advance what shall be talked about and keep discussion limited to those few issues! Unfortunately, although such an approach may ease the therapist's distress, issues of theater are often forced underground, only to reappear in less auspicious places. To address these concerns, I begin with the therapists' tasks of listening to and intervening around political and family issues, which are usually the easiest to understand.

Listening to and intervening in issues of politics and family.   Following the structure I described earlier, the opening issues of a community meeting are often political and familial in nature. Saying hello, making announcements, and discussing changes in the hospital or among the staff are of this nature, as are many of the issues that patients and staff may raise after the introduction. For instance

> About 10 minutes into a community meeting Ms. A, a tall, elderly woman, asked the therapist "What do you do with people who change television stations?" The therapist was puzzled and asked the woman to tell the community what had been happening. In an irate manner she described how Bob, a new adolescent patient on the unit, walked into the living room where she and a number of other patients were watching television, switched channels, watched for a few moments, and then left.

This complaint has the earmarks of politics and family: concern about television-viewing policy and the treatment of fellow patients. The therapist makes one intervention that serves two purposes. The first is to invite clarification and further discussion of the matter; the second is to invite

---

[3] As I indicate later, much of what is said about therapist-leaders also applies to staff behavior in the community meeting.

the woman to include the whole community in the discussion and not just the therapist. More listening is required by the therapist, staff, and patients if this woman's complaint is to be understood and adequately addressed. The meeting continued

> The therapist listened quietly for a few moments to see if Ms. A had more to say. She said nothing. The meeting felt quite uncomfortable. The therapist noted the discomfort and asked if others had something to add to Ms. A's story. Several people mumbled under their breath. The therapist encouraged them to speak up. Mr. B, a member of the television-watching group, yelled, "Bob is out of control. He shouldn't be allowed to do those things." Several others followed suit, complaining about Bob changing the channels.
>
> Finally Bob spoke up in his own defense. He argued that "those old people" were all busy talking and not really watching the show: "So I just flipped through the stations." Bob's comments created some more irritation, but they also led to further discussion by both staff and patients, and he managed to garner some support from other patients who felt that Ms. A and her friends dominated the television. A staff person clarified that the television was available to all patients and that, when viewing it, patients should consider other people's needs. Some patients and staff suggested that Bob ask people sitting near the television if they are watching before he switches channels. Others asked that Ms. A's group consider other people's wishes.

In this phase of the meeting the complaint was elaborated and discussed fairly thoroughly, sometimes in a clear manner and sometimes in a confusing manner. The therapist's first intervention was to remain silent. That silence was important because it informed her that Ms. A had nothing more to say at that point, and it also informed her of the degree of tension in the community around this incident. That led to her second intervention, inviting further discussion of the conflict and thus enabling a number of otherwise reluctant patients to express their concerns.

In summary, the therapist's interventions up to this point had the primary purpose and effect of allowing the conflict to be elaborated, of encouraging greater participation by patients and staff alike, and of leading to potential solutions to a political and family problem. Serendipitously and importantly, she also increased a sense of trust and safety by her willingness to hear what members wanted to say. The meeting continued

> Ms. A and Bob reluctantly agreed to the suggestions of the patients and staff, and the meeting moved on at a sluggish pace. The therapist realized

that the crisis was not yet finished. She continued to listen. One troubled and confused patient, Mr. C, asked to say a poem he had created. He stood up and spoke of peace and beauty that, in a world of war, could only be gained by talking to God, the supreme authority. Then he sat down. Ms. D raised her hand. "Tell me doctor, what do we do if Bob changes the stations and we tell him we're watching and he won't listen?" she asked, stumbling over her words. One of the nursing staff recognized the need for intervention from "above" and said that she should report the difficulty to the nurse in charge. Ms. D said "Thank you." The meeting settled down, the matter seemed resolved, and the members turned to other things.

Sometimes, open discussion of political and family concerns and the resolution of conflicts among the members constitute a sufficient response to the dilemmas that patients and staff raise at a community meeting. Patients learn the value of open discussion, gain some capacity to manage their impulses, and learn to live with others. The primary interventions of therapists are those that facilitate further dialogue, clarify what is being discussed, and set limits on disruptive behavior.

In our example, however, these interventions (although helpful and necessary) were not sufficient. After discussing a number of other issues that were similar in nature to the original conflict, the patients returned to talking about Bob and the television

Seemingly out of the blue, and after a period of lively dialogue, Ms. D said, "I don't think we should talk to the nurse in charge," slurring her words under the influence of her medication. "You, doctor," she said, pointing at the therapist, "should throw Bob out of the hospital." She then left the meeting. The therapist realized, as she had been suspecting for some time, that this was more than just a conflict over viewing television. This was more than just a case of rational political and family conflict. The real concerns of the patients had not yet been addressed.

To help the patients at this point, it was imperative that the therapist and staff also think of the community meeting as theater and intervene in ways that would make the message of the theater clear. In brief, therapists had to address not merely what the political and family issues denoted but also what they connoted.

Listening to and intervening around issues of theater. As the meeting continued, the therapist recalled pieces of information that she had been given about the hospital community before the meeting began. She had learned that numbers of patients, especially members of the television group, were very upset with Bob. She also had learned that the staff were feeling somewhat frazzled because of new admissions and a shortage of staff. Numbers of staff members were on vacation. She also remembered comments made by the patients during the first part of the meeting. She recalled Mr. B's concern about control, Bob's comment that the old people weren't really paying attention, Mr. C's psychotic calling on the supreme authority to bring peace, and Ms. D's frustration about being asked to speak to the nurse in charge and her plea that the therapist get rid of Bob. The therapist also noted her own emotional state during the meeting. Initially she felt that things were going quite well and that the members were dealing effectively with a fairly routine conflict. As time passed she felt more and more frustrated, unable to satisfy the patients' needs, especially Ms. D's, and was surprised how relieved she felt when Ms. D left the meeting. On the basis of these data, she hypothesized that the patients may have been talking, in derivative and metaphorical terms, about feelings (most likely angry ones) that they were having towards the staff. The meeting continued

When Ms. D left, a member of staff followed her to make sure she was safe. The meeting became very quiet. Then Polly, a rather sensitive teenager, said, "Penny," calling Ms. D by her first name, "has been pissed all day at everyone; it's a real pain." The therapist intervened, seeing yet another scapegoat being created. "Maybe Ms. D is not the only one who's pissed. I know that as a staff we have not been as available recently as usual." Polly retorted, "Bloody shrink talk!" "Naw," said Bob. "Penny got very pissed when she tried to talk to [a nurse] about me, and she couldn't find her. I remember, because I laughed at her."

Slowly the conversation shifted, and others talked about how frustrated they felt at this particular nurse when they couldn't find her. The nurse listened quietly. She was tempted to defend herself, given how frazzled she felt. Instead, she acknowledged the members' frustration and the fact that she had not been as available as she normally was. The patients accepted her comments and agreed, and then they began to attack other staff not present. The therapist intervened again, saying, "None of us are as available at this time as we usually are, including me. It's not surprising that you are taking it out on each other and on absent staff." After this intervention the accusations slowed down, and patients became able to talk about the frustration, anger, and fear they experienced during the summer vacation period. Fear became the predominant theme—fear that they would not be given good treatment and fear that there was no one in charge.

The message of the community meeting drama had been deciphered and understood, at least enough to enable the patients to acknowledge their feelings and recognize that under the circumstances they made sense. The projection of those feelings onto others and the accompanying scapegoating were reduced. The earlier political- and family-level conflicts also lost much of their sting. The therapist had allowed the members to give voice to what Langs (1978) called their adaptive task and Ezriel (1950) called the common group tension.

Several aspects of listening to what the political and family issues of a community meeting connote are illustrated or implied in this clinical example. First, therapists listen to political, family, and theater levels at the same time and throughout the whole meeting. Second, to determine what the political and family communications connote, therapists listen to the data from a variety of sources and from a variety of angles, including data acquired before and during the meeting, the flow of topics during the meeting, and their own experience of the meeting (Rice and Rutan 1987; Langs 1978). From these data, hypotheses are made about what the communications connote. The hypothesis best supported by the data leads to an intervention. Third, the interventions that clinical experience suggests are most helpful are those addressed to here-and-now events that make sense of current experience. They are also groupwide in nature and not focused on particular individuals (Kibel 1978; Winer and Lewis 1984). It is important to note, however, that interpretations are not just vague general statements about the community. Such statements often generate further anger, frustration, and regression among the members. Rather, they are statements directed toward specific active attitudes, which are probably preconscious, about therapists and staff. Finally, it is important for therapists and staff to be willing to tolerate and permit criticism of themselves during the process of listening, without becoming either masochistic or overly defensive. In the example this was illustrated by the response of the nurse.

During the Sturm und Drang of the community meeting, therapists must also pay attention to individual members. Clearly, during a community meeting therapists cannot listen to individual communications as carefully nor with as much attention to the details as they can during individual or group therapy. But therapists do need to listen to individuals well enough to understand their communications as giving voice to the common group tension. This was illustrated in the clinical example above when the therapist recalled the communications of various members. Therapists also need to listen to the communication of individuals to be alerted to how they are responding to the drama of the meeting with its powerful regressive pulls. When Ms. D left the meeting it was important that a staff member was available to check her condition. Ms. D's behavior was an expression of her personal anger and frustration at the unavailability of the staff, and in that sense it was in tune with the common group tension. But it was also quite possible that Ms. D was having difficulty with impulse control, was beginning to fragment and seriously regress, and may have needed special attention to help her contain that process. Further discussion of the topic in individual and group therapy may help Ms. D benefit from that regressive struggle.

The role of staff.   Although staff members carry less responsibility for the meeting than the designated therapist-leaders, their role has striking similarities to that of the therapist-leaders. The staff also has the responsibility of listening carefully to the three levels of the patients' communications and of responding accordingly. On occasion staff members, as representatives of various staff subsystems such as group therapy, medical, and nursing, may be called on to speak in those political and professional roles. On other occasions they may be called on to address conflicts one or more patients may have with them. The staff will have to use clinical judgment in deciding how much of the conflict to address in the community meeting and how much to address elsewhere. For instance, if a patient is angry about an event in individual therapy and raises it with the individual therapist during a community meeting, it will probably be most helpful for the therapist to acknowledge the importance of the subject and suggest that they discuss it in more detail during the next session. On the other hand, a conflict with another therapist that directly affects a number of patients and their life in the community is probably best addressed more fully and openly in the meeting. On yet other occasions, staff, such as the nurse in the example, may have to address more subtle and covert messages from the patients. Finally, and not infrequently, staff may have to address all of the above levels of communication within a single issue.

To make the role of staff members more effective, it is important that the therapist-leaders and staff have an opportunity to talk about the community meeting between sessions, preferably immediately after a meeting. This talk enables staff to express their understanding of the meeting and clarify misunderstandings, and it becomes an effective tool to train new staff in how to listen and participate in a community meeting.

Summary

I view the community meeting as the central treatment group of the psychiatric hospital. It is the meeting where the hospital culture, values, and practices are passed on from one patient generation to the next; the place where all other treatments and various formal and informal meetings between and among the staff and patients come together; and a stage on which the unconscious and irrational inner worlds of the participants, as well as their mature, conscious, and rational worlds, are played out.

In the community meeting patients can learn much about working in an institution and about living with others, skills in which many of them often have major deficits. It is also a place where interpersonal conflicts can be addressed and where the sometimes-fearsome projections of the community members can be contained and understood, thus reducing acting out on the floors or grounds of the hospital.

Because of its centrality, the community meeting can contribute significantly to the success of other treatments and to the creation of a hospital atmosphere that is conducive to healing. However, with its tendency to split into smaller groups, to reinforce individual projections, and to threaten individual identities, the community meeting can also be a potent antitherapeutic force if *not* well structured and led.

Thus it is important that the community meeting contracts be clear and that its frame be well maintained. It is also important that leader-therapists and staff listen to and address issues of politics, family, and theater and that they are attuned to both what the members' interactions and communications denote and what they connote.

References

Almond R: The Zar Cult of Ethiopia, in The Healing Community: Dynamics of the Therapeutic Milieu. New York, Jason Aronson, 1974, pp 161–179

Bergman MS: The Anatomy of Loving. New York, Columbia University Press, 1987

Bion WR: Experiences in Groups. New York, Basic Books, 1959

Buber M: I and Thou. New York, Charles Scribners Sons, 1958

Ellenberger HF: The Discovery of the Unconscious: The History and Evolution of Dynamic Psychiatry. New York, Basic Books, 1970

Ezriel H: A psychoanalytic approach to group treatment. Br J Med Psychol 23:59–74, 1950

Foulkes SH: Therapeutic Group Analysis. New York, International Universities Press, 1977

Greene LR, Morrison TL, Tischler R, et al: Aspects of identification in the large group. J Soc Psychol 111:91–97, 1980

Jones M: The Therapeutic Community. New York, Basic Books, 1953

Kernberg O: Regression in groups, in Internal World and External Reality: Object Relations Theory Applied. New York, Jason Aronson, 1980, pp 211–273

Kibel HD: The rationale for the use of group psychotherapy on a short-term unit. Int J Group Psychother 28:339–358, 1978

Kindts P, Verhaest S: Le "community meeting" dan la communauté thérapeutique. Acta Psychiat Belg 80:295–306, 1980

Kirsch J, Kroll J, Gross B, et al: Inpatient community meeting: problems and purposes. Br J Med Psychol 54:35–40, 1981

Langs R: The Listening Process. New York, Jason Aronson, 1978

Main TF: The hospital as a therapeutic institution. Bull Menninger Clin 10:66–70, 1946

Mann J: Time-Limited Psychotherapy. Cambridge, MA, Harvard University Press, 1973

McMillan SD: An application of Turquet's basic-assumption oneness to the analysis of a group in search of utopia. Human Relations 34:475–490, 1981

Morrison TL, Greene LR, Tischler R, et al: Manifestations of splitting in the large group. J Soc Psychol 125:601–611, 1985

Pfister O: Instincktive Psychoanalyse unter de Navaho-Indianern. Imago 18:81–109, 1932

Raguenau, Father: The Jesuit relations and allied documents, in The Discovery of the Unconscious, Vol 8. Edited by Ellenberger HE. 1897, pp 260–262

Rice CA, Rutan JS: The charismatic leader: asset or liability. Psychotherapy: Theory, Research and Practice 18:487–492, 1981

Rice CA, Rutan JS: Inpatient Group Psychotherapy: A Psychodynamic Perspective. New York, Macmillan, 1987

Stevenson MC: The Zuni Indians: their mythology, esoteric fraternities and ceremonials. Annual Report of the Bureau of American Ethnology, Vol 23. Washington, DC, Smithsonian Institution, 1901–1902, pp 3–106

Turquet PM: Leadership: the individual and the group, in Analysis of Groups: Contributions to Theory, Research and Practice. Edited by Gibbard GS, Hartman JJ, Mann RD. London, Jossey-Bass, 1974, pp 349–371

Turquet P: Threats to identity in large groups, in The Large Group: Dynamics and Therapy. Edited by Kreeger L. Itasca, IL, F. E. Peacock, 1975, pp 87–114

von Bertalanffy L: General Systems Theory: Foundations, Development, Applications. New York, George Braziller, 1968

Winer JA, Lewis L: Interpretive psychotherapy in the inpatient community meeting. Psychiatry 47:333–341, 1984

CHAPTER 7

Groups in the Day Hospital

Lawrence L. Kennedy, M.D.

Historical Background

The first psychiatric day hospital, or "hospital without beds," was begun in Moscow in 1933. Dzhagarov (1937) wrote of his experience in starting a program, consisting mostly of work therapy. He treated 80 patients at a time for an average duration of 2 months. It is interesting to note that the program was begun because of a bed shortage and inadequate funding in a fairly typical large institution for psychotic patients. These conditions approximate the current economic climate in the delivery of mental health care in the United States.

The first known psychiatric day hospital in the Western hemisphere was developed by D. Ewen Cameron at the Allan Memorial Institute of Psychiatry in Montreal, Canada, in 1947 (Cameron 1947). Cameron presented his ideas about "an experimental form of hospitalization for psychiatric patients" at a meeting of the American Psychiatric Association in New York in May 1947. At that time, he indicated that psychiatry had taken over many ideas from other areas of medicine in the development of psychiatric hospitals. Although he found that some of these ideas were useful, he recognized that sometimes what applied to hospitals treating physical illness did not apply to a hospital treating psychiatric illness: "a hospital is a place where the patient goes to bed; a hospital is a place where a patient stays until he is well, or as well as the doctor can make him, and a hospital is a place where only the patient is treated" (Cameron 1947, p. 60). Cameron was well suited to be the dynamic force behind the discovery of day programs. He had studied the psychobiological approach of Adolph Meyer and was responsible for a number of innovative approaches in psychiatry. These are described in a paper by Goldman and Arvanitakis (1981), who indicated that

The Allan Memorial Institute under Doctor Cameron was the first open psychiatric hospital in Canada. Side by side with the open hospital, he emphasized the importance of admitting only voluntary patients. These two developments called forth new treatment approaches which do not rely on unbreakable glass, barred windows and locked wards. These modalities would include psychopharmacology and physical therapies, psychosocial approaches emphasizing group integration, and creative use of hospital architectural design to advance therapeutic goals. (p. 366)

Goldman and Arvanitakis (1981) saw Cameron's interest in psychiatric hospital architecture and his ideas about the day hospital as coming together in the construction of the original T-shaped wing of the Allan Memorial Institute built in 1954 under his auspices:

The day hospital contained in one of the wings of the main building has, besides a living space marked by the absence of beds, other important environmental aspects that should be considered. Furnishings resemble those of a human setting with drapes on the windows, comfortable furniture, objects breakable or otherwise being present, and so on. This ambiance is designed to beckon the patient toward full and mature living and to stimulate positive expectations that he will behave responsibly, concepts that Cameron originally delineated. By definition there are open doors in the day hospital, an environmental element that presupposes a free individual who seeks treatment voluntarily, not a wild beast who needs to be caged. (p. 366)

Cameron (1947) also believed that the mental patient often did not require 24-hour care. A day hospital program was similar to ordinary life in that the patient came to treatment only during the day, just as he or she might attend work. Separation from environment and relationships was also not seen as essential. As a matter of fact, Cameron (1947) stated that "the Day Hospital has apparently the additional advantage that to go home each night and to return each morning seems to act as a daily reaffirmation of the fact that the patient is there on a voluntary basis" (p. 62). He emphasized the point that no psychiatric patient should be seen as existing except in the context of the patient's being a member of his or her family and of society. This meant that families should be a part of the treatment. Group programs and the emphasis on group psychological approaches were introduced early.

An important phase in the development of the day hospital also took place in England, where Joshua Bierer (1964) began the Marlborough

Day Hospital. Bierer was interested in social treatment of mentally ill patients and started community-based social clubs.

Moll (1953, 1957) developed a day hospital program in the Montreal General Hospital in 1950. He, too, formulated his program using Cameron's ideas.

In 1949 a day hospital program was founded at the Menninger Clinic in Topeka, Kansas (Barnard et al. 1952), after staff members from the clinic visited the Cameron program. This program followed the concept of "milieu therapy" as it had been developed at the Menninger Hospital under William C. Menninger (1936). In this program the day hospital was simply an extension of the inpatient psychiatric treatment. Part of the inpatient treatment included a wide variety of activity therapies that were individually prescribed by the patients' psychiatrists. The day hospital patients attended these same activity programs and mixed with the inpatients. This provided a useful transition for the inpatients to life in the community. Reports on this program also noted that the indications for day hospitalization were unrelated to any specific diagnostic categories. The Menninger program also occasionally included family members in the therapeutic activities. This provided the family with a better understanding of treatment and facilitated the patient's return home.

The next major push in the development of day hospital programs in the United States came with the passage of the Mental Health Centers Act of 1963. This congressional act required day hospital programs to be a part of community mental health centers.

Philosophy

The philosophical underpinnings of the day hospital programs have varied widely. This has led to a profusion of confusing but often creative developments in partial hospitalization. One philosophical issue that both facilitated and impeded the development of the day hospital was an antihospital bias in the early days of the community mental health center development. The deinstitutionalization of the 1950s and 1960s in the United States and the development of community mental health centers had as their philosophical bases the belief that individuals could be treated earlier in mental health centers and in their own communities and thereby prevent hospitalization. The community mental health center movement was, in a sense, not only an antihospital movement but also an antipsychiatry movement. Many day hospitals viewed themselves almost as adversaries of inpatient units. Hospitalization was viewed as something that destroyed the spirit and alienated mentally ill patients from society.

Zwerling and Wilder (1964) found that day hospitalization was an appropriate alternative to 24-hour hospitalization for seriously ill mental patients. Their study showed that two-thirds of a group of newly admitted inpatients who were randomly assigned to a day hospital were actually accepted for treatment at the day hospital. The remaining one-third were rejected and treated on an inpatient basis. Of the patients accepted for treatment at the day hospital, three-fifths never required boarding on the inpatient service. Such studies seemed to promote the idea that hospitalization was not appropriate or at least not necessary for many patients. In some ways this idea generated an ongoing split between day hospitals and inpatient units that exists to the present time. Each program has seemed to guard its own territory, and there are still many indications that day hospitals have been underutilized.

It is probably true that patients' strengths are emphasized more in the day hospital, which requires more active participation of the patient from the beginning. This emphasis on strengths may be productive and useful to patients who are able to respond to such expectations, and it can counter the potential negative effects of full hospitalization—regression, dependency, and isolation.

Astrachan et al. (1970) delineated several primary tasks of the day hospital: 1) to provide an alternative to 24-hour hospitalization, 2) to provide a transitional-care setting that has the task of facilitating the reentry into the community of previously hospitalized patients, and 3) to provide a structure that delivers those psychiatric services that the community defines as an overriding public need.

Once a day hospital has defined its primary task, it can then go about the process of deciding what type of treatment, staff, and other programs it may need. For example, in designing a day hospital as an alternative to full-time hospitalization, it is important to provide the variety of treatments that are included in the traditional psychiatric hospital. Programs that emphasize group treatment, family therapy, and medication are important. Also, the ready availability of a hospital unit is obviously essential for such programs. Day hospitals that have the primary task of facilitating the patient's transition into the community may need quite different programs. For example, in such a program much effort is placed on resocialization and rehabilitation activities, including vocational programs. There is less need for medical intervention in this setting.

The "Group" Milieu

Maxwell Jones's concept (1953) of "the therapeutic community" was developed in mental hospitals but soon taken over by day hospitals. He emphasized altering the traditional barrier between staff and patients by bringing patients into more active participation in the development of their treatment programs and in the ongoing operation of hospital units. This emphasis on the importance of the social environment of the hospital has carried over into day hospitals.

Most day hospitals, through efforts such as the therapeutic community and the use of groups and patient government activities, emphasize the importance of the patients' belonging to a group and a culture within the day hospital. Considerable emphasis is placed on helping newly admitted patients to become integrated into the community, helping those being discharged to prepare for their leave, and helping the entire group to experience its own reactions to such comings and goings. A major problem of most psychiatrically disabled individuals has to do with their isolation. The therapeutic milieu of the day hospital aims to engage the patient in productive social encounters.

Group Approaches

A number of authors have attempted to develop a theoretical perspective regarding the use of groups in partial-hospitalization programs. Fidler (1975) described the development of multimodel groups within a day hospital with emphasis placed on maintaining the integrity of a small group throughout the program treatment day. The patients moved from one group to another throughout the day. The group to which the patient was assigned at admission was maintained with the same membership, and the patient remained in this group until discharge. Fidler believed that this provided a high level of intense cohesion in the group treatment experience. DiBella et al. (1982) stated, "Partial hospitalization programs by their definition are a group, and the use of the group as a treatment method implies a certain theoretical belief about the origin of psychological problems and how they are best approached in treatment" (p. 59). They listed advantages of group treatment:

1. The individual has the opportunity to receive support not only from the therapist but from a number of others as well.

2. Groups give greater opportunity to reduce inappropriate dysfunctional interactions (e.g., shyness, silence, and withdrawal) with people who are not professional psychotherapists.
3. The group provides an excellent opportunity for reality testing.
4. Groups provide an immediate opportunity for individual processing of information that has just been given in the group.
5. Groups provide an opportunity for experimentation and practice in the assumption of various roles.
6. The group experience provides multiple behavior models with which the group member can identify.
7. The reality orientation of the group is strong because transferences are kept in check.
8. There is some dilution of countertransferential reactions by the use of the group treatment method.
9. Groups permit the conservation of financial resources and greater efficiency of staff time.

DiBella et al. (1982) also discussed the advantage of "innerconnected groups," a series of group events that may help to intensify treatment and provide a variety of experiences for the patient. Innerconnected groups might include various-sized groups, vocational groups, art and music groups, and various social and recreational groups.

DeChant and Heil (1982) attempted to develop a theoretical framework for the planning of groups in partial-hospitalization programs. They described a program in which multilevel psychotherapy groups function as an integrative core to a range of therapeutic skills. Washburn and Conrad (1978) described a variety of group programs within a day hospital structure, including groups with recreational, social, rehabilitative, and psychological approaches.

Almost any type of group is possible within a day hospital. Groups may range from insight-oriented expressive therapy groups to clearly task-oriented or educational groups. A task group, for example, might focus on the development of knowledge about community agencies or learning a craft or cooking skill. Other groups may be purely social or recreational in nature, such as exercise groups or volleyball and bowling groups. Some groups may be taught in an educational fashion and might include classes about the side effects of medication, orientation programs for job-seeking skills, or classes in sexuality. The difficulty is in knowing how many and what type of groups are needed in any one day hospital. It is clear, however, that group-focused treatment is a mainstay of day hospitals.

Group Psychotherapy

Group therapy is a method par excellence for the day hospital in that groups clearly replicate the problems encountered by their member-patients in everyday life. The central issue in all such groups is the issue of dependency versus autonomy. Group therapy offers a social-psychological setting in which such issues can be addressed with one's peers.

Day hospitals frequently have as a major purpose the facilitation of transition to community life. Hence, the patients are engaged in struggles not only to separate themselves from the hospital experience where they felt safely cared for, but also to begin gradually to take on an array of adult life tasks. Day hospitals provide rich opportunities for these individuals, who may be half-time patients and half-time citizens of society at large. This status gives them many opportunities to practice individuation attempts (Crafoord 1977). Crafoord described the atmosphere of a day hospital in Sweden for adolescents that is similar to the psychological phenomenon of a transitional object as described by Winnicott (1953). Patients know the day hospital exists and that they can come to it and then leave, gathering strength over time. This provides a powerful tool for maturation. As Crafoord (1977) stated:

> The staff members of the day hospital or even the physical structure itself become a transitional object for the patient—a mother image without the threatening characteristics of a real mother, an object the patient may love, interject, toss around, spit out, and take in again. It offers the possibility of re-enacting the experience of separation over and over, enabling self- and object-images to become integrated in ego boundaries to acquire stability. (p. 395)

In groups of 8 to 10 patients, often with cotherapists, patients view an array of behaviors related to their stirrings for independence. The group has the opportunity to observe the new member coming in who may just be leaving the hospital and may still be struggling with anxiety over imminent separation from the hospital staff, as well as the preparation of other members getting ready to terminate from the day hospital. This latter group are individuals who usually have gradually taken on responsibilities such as a job, an apartment, school, and new relationships. With a good mix of patients at both ends of the spectrum, such groups provide a powerful opportunity for patients to observe one another's behavior, as if looking into many mirrors while examining their own difficulties. The patient group takes on a strong role in providing support and feedback to its members. One such form of patients assisting other patients has to do with treatment monitoring. The patients become aware of each other's potential for suicidal preoccupations, for noncompliance with medication, for withdrawal, and for a whole array of symptomatic behaviors. The patient group can pick up rapidly on these symptoms and actively address them as treatment issues. The following case examples illustrate how effective members can be in confronting others:

Case 1

Ms. A, a young borderline woman who was apt to have great difficulties with her weekends, was confronted by another member over whether or not she had been drinking and abusing drugs on the weekend. Although initially angry about the confrontation, Ms. A began to cry and indicated that she had had a particularly difficult weekend and had felt lost and confused. Other patients joined in to challenge her to more carefully plan her weekends and use available backup services. The group also suggested that Ms. A might require a short rehospitalization to get herself under control.

Case 2

In another group, Mr. B, a young man who had recently left the hospital after a serious depression and suicide attempt, recounted an argument he had had with his father over money. Other members described similar difficulties and indicated how difficult it was to be dependent on one's parents and at the same time to be an adult and a psychiatric patient.

The theme in Cases 1 and 2—the painful dependency of patienthood—is a recurrent and never-ending issue in such groups because young, able-bodied, adult psychiatric patients are particularly apt to experience extreme guilt over having to remain in a dependent relationship with their parents. Also, the patients in such groups may have been hospitalized together and may have observed one another undergoing episodes of serious regression. This may help them share many experiences of which they are deeply ashamed. The groups become particularly useful in helping members assess their readiness to take new steps such as leaving a halfway house, starting volunteer work, contemplating school, getting a job, or moving to an apartment. All such steps toward autonomy can be worked and reworked by the membership.

These groups provide a particularly valuable function for members in periods of crisis. If possible, the patient should return to his or her day hospital therapy group while hospitalized. Members in the group can focus their attention on the incidents leading up to the hospitalization. Also, the patient need not lose his or her membership because of rehospitalization, and this can facilitate the transfer back to the day hospital.

Because many day hospital patients are vulnerable to episodic regressions, it is particularly useful for groups to explore the array of issues that may lead to crisis. All group members have an opportunity to learn about crisis "prevention." In those situations where it is not possible for the patient to continue in the group while rehospitalized, members view the loss of a fellow group member as a traumatic event of which they cannot gain a good understanding unless the patient continues in the group while hospitalized or returns to the group fairly soon after discharge from the hospital. Realities such as crisis rehospitalizations are part of the daily life of many psychiatric patients, and having an opportunity to evaluate them in a day hospital setting is a uniquely constructive experience.

The patients in day hospital group therapies have multiple contacts with one another in various other group activities. Away from the day hospital, they may get together socially or often may even live together in settings such as halfway houses. Groups provide an opportunity for patients to address relationship issues in their community. Patients can be encouraged to raise problems that have occurred in their relationships with other patients. For example, a patient may have sought out another individual when feeling suicidal and received some advice. In the group setting, such interventions can be discussed and patients can learn what has been helpful and what has not been helpful. The following case example illustrates how outside behavior may be discussed in the group and be of benefit to a member:

Case 3

Several group members were able to discuss with Ms. C a problem that they experienced with her in the halfway house, where she had been crying a great deal for several days and seeking attention from everyone. They were able to address directly their frustration and irritation with her and the fact that no matter what they did nothing seemed to help. They told her that she seemed intent on rejecting all advice and support, as if to make everyone in the house miserable. The patient was shocked and angry to hear this and in an angry outburst walked out of the group. In the next several sessions, the group was able to continue to discuss with Ms. C their frustration with her inability to receive help and support from others and yet to

remain angry and to feel left out. With continued work of the group, Ms.
C was able to take this issue to her psychotherapist and to work on it there
as well as in her family meetings, where similar behavior between Ms. C and
her parents was frequently displayed.

In some day hospitals there is a mixed population of patients with serious chronic illnesses such as schizophrenia and patients with borderline
conditions who function at a higher level. It may be valuable to separate
the patients into higher- and lower-functioning therapy groups, as Yalom
(1983) recommended for inpatient group psychotherapy. It is possible,
however, to place both higher- and lower-functioning patients in the same
groups, as long as the lower-functioning patients are not so psychotically
disorganized that they are disruptive to the group and as long as the
group experience is not too intensely stimulating for them. In such
groups, I have found that less ill patients can be very supportive in promoting the assimilation of sicker patients into the group, thereby promoting higher levels of behavior and greater socialization. But one must
always be on the lookout that the sicker patients are protected to some
extent. In this case, the therapist may need to play a more active role. If
there is a mix of patient ages, one may wish to put younger adult patients
in separate groups from older patients. This way, patients are in groups
in which life tasks are similar, although individual diagnoses may vary.

Rosie and Azim (1990) described the use of large-group psychotherapy
in a day treatment program in Edmonton, Canada. All patients and staff
in this program attend a large group meeting daily with a total number
of 50 to 55 people. The group is conducted "on the premise that it reflects
the approach taken in the total program; that is, the promotion of a 'good
enough' environment for insight-oriented, interpretative work to take
place" (p. 311). A psychiatrist functions as the designated leader of the
group, and group-as-a-whole phenomena as well as individual transference phenomena are explored and interpreted within this setting. In addition, the program uses a number of other forms of group treatment.
These authors believe that the large group may offer particular help to
new patients "to remain in the background while dealing with anxiety,
thus learning that the group is safe until they are ready to take risks and
to participate actively instead of continuing to learn vicariously" (Rosie
and Azim 1990, p. 318). They feel that the large-group setting allows for
an array of individual issues to emerge and for patients to rapidly identify
common concerns. Also, they see this large-group setting as an excellent
opportunity for trainees to observe group psychotherapy in process.

Behavioral Approaches

Although many day hospitals operate within a psychodynamic framework, others use behavior modification techniques. As Eckman (1978) stated, "The goal of behaviorally oriented treatment techniques is to alter the patient's primary presenting problems rather than to directly bring about a change in personality or to treat underlying conflicts" (p. 26). Such behavioral techniques are particularly applicable for many chronic patients, who are apt to be lacking in a wide variety of daily living skills. Some of the common behavioral techniques include specifying individual goals, assertiveness training, desensitization, anxiety management training, token economies, and educational workshops aimed at improving daily living skills.

Liberman et al. (1977) developed a day program to provide training and social and daily living skills for patients. The program was described as "personal effectiveness" training, and patients learned skills such as improving the expression of affects, initiating and maintaining conversation, conducting job interviews, and expressing emotions such as sadness, anger, affection, criticism, and praise. The biweekly training was usually carried out in small groups of 8 to 10 patients. Patients were given considerable feedback about their improvement and skills and were encouraged to practice their skills away from the training sessions. Lamb (1976), Hersen and Luber (1977), and Carmichael (1964) all emphasized teaching day hospital patients skills that could be actively used in daily life. DiBella et al. (1982) indicated the importance of a variety of skills groups for day hospital programs and mentioned the teaching of skills such as meal preparation, health care, personal finance, and social skills. There appear to be particular advantages to conducting this kind of training in small groups with as few as four to five patients and one or two staff members. Regular membership in the group eases the discomfort among individuals and tends to create an atmosphere in which people can practice what might otherwise appear to be embarrassingly simple behaviors. Patients may gradually lose some of their inhibitions when they find that others suffer from similar difficulties.

Medication Groups

Goldman (1987) and others (e.g., Perry 1990) described the use of medication groups in the day hospital. Patients in medication groups can share their symptoms, experiences with various medications, troubling problems with side effects, and potential difficulties with the drugs, for example, tardive dyskinesia. Such discussions facilitate compliance and give the patients more control over their treatment. The following example illustrates the usefulness of such a group for a schizophrenic patient:

Case 4

Mr. D, a 37-year-old chronic schizophrenic patient, admitted to hearing voices for the first time known to any clinical staff. After hearing several other patients talk about their hallucinations, he shared his own experiences and indicated considerable relief at being able to tell what he felt was shameful and humiliating.

Family Groups

Because it is not unusual for patients in day hospitals to be simultaneously living with their families, it is particularly important for families to be brought actively into the treatment. Henisz (1984) described the use of multiple family group therapy in a partial-hospitalization setting. He saw such a group as a bridge between the hospital and the outside world:

The patient and his/her family can no longer exist in the isolation of their own family's sub-group; they must interact with outsiders. Because outsiders are included in the group, reality testing is greater, distortions and aberrant behaviors within an individual family are commented on and challenged, and changes in behavior are expected by the group. (p. 45)

Griefen and Lawton (1979) described the development of parents' groups in a day hospital setting. They saw two main reasons for initiating such groups: 1) to provide support and information to parents and to give the parents the experience that they were all struggling with similar problems and 2) to provide specific information about the program to the parents. These groups were closed, short term, educationally oriented.

Activity Groups

Activity programs for chronically ill patients may use smaller groups than usual with simplified tasks that are repetitive in nature and not excessively demanding.

Fullilove et al. (1985) emphasized the value of task-oriented groups for day hospital patients. The concentration and performance of individuals in these groups gradually improved, as did their involvement in the group. The authors stated that

> Task-oriented groups focus the interaction of the members on the accomplishment of a common goal. They can be geared to an appropriate level within the range of development. Thus the regressed state of the acutely psychotic patient is addressed through an activity that is sensimotor and individually implemented, a rough parallel to the infant's early sensorimotor play. Stimulation to language, cognition, and social functioning is an outgrowth of this attention to primary levels of developmental experience. (p. 998)

In another program for chronically mentally ill patients, Maniacci (1988) described a language skills group. The purpose of this group was to "teach clients the requisite skills for clear communication (both written and verbal), to teach them to better differentiate and organize incoming information, and to provide them with the opportunity to practice constructive interactions" (p. 129). In this group patients were involved in developing basic writing skills in order to "communicate and process information better." They studied grammar, rewriting, and reading.

In another interesting program for chronically ill psychiatric patients (Grillo-DiDemenico 1990), an educational occupational issues group was formed to help patients learn basic occupational precepts. The program analyzed businesses and organizations to help patients understand what was expected of them as workers or recipients of social services. The authors felt that these patients had not obtained this knowledge and that the lack of this information added to their failures in negotiating with various agencies.

Piran and Kaplan (1990) developed a day hospital program for patients with eating disorders in Toronto, Canada, that had a strong emphasis on group therapies. As a matter of fact, one-to-one interactions with patients were avoided if possible, and no individual psychotherapy was provided. The primary goal of the program, which was moderately successful, was to normalize eating behavior.

Staff members working in day hospital settings may experience themselves as always being on the firing line compared with staff members in inpatient settings. The day hospital staff must be always alert to the potential for serious regressive behavior such as drug abuse or suicide. This requires a degree of attention that becomes stressful when there are a large number of patients in the program acting out at any one time. Day hospital teams need to have plenty of opportunity to process their work with patients as well as to examine their own interrelationships so that they do not interfere with the work of the patients. Such open discussions among staff are an essential component of any day hospital program that is engaged in intensive treatment. There is always a high potential for countertransference problems in the staff, and an atmosphere that promotes nonjudgmental sharing of feelings and concerns may help to relieve staff anxiety and avoid the staff's acting in nontherapeutic ways with patients. In some day hospital programs, staff arrange periodic "process" meetings in which all daily business is set aside and the staff examines its own working relationships. Sometimes, if difficulties become too great to be handled by the teams themselves, they may need outside consultation. This should be viewed as an acceptable activity, not as evidence of failure. Indeed, it is essential that staff accept that their problems can be solved in open discussion, because this is the model emphasized in various psychotherapeutic activities within the day hospital itself. The following case example illustrates such a staff process group:

Case 5

> In one team, a staff member had taken on an increasingly significant role as the team "strong man" who could always deal with the most difficult patients. The team leader as well as other staff members tended to go along with this notion and frequently assigned the problem patients to this person. This left all the other team members feeling inadequate and diminished, as if most of the clinical skill resided in one individual. In a series of discussions the team was able to recognize the extent to which they had all participated in overly qualifying one member while devaluing all the others. This led to a useful redistribution of patients and considerable growth in the entire team. The strong man initially felt slighted but later indicated what a relief it was to not always be seen as the major strength within a team. He shared with his teammates experiences in his family in which everyone characteristically turned to him during times of difficulty or crisis.

Day Hospital Boundaries

Frequently, day hospitals are one portion or subsystem of a larger comprehensive center, and their patients may use services in many other components of this system. These may include inpatient services during periods of crisis, alcohol and drug programs, outpatient clinics, aftercare clinics, and a host of community agencies that provide services to patients, such as public assistance, vocational rehabilitation, psychosocial centers, and halfway houses. Day hospitals, because they lie between larger and often more fiscally dominating systems of the hospital and the community, are often subject to a wide array of intergroup pressures and boundary issues that affect the staff, the program, and the patients. For example, conflict may arise in the process of transfer of patients from the inpatient setting to the day hospital. Does the day hospital staff control this boundary? Or does the hospital staff simply move patients when they feel the patients are ready to be transferred? If the day hospital staff does not have any control over the admissions and decisions as to who they could best treat, they are apt to feel constantly undermined and suffer from an inability to function autonomously. The day hospital staff may suspiciously view hospital staff as sending them their unwanted patients or project onto the hospital staff feelings of inadequacy, thereby enhancing the feeling that they are devalued by the inpatient staff. Intergroup phenomena between the two groups become particularly striking when there are transfers of difficult patients, as the following case example illustrates:

Case 6

Ms. E, who had been a day hospital patient for several years, was transferred to an inpatient unit after a period of debilitating regression. She had not taken her medication for over a week. Ms. E was often abrasive and demanding, and she created considerable stress in the inpatient unit because of her intrusive attitude. She pushed constantly to leave the hospital. When the inpatient unit felt that she was ready to leave, they referred her to the day hospital. However, the day hospital staff felt that there were important issues unsettled with the patient. The inpatient staff accused the day hospital staff of not wanting to take her back. Although the day hospital staff were aware of their own reluctances and countertransference with this patient because they had worked with her for a number of years, they continued to have difficulty in clarifying to the inpatient staff exactly what they felt needed to be accomplished before the patient moved out of the hospital. Ms. E began to make repeated calls, sometimes three or four times a day, to various day hospital staff, attempting to browbeat them into admitting her. The day hospital staff finally concluded that they would not respond to these calls but instead would notify the inpatient team of the patient's behavior. Several meetings were held between the day hospital team and the inpatient team to sort through the many feelings arising around this particular patient. A successful transfer of the patient was made.

The day hospital sits in a particularly vulnerable position. The fact that many of its patients come from inpatient units means that the day hospital staff must depend on those units to make referrals to them. They must also act responsibly in expediting the patient's transfer but at the same time be sufficiently protective of patients to recognize whether the patients can tolerate the less-structured environment of the day hospital. Hence, it becomes very important for day hospital staff to be aware of intergroup phenomena.

Handling boundary difficulties by creating various rules, procedures, and delay mechanisms does not work as well as engaging in interaction at the boundaries toward mutually satisfying and collaborative decisions. It is exactly with such boundaries that the patient must engage in his or her task of transferring from one group of staff and becoming engaged with another group. Such transfer processes have a powerful impact on patients and can provide very useful opportunities for learning, provided that the staff are aware and keenly interested when the patient examines his or her reactions to such movement. Being aware of some of their own transfer-related issues may aid the staff in helping patients move from one group to another and from one level of treatment to another along the continuum of care.

In sum, group process and group therapy play a major role in developing and sustaining the treatment environment in a day hospital. For many patients, the model offers a beneficial alternative at a very difficult life moment.

References

Astrachan BM, Flynn HR, Geller JD, et al: Systems approach to day hospitalization. Arch Gen Psychiatry 22:550–559, 1970

Barnard RI, Robbins LL, Tetzlaff FM: The day hospital as an extension of psychiatric treatment. Bull Menninger Clin 16:50–56, 1952

Bierer J: The Marlborough experiment, in Handbook of Community Psychiatry. Edited by Bellak L. New York, Grune & Stratton, 1964, pp 221–247

Cameron DE: The day hospital: an experimental form of hospitalization for psychiatric patients. Modern Hospital 69(3):60–62, 1947

Carmichael D: Day hospital program with emphasis on translatable skills, in Day Care of Psychiatric Patients. Edited by Epps RL, Hanes LD. Springfield, IL, Charles C Thomas, 1964, pp 66–78

Crafoord C: Day hospital treatment for borderline patients: the institution as transitional object, in Borderline Personality Disorders. Edited by Hartocolis P. New York, International Universities Press, 1977, pp 385–397

DeChant B, Heil RA: The hub of the wheel: core group psychotherapy and its integrative function in the partial hospital, in Proceedings of the Annual Conference on Partial Hospitalization. Boston, MA, The American Association for Partial Hospitalization, 1982, pp 61–72

DiBella GAW, Weitz GW, Poynter-Berg D, et al: Handbook of Partial Hospitalization. New York, Brunner/Mazel, 1982

Dzhagarov MA: Experience in organizing a day hospital for mental patients. Neuropathology Psychiatry 6:137–147, 1937

Eckman TA: Behavioral approaches to partial hospitalization, in Partial Hospitalization, A Current Perspective. Edited by Luber RF. New York, Plenum, 1978, pp 21–47

Fidler JW: The day hospital: a multi-model group therapy, in Group Therapy. Edited by Wolberg LR. New York, Stratton International Medical Book Corp, 1975, pp 38–49

Fullilove MT, Pacheco O, Fourchard C: Task-oriented group in a day hospital. Journal of the National Medical Association 77:995–998, 1985

Goldman DL: The uses of a medication group in a day hospital. International Journal of Partial Hospitalization 4:127–136, 1987

Goldman DL, Arvanitakis K: D. Ewen Cameron's day hospital and the day hospital movement. Can J Psychiatry 26:365–368, 1981

Griefen MW, Lawton RK: Parents' groups at partial hospital, in Proceedings of the Annual Conference on Partial Hospitalization. Boston, MA, The American Association for Partial Hospitalization, 1979, pp 104–114

Grillo-DiDemenico B: An educational occupational issues group for the chronic psychiatric patient, in Group Work With the Emotionally Disabled. Edited by Levine B. New York, Hawthorn, 1990, pp 113–127

Henisz JE: Psychotherapeutic Management in the Day Program. Springfield, IL, Charles C Thomas, 1984

Hersen M, Luber RF: Use of group psychotherapy in a partial hospitalization service: the remediation of basic skill deficits. Int J Group Psychother 27:361–376, 1977

Jones M: The Therapeutic Community. New York, Basic Books, 1953

Lamb HR: An education model for teaching living skills to long-term patients. Hosp Community Psychiatry 2:875–877, 1976

Liberman RP, Fearn CH, Roberts DJ, et al: The credit-incentive system: motivating the participation of patients in a day hospital. British Journal of Social and Clinical Psychology 16:85–94, 1977

Maniacci MP: Language skills group: a psychoeducational group treatment approach. Individual Psychology 44:129–137, 1988

Menninger WC: Psychiatric hospital therapy designed to meet unconscious needs. Am J Psychiatry 93:347–360, 1936

Moll AE: Psychiatric service in a general hospital with special reference to a day treatment unit. Am J Psychiatry 109:774–776, 1953

Moll AE: Psychiatric night treatment unit in a general hospital. Am J Psychiatry 113:722–727, 1957

Perry EK: Personal communication (in Shekleer-Wolfson L, Woodside DB: Family therapy), in A Day Hospital Group Treatment Program for Anorexia Nervosa and Bulimia Nervosa. Edited by Piran N, Kaplan A. New York, Brunner/Mazel, 1990, pp 79–109

Piran N, Kaplan A (eds): A Day Hospital Group Treatment Program for Anorexia Nervosa and Bulimia Nervosa. New York, Brunner/Mazel, 1990

Rosie JS, Azim HFA: Large-group psychotherapy in a day treatment program. Int J Psychother 40:305–321, 1990

Washburn S, Conrad M: Organization of the therapeutic milieu in the partial hospital, in Partial Hospitalization, A Current Perspective. Edited by Luber RF. New York, Plenum, 1978, pp 47–70

Winnicott DW: Transitional objects and transitional phenomena: a study of the first not-me position. Int J Psychoanal 34:1–9, 1953

Yalom I (ed): Inpatient Group Psychotherapy. New York, Basic Books, 1983

Zwerling I, Wilder JF: An evaluation of the applicability of the day hospital in treatment of acutely disturbed patients. Israeli Annals of Psychiatry and Related Disciplines 2:162–185, 1964

CHAPTER 8

Medication Groups

David W. Brook, M.D.

Introduction

Successful therapy of major mental illnesses is a monumental challenge for modern medicine and society. Current techniques have been inadequate because many patients receive poor treatment or no treatment at all. A variety of economic, social, and medical shortcomings contribute to the appalling lack of treatment. First, fewer state facilities are available, and funding for this purpose is more insufficient than ever. Second, despite the great progress in neurobiology over the last 15 to 20 years, the biological aspects of the major mental illnesses are still barely understood. Third, compliance with recommended therapeutic regimens has been difficult to obtain and maintain for large groups of patients. Fourth, current treatment methods have proven to be inadequate for many patients, who continue to be refractory to psychopharmacotherapy, despite the rapid advancements in the field. Finally, because of problems with funding and labor distribution, extending the benefits of the latest treatment to a large percentage of sick, poor, and hard-to-reach patients has been difficult.

There remain a vast number of inadequately treated patients. These patients are most glaringly noticeable in large cities, where deinstitutionalization policies, poor care, and insufficiently funded treatment programs make the growing street presence of such patients obvious and disturbing. It has been estimated that up to two-thirds of the homeless population may suffer from mental illness (Lamb et al. 1992).

Because of the great number of inadequately treated, hard-to-reach

---

This chapter is based on work done in the Psychiatric Clinic of the Mount Sinai Medical Center, New York, New York.

patients, Mount Sinai Hospital's psychiatric clinic in New York has reintroduced a novel form of group treatment for medicated, seriously ill
patients. In this chapter, I describe these medication groups and our experiences with them and discuss the theoretical rationale behind, and
techniques for, the use of these groups. Although we are aware of the
inherent limitations of any one program, this one is described as a model
that can be modified or extended by other systems as appropriate. Other
models are referenced in the "Additional Readings" at the end of this
chapter.

Literature Review and Brief History

Group psychotherapy has been used to treat severely and chronically ill
psychiatric outpatients for decades (Battegay and von Marschall 1978;
Hellerstein and Meehan 1987; Lesser and Friedman 1980). However,
the deliberate combination of groups with psychopharmacotherapy did
not gain popularity until the 1970s. The development of more effective
medications has been the key to the growing amount of attention paid
to this format. Also a factor was the successful adaptation of group techniques to the treatment of medicated patients on inpatient units (Kanas
et al. 1980; Kibel 1987; Rice and Rutan 1987; Yalom 1983).[1]

Early experimenters with medication groups and group treatment of
seriously mentally ill patients attempted to gratify oral dependent needs
in the group setting, feeding the patients as well as dispensing medication. Their goals included lessened isolation, increased communication,
and improved emotional expression (Isenberg et al. 1974; Payn 1974).
Other researchers used the groups to monitor the clinic patients' medication usage. Although these groups discussed everyday problems, a psychiatric resident checked each patient's medications individually (Alden
et al. 1979; Covi et al. 1976; Malhotra and Olgiatf 1977; O'Brien 1977).
Diagnoses were heterogeneous, and the groups were conducted in a relatively unstructured manner. Cohen and Amdur (1981) further evolved
the group technique, using the setting to educate patients about medications and hence avoiding interpersonal group processes. Later researchers combined medication with group support to enhance self-identity,
and the group leaders role-played to lessen anxiety about psychotic symp-

---

[1] Of particular note is the work of Hogarty et al. (1974) in the development of
psychoeducational and sociotherapy techniques.

toms (Larkin 1982; Moffic 1982). Diamond and Little (1984) had patients share experiences with medication in an unstructured group setting, while validating and reality testing. They also used the setting to give a psychiatric lecture about medications, followed by a question-and-answer period.

Far from having a single accepted doctrine, many authors have debated and refined combining of medications with psychotherapy in various settings (Beitman et al. 1984; Gutheil 1982; Karasu 1982; Kymissis 1978; Ostow 1983). Astigueta (1983) and Ostow (1979) examined the combination of group psychotherapy with psychopharmacotherapy from a psychodynamic viewpoint. Rodenhauser (1989) noted the possibility of engendering group denial and aggression when using medications in groups. Conversely, Fink (1989) noted an increasing recognition among professionals of the benefits of combined treatments and approaches for patients and pointed out the prejudices against using such techniques.

Resistances to the Use of Medication Groups

Medication groups were not widely used in the past because of several basic misconceptions. Some therapists perceived them as unsuccessful; others, as too difficult to conduct. In most cases, the difficulties arose not from the group format, but from poor techniques.

One common and debilitating mistake that decreased group effectiveness was that although medications were dispensed concurrently to patients in groups, the focus of the session remained on the group processes and interactions, rather than on the medications or the group's interactions regarding medications. Ordinarily in these groups, many patients were not on the same medication, and some were not on any medication. Therefore, compliance was not enhanced enough for effective treatment (Boza et al. 1987). In addition, the use of medication was generally and mistakenly viewed as an adjunct to the group psychotherapy rather than as the primary or coequal treatment that it actually was for many patients. This attitude of therapists and patients also had an adverse effect on compliance.

For many reasons, severely ill psychiatric patients often have difficulty taking effective medications on a regular schedule (Babiker 1987). Some patients experience uncomfortable side effects, such as parkinsonian symptoms. At the extreme a few patients may develop movement disorders such as tardive dyskinesia, akathisia, or dystonia. Many patients feel neglected and uncared for despite the best treatment efforts, and they may, on that account, take medications incorrectly or not at all. Others, particularly those suffering from psychotic disorders, often include their doctors or group leaders, other group members, and/or their medications in their paranoid delusions, believing that people and medications are part of a plot to harm them. Finally, certain sociocultural beliefs and attitudes may support patient resistance to taking medication as prescribed.

Goals of Medication Groups

The goals of medication groups are

1. To combine group psychotherapy with pharmacotherapy to increase patient compliance with medications and to decrease incidents of rehospitalization
2. To provide a close, ongoing assessment of large numbers of patients on medications and to do so in a manner that makes better use of staff time and reaches more patients
3. To help patients learn more about the main effects and side effects of medications
4. To provide a forum for discussion of medications and the risk of relapse
5. To present medications as the primary means by which patients can obtain and establish control over their lives
6. To educate patients about their illnesses
7. To discuss issues of coping with the stresses of daily life
8. To decrease patient isolation and increase socialization through practicing interactional skills in a group setting
9. To provide a supportive and cathartic interactional environment for patients to express their feelings
10. To provide a trial of group psychotherapy to allow for the eventual transition of appropriate patients to more dynamic therapy groups

Treatment Planning and Patient Selection

The treatment team diagnostically evaluates each patient according to DSM-III-R criteria (American Psychiatric Association 1987) to achieve an integrated understanding of each patient's ability to function in and benefit from a group treatment setting. Psychodynamic, educational, social, familial, psychobiological-genetic, and phenomenological aspects of each patient's life are examined. The history of prior treatment is also studied, especially past responses to medications and group therapy. Often, neuropsychological consultation and other consultations are helpful before starting the patient in the group.

At this point, the treatment team formulates a plan of therapy for each patient, relying on the assessment of the dimensions summarized above. Decisions about which patient joins which group are made during each patient's first few individual preparatory sessions. In addition to selecting the most likely suitable group (or, as the case may be, no group at all), the treatment team may recommend concurrent individual short- or long-term therapy, vocational rehabilitation, or other socialization experiences. A rigorous assessment is conducted to recommend specific medications and appropriate laboratory tests.

The decision regarding placement of each patient in a particular group primarily is based on what most benefits the patient, but the treatment team also considers which patients will best "fit" in each group with the minimal disruption of group processes and with the fewest detrimental effects on group members. The professional qualities and abilities of the particular group leaders are considered, especially in terms of understanding and guiding group interactions. Some group leaders interact more therapeutically with certain types of patients and groups of patients than with others.

At Mount Sinai, *all* outpatients for whom psychopharmacotherapy is a primary treatment modality are placed in medication groups, unless there is a specific contraindication. In most cases, groups are composed of diagnostically similar patients. Although grouping patients according to similar diagnostic criteria seems to be most effective, this needs to be tested empirically. The practice at Mount Sinai has been to treat patients with schizophrenia and affective disorders in separate groups. All patients in each group have the same diagnosis, and all are on similar medications.

Group Organization

All groups accept new patients as they enter the clinic, achieving a constant attendance of about 12 to 15 group members at each weekly meeting. Some short-term patients may join, but because groups are long term, a critical mass of at least six to seven long-term patients is necessary, especially considering the poor attendance at most clinics. Because patients are scheduled to attend only every third or fourth week, and because attendance may be irregular, the total number of patients in each group—say, the Tuesday 10 A.M. schizophrenic group—is set at about 60 people. Groups contain men and women, and members vary widely in age, from 20 years old on up. Although Mount Sinai has not yet tried adolescent medication groups, it appears likely that such groups should be age limited because of the special developmental issues arising in treating children and adolescents.

All the groups for schizophrenic patients are held on one day and all the groups for patients with affective disorders are held on another, so patients in the waiting room see other patients with similar diagnoses, as well as other people in their group. The knowledge that other people with similar symptoms and illnesses are being treated in the same manner is in itself supportive and therapeutic. In the actual group discussions, patients often allude to people and occurrences observed in the waiting room.

Each group is led by two or three coleaders, including one or two psychiatric residents, and a psychiatric nurse or social worker. The leaders conduct several sessions of different groups on a weekly basis. Each member attends a 1-hour group session once every 3 or 4 weeks. The format is flexible and determined by the leaders. (For more information on group format, see Chapter 4.)

Because patients can attend the groups irregularly and inconsistently as long as they attend at a minimum frequency, the leaders must learn to moderate the inevitable strain on cohesion and group identity brought on by shifting weekly membership. With time, all the members of one group—that Tuesday 10 A.M. schizophrenic group, for example—come to know one another.

It is advisable to limit the number of members with psychogeriatric problems in each group. Other relative contraindications include active suicide attempts, violent acts, severe substance abuse and/or dependence, acute psychosis, or an inability to care for oneself (i.e., severe enough to warrant hospitalization). Such contraindications are contingent on the needs and abilities of the particular patient and on the particular group. It should be noted, however, that behavior deviating greatly from the group norm becomes the focus of resistance and can interfere with compliance and the group process.

Preparation of Patients

To help patients succeed in the program, they are carefully prepared in two or three individual sessions before beginning group therapy. The therapeutic contract is discussed with each patient individually (as well as collectively in the group), but with different emphases than the contract for psychodynamic group therapy. The importance of taking medications as prescribed is explicitly detailed.

Patients are told that physical contact of any kind between group members is prohibited. Confidentiality of material disclosed during group sessions is encouraged, but patients are to understand that staff members may discuss the patients' problems and improvement with other staff. Patients are told that individual sessions are always available during the course of the group as deemed necessary by either the leaders or the patient. Lastly, patients are instructed that continuing medication treatment is necessary to join and remain in the group. Details about prescriptions, side effects, laboratory tests, and the expectation that patients will discuss their use of, and feelings toward, medication are clarified at this time. Patients require instruction regarding appropriate group participation. They should be encouraged to listen to fellow group members (not just to staff) and to respond honestly and thoughtfully to one another.

First Group Sessions

During the first group session, the leader should state, preferably near the beginning, that the major reason each member is in the group is because each is taking medication as an integral part of treatment. The leader should further state that medication has been effective for treatment of their illnesses and is expected to help each member improve symptomatically, in interpersonal functioning, in relationships, and in the quality of life. Consistently using a medically oriented approach like this should increase group cohesion and focus on the necessity of correctly taking medications. One technique is to have each patient or the leader mention the medications taken by everyone. If this course is taken, the group process might undergo regression, but for patients already quite regressed, this process may engender trust that the leader knows how to help people. The result for these patients may be an increased sense of group support. These patients are more dependent, leader focused, and less able to relate to one another in an interactive manner than are patients in ordinary, more uncovering outpatient groups. In later sessions interpretations and interventions can be directed toward gradually reducing the patients' dependence on the leader and increasing group interactions. However, the group will always remain substantially focused on the leader.

Patient Concerns

One of the first patient concerns to arise in the group is the fear of decreased attention because of the group setting. They worry, understandably, that the setting results in decreased staff ability to effectively allay their complaints, difficulties, and fears. Another difficulty arising from apprehensions about the setting is that patients fear having less therapeutic input from the leaders. Patient ambivalence toward taking medication, despite its clear necessity and effectiveness for treatment of their illnesses, can be stubborn and troublesome. Their ambivalence may be a reflection of paranoid thinking, a lack of understanding, unsuccessful or disturbing prior experiences with medication, or unconscious conflicts. It may also reflect patients' reasonable fears about using potent medication.

As part of its ultimate goals, the medication group must help patients understand and cope with such concerns. The concerns are best handled by establishing a clear structure for each group and for the program as a whole, with clear treatment and rehabilitative goals for every individual. The leader should emphasize that each patient receives "first class" treatment and that the medication group is not just an integral part of the patient's treatment plan but also is a treatment of choice. Finally, the leader should reiterate, as often as necessary, that combining group process with medications is effective and appropriate.

Techniques

All the major goals detailed in this chapter (assessment of symptoms and current functioning, reduction of dependence, increased compliance, and enhancement of group interactions) can be accomplished with a group-centered approach (Stein and Kibel 1984). Leadership techniques should be modified according to the needs of the members to include behavioral, psychoeducational, and cognitive elements.

The recognition and utilization of unconscious processes, such as transferences, psychological group roles, defenses, and resistances, remain crucial aspects of working with medication group dynamics. Knowledge of unconscious processes enhances the therapist's and group leader's ability to intervene effectively. The ability to intervene with the proper mix of behavioral, educational, supportive, and psychodynamically based interventions depends on an understanding of group interaction, as well as an understanding of unconscious process. Finally, the leaders should recognize and explain phenomena such as denial, scapegoating, rationalization, and other unconscious group processes to clarify interactions and feelings in the group. This clarification can be best be accomplished with a group-centered approach, studying both the group process and the individual members' contributions to this process.

The group leader should actively involve the members in discussing their medications. Referring specifically and often to medications or to patients' feelings and thoughts about their medications will help accomplish this. Group members should be encouraged to discuss the medication issues themselves. If extraneous issues arise in their discussions, the leader should redirect the group's focus onto medications. The group is the main therapeutic tool in enabling the members to discuss and implement the most effective use of their psychopharmacological treatment. The leaders point out, through the improving group interactions, the ways in which the medication is helping the patients. Medication is the vital primary focus of the group, and all fears about it must be allayed, all queries answered, and all discussion encouraged.

In addition to the focus on medications, the leader may choose group-centered interventions to focus on the other group goals—independence, social functioning, and so on—noted previously. The amount by which the leader attempts to reduce dependence and to help shift the group to a more interactive mode of functioning depends on the specific group's composition, goals, and level of functioning. An example of this continual effort to increase independence is seen in the following fragment of an ongoing group session:

Case 1

Ms. A, a paranoid schizophrenic patient, was detailing how angry she became when forced to wait in line at the cardiology clinic. Mr. B, a patient with a schizophreniform disorder and periods of psychotic decompensation, responded by relating how his dentist had become ill during his major dental reconstructive work and was unable to continue the repairs. Mr. C, who was also schizophrenic, walked into the session saying he was late because he couldn't get through the cashier's line soon enough to be on time.

At that point, a group coleader said that it sounded as though people believed the staff was not taking satisfactory care of them. Ms. D, a schizophrenic patient who was on high doses of neuroleptics and who had a history of extrapyramidal side effects, said angrily that she felt the staff members were using the patients as guinea pigs. Then Mr. E, who also had a schizophreniform disorder and also was taking neuroleptics, intervened. He was one of the few group members who, from time to time, filled the group role of "assistant leader." He stated that he believed the doctors knew their duty and the staff really did care for the patients. He led a review of everyone's medications to prove his point, calling on other group members in the process. Several group members then proceeded to add that although they didn't enjoy taking the medications, they would continue because the medications were helpful. The mood of the group changed sharply and became less angry and depressed.

In subsequent sessions, group members became more interested and open in exploring their feelings about needing to take medications, and they showed an increased interest in the effects of their medications. All these changes led to increased compliance with the medicine treatments, the central objective of the group.

The group may resist focusing on issues concerning the use and effects of medications both in the group and in each patient's daily life. Patients do, of course, discuss material not directly related to medications in a nonresistant manner. Discussion of psychoeducational issues, in particular those that help patients learn more about their illnesses and about coping techniques, is a productive use of group time. Through the group-centered interventions, the leader should try to help maintain the focus on the immediate concerns in the group and in the group members' lives. Excessive focus on individual psychodynamics should be avoided. The leader might explain, for example, that a patient talks about his childhood relationship with his mother (with whom he has no current contact) because complaining about the injustices of the past is easier than taking constructive, if difficult and painful, actions in the present. Such actions, of course, include the continued, regular use of his medicine, which will likely be of benefit despite continued side effects and despite his doubts about its effectiveness. The timing of such an intervention must be appropriate, and a short and concise intervention is likely to be more effective than a long-winded theoretical explanation.

Because most seriously ill patients have a severely limited ability to communicate and relate, the interactions in the group are helpful in igniting discussions of symptoms, interactional and functional difficulties, and the problems of daily life. For example, a patient related her difficulty in asserting herself to express opinions in the sessions. The coleader asked if other group members had similar difficulties, both in the group and in the world. This led to a general discussion of the assertiveness difficulties of several of the patients. A male patient then remarked how occasionally he was lazy and did not take his medication as he knew was best. Thus the theme of behaving positively to assert and help oneself was raised and discussed. After this exchange, both of these patients became more active in group meetings and more compliant in taking their medications.

The primary focus always is medications. During the course of group sessions, each member's medication side effects and functioning must be assessed. In the tangents of group discussion, medical, psychological, and dynamic issues may become the focus. Nevertheless, the primary goal remains helping the patients to use their medications effectively. This can be accomplished with the techniques stated earlier (i.e., direct discussion of medications, brief explorations of effects, and mutual support through shared experiences). The group is an aid to the medicine, not vice versa.

Use of Institutional Transference

Patients who have been in one clinic for an extended time tend to develop strong transference feelings to the institution, often relying on it as a parental surrogate. This institutional transference can be used by the group leader to enhance cohesion, help new members adjust, and help current members weather episodes of exacerbation and illness. Compassionate and empathic use of institutional transference can also increase group interaction and lessen attachment to the leaders. Occasionally, accomplishing the goal of patient independence is undesirable because some patients need the attachment and dependency. If a leader attempts to motivate such patients to interaction and independence, increased anxiety, poorer functioning outside the group, self-destructive acts, and even psychotic decompensation may ensue.[2]

---

[2] In medication groups, as in other groups, a patient's level and mode of functioning in the group are indicative of his or her level and mode of functioning outside the group.

Use of Individual Sessions

An important goal of the medication group is to update the assessment of each patient's functioning and mental status. If this cannot be accomplished during the group session, patients can be seen in brief post-group individual sessions or in regular concurrent ones. In addition, some patients specifically benefit from regular individual and/or psychodynamic group psychotherapy sessions. Concurrent treatment complements and rarely interferes with the process and goals of the medication group.

Concurrent individual sessions with the leaders are useful in decreasing resistances and weathering recurrent psychotic episodes. Such episodes, individual and terrifying, are difficult to approach and treat in the group. Deciding whether the patient should be seen by one leader or the coleaders together depends primarily on staff time, but also on the circumstances of each patient and transference issues. Individual sessions are helpful when they contribute to the patient's interacting with the group and to compliance with medication treatments. They interfere when the patient uses them to avoid active group participation and interaction. Occasionally, the dyadic attachment between therapist and patient becomes too intense for patients to tolerate; in reaction, symptomatology increases, as does resistance to treatment. The group leader must travel a fine line to make effective use of individual sessions. Because severely ill patients often have immense difficulty in maintaining satisfactory object relationships, the therapist's sensitivity and skill are vital, and patient setbacks become common. The best approach is to use concurrent individual sessions for most patients only in periods of decompensation or trying life circumstances.

Supervision

Efficient supervision is necessary for the therapeutic effectiveness of medication groups. At Mount Sinai, group supervisory sessions with the entire staff are scheduled on a monthly basis and are jointly led by an experienced group psychotherapist and the chief of the outpatient department. In addition, consultations with senior psychopharmacologists are available for group leaders.

The primary goal of supervision is to teach group leaders to combine the effectiveness of the group processes with the therapeutic effects of medications to enhance compliance and to improve the treatment of a difficult patient population. Leaders are educated in the use of task-oriented group processes, innovative concurrent treatments, and techniques (behavioral, cognitive, and psychoeducational) relevant to treatment of the severely ill. In addition, they are taught to select, assign, and prepare patients for group therapy and to evaluate patients within the group process. Finally, the group leaders discuss countertransference problems arising during the course of medication groups. There are three basic types of countertransference problems: boredom stemming from patient poverty of ideation and affect; frustration caused by demanding and difficult patients; and lack of focus because of the hallucinations, delusions, and residual thought disorders of many patients.

The supervisory sessions often parallel the patient groups because they are similarly structured, task oriented, and conducted in a supportive manner with the focus on interaction as well as issues. An intriguing and fruitful area for exploration is the relationship, in and out of medication groups, of the coleaders. Treatment issues are often a springboard to interaction and open discussion. Exploration by coleaders during the supervisory session of areas of agreement, disagreement, or misunderstanding results in better treatment for patients. Group leaders learn by example (as well as instruction) to develop independence and skill in treating their patients.

Conclusions

In the past few years there has been a surge of professional interest in medication groups. The Mount Sinai Psychiatry Department's experience with these groups illustrates their advantages. As the hospital's clinic population increased, the staff found medication groups to be both a more efficient use of professional time and a more effective form of treatment. Initially skeptical, the staff observed increased patient compliance, more regular clinic attendance, and less severe and less frequent episodes of decompensation when medication groups were used. The group process offered patients education, mutual support, an opportunity to practice socialization, decreased isolation, and a haven to express their feelings and reveal their fears without the worry of rejection. With time the medication group became the patients' treatment of choice. Patient compliance with medication usage has substantially increased.

Controlled outcome studies are now necessary to confirm the utility of medication groups, but clinical experience thus far supports medication groups as an effective method of treatment for an inadequately treated population of patients.

References

Alden AR, Weddington WW Jr, Jacobson C, et al: Group aftercare for chronic schizophrenia. J Clin Psychiatry 40:249–252, 1979

American Psychiatric Association: Diagnostic and Statistical Manual of Mental Disorders, 3rd Edition, Revised. Washington, DC, American Psychiatric Association, 1987

Astigueta FD: Integrating psychopharmacology and contemporary psychoanalytic group psychotherapy. Small Group Behavior 14:261–268, 1983

Babiker IE: Noncompliance in schizophrenia. Psychiatr Dev 4:329–337, 1987

Battegay R, von Marschall R: Results of long-term psychotherapy with schizophrenics. Compr Psychiatry 19:349–353, 1978

Beitman BD, Chiles J, Carlin A: The pharmacotherapy-psychotherapy triangle: psychiatrist, nonmedical psychotherapist, and patient. J Clin Psychiatry 45:458–459, 1984

Boza RA, Milanes F, Slater V, et al: Patient noncompliance. Behavior patterns underlying a patient's failure to follow doctor's orders. Postgrad Med 81(4):163–170, 1987

Cohen M, Amdur MA: Medication group for psychiatric patients. Am J Nursing 81:343–345, 1981

Covi L, Lipman RS, Alarson RD, et al: Drug and psychotherapy interactions in depression. Am J Psychiatry 133:502–508, 1976

Diamond RJ, Little ML: Utilization of patient expertise in medication groups. Psychiatr Q 56:13–19, 1984

Fink PJ: The marriage of psychobiology and psychotherapy: a discussion of the papers by Rodenhauser, and Zaslav and Kalb. Int J Group Psychother 39:469–474, 1989

Gutheil TG: The psychology of psychopharmacology. Bull Menninger Clin 46:321–330, 1982

Hellerstein DJ, Meehan B: Outpatient group therapy for schizophrenic substance abusers. Am J Psychiatry 144:1337–1339, 1987

Hogarty G, Goldberg SE, Schooler NR, et al: Drugs and sociotherapy in the aftercare of schizophrenic patients, II: two year relapse rates. Arch Gen Psychiatry 31:603–609, 1974

Isenberg PL, Mahnke MW, Shields WE Jr: Medication groups for continuing care. Hosp Community Psychiatry 25:517–519, 1974

Kanas N, Rogers M, Kreth E, et al: The effectiveness of group psychotherapy during the first three weeks of hospitalization: a controlled study. J Nerv Ment Dis 168:487–492, 1980

Karasu TB: Psychotherapy and pharmacotherapy: toward an integrative model. Am J Psychiatry 139:1102–1113, 1982

Kibel HD: Contributions of the group psychotherapist to education on the psychiatric unit: teaching through group dynamics. Int J Group Psychotherapy 37:3–29, 1987

Kymissis P: Pharmacotherapy combined with analytically oriented group therapy, in Group Therapy. Edited by Wolberg L, Aronson M. New York, Stratton Intercontinental Book Corp, 1978, pp 131–139

Lamb HR, Bacharach LL, Kass FI (eds): Treating the Homeless Mentally Ill: A Task Force Report of the American Psychiatric Association. Washington, DC, American Psychiatric Association, 1992

Larkin AR: What's a medication group? J Psychosoc Nurs Ment Health Serv 20(2):35–37, 1982

Lesser IM, Friedman CTH: Beyond medications: group therapy for the chronic psychiatric patient. Int J Group Psychotherapy 30:187–199, 1980

Malhotra HK, Olgiatf SG: Fluphenazine therapy in groups. Compr Psychiatry 18:89–92, 1977

Moffic HS: A preliminary report on effects of initiating medication groups at a mental health clinic. Hosp Community Psychiatry 33:387, 1982

O'Brien CP: Group therapy of schizophrenia. Current Psychiatric Therapies 17:149–154, 1977

Ostow M (ed): The Psychodynamic Approach to Drug Therapy. New York, Psychoanalytic Research and Development Fund, 1979

Ostow M: Interactions of psychotherapy and pharmacotherapy (letter). Am J Psychiatry 140:370–371, 1983

Payn SB: Reaching chronic schizophrenic patients with group pharmacotherapy. Int J Group Psychother 24:25–31, 1974

Rice C, Rutan JS: Inpatient Group Psychotherapy: A Psychodynamic Perspective. New York, Macmillan, 1987

Rodenhauser P: Group psychotherapy and pharmacotherapy: psychodynamic considerations. Int J Group Psychother 39:445–456, 1989

Stein A, Kibel HD: A group dynamic peer interaction approach to group psychotherapy. Int J Group Psychother 34:315–333, 1984

Yalom ID: Inpatient Group Psychotherapy. New York, Basic Books, 1983

Additional Readings

Alonso A: The Quiet Profession: Supervisors of Psychotherapy. New York, Macmillan, 1985

Davenport YB, Ebert MH, Adland ML, et al: Couples group therapy as an adjunct to lithium maintenance of the manic patient. Am J Orthopsychiatry 47:495–502, 1977

Herz MI, Spitzer RL, Gibbon M, et al: Individual versus group aftercare treatment. Am J Psychiatry 131:808–812, 1974

Katz-Garris L: Group-oriented therapy with psychiatrically disabled persons, in Group Psychotherapy and Counseling With Special Populations. Edited by Seligman M. Baltimore, MD, University Park Press, 1982, pp 245–265

Neizo B, Murphy MK: Medication groups on an acute psychiatric unit. Perspect Psychiatr Care 21(2):70–73, 1983

Ringler KE, Whitman HH, Gustafson JP, et al: Technical advances in leading a cancer patient group. Int J Group Psychother 31:329–344, 1981

Shakir SA, Volkmar FR, Bacon S, et al: Group psychotherapy as an adjunct to lithium maintenance. Am J Psychiatry 136:455–456, 1979

Vinogradov S, Yalom ID: A Concise Guide to Group Psychotherapy. Washington, DC, American Psychiatric Press, 1989

Weissman MM, Klerman GL, Prusoff BA, et al: Depressed outpatients: results one year after treatment with drugs and/or interpersonal psychotherapy. Arch Gen Psychiatry 38:51–55, 1981

CHAPTER 9

Staff Support Groups for High-Stress Facilities

Marguerite S. Lederberg, M.D.

Historical Trends in Staff Stress

The awareness that medical personnel experience stresses great enough to benefit from intervention is a comparatively recent development. In the nineteenth and early twentieth centuries, medical institutions were often staffed by religious people for whom the demands of caregiving were buttressed by their faith and their vows of obedience and service. The nearly 50 years since World War II have seen the development of the idealized lay caregiver, paralleling the remarkable medical and technological advances of that era. However, with the 1960s came a technological "backlash"; people's inflated expectations of medicine were not met, and the problems of poorly controlled technology became evident. This led to an emphasis on the behavioral, emotional, and moral shortcomings of medical staff. It was not until the 1970s that the plight of medical caregivers began to be viewed with curiosity and compassion. The avalanche of publications that followed Maslach's early work (Freudenberger 1974; Maslach 1976, 1979) on burnout addressed the needs of caregivers. Fox's conference on "The Human Condition of Health Professionals" is a particularly thoughtful exposition of this new attitude (Fox 1980). In the 1980s researchers dealing with the psychological consequences of disasters studied health care workers alongside the identified victims, sometimes finding comparable levels of stress responses in both groups (Wilkinson 1983). Emergency personnel have been labeled "secondary victims" (D. R. Jones 1985) or "tertiary victims" (Taylor 1987), and further studies of their responses are viewed as an integral part of trauma studies (McFarlane 1984; Raphael 1987).

The Anatomy of High Stress in Medical Settings

General Considerations

The need for organizational factors, such as adequate staffing, decent physical conditions, competent leadership, and clear job descriptions, is evident and universal, but this need is not always met in highly stressed working environments. Intense and repeated exposures to mutilation and suffering leave the staff feeling pain, sadness, fear, and revulsion. These feelings in turn may engender shame and guilt. Young staff members are frequently exposed to death, resulting in a premature loss of the sense of invulnerability and a painful awareness of personal mortality. The arbitrariness of human suffering can cause a deep questioning of personal value systems. Frequent poor outcomes undermine the professionals' self-esteem and promote feelings of helplessness, failure, and futility. Further attacks on self-esteem come from fear of failure, anxiety, and fatigue. Survivor guilt, much of it unconscious, is pervasive. Ethical dilemmas are increasingly brought into prominence and force staff to confront ambiguity and irreducible conflicts. In the increasingly frequent situations where staff are exposed to personal risk, fear and anxiety can lead to anger and bitterness. More angry responses may emerge when staff bear the brunt of irrational social responses of blame or idealization.

Setting-Specific Issues

Although the reactions described above have a certain universality, the emphasis varies in different settings. The effect of intimate exposure to death was first discussed in detail in the thanatology literature (Kubler-Ross 1969; Vachon 1978; Vachon et al. 1978), was expanded on by Campbell (1980), and remains central to hospice workers' experience (Munley 1985; Woolley et al. 1989). Special-care units (coronary, pulmonary, neurological, and pediatric intensive-care units) were among the earliest to explore the effects of highly pressured settings on staff functioning and morale (Cassem and Hackett 1975, 1979). Studies of dialysis units focused on staff difficulty in dealing with patient passivity, dependence, and chronic suicidality and on problems in setting boundaries because of the prolonged patient-staff contact (De-Nour and Czaczkes 1968). On burn units, not only the exposure to pain and disfigurement but, even more, the necessity of inflicting pain during treatment are recurrent issues (Quinley and Bernstein 1971). These issues are echoed on cancer wards, where the toxicity of treatment can be quite corrosive to staff morale, and decisions about how aggressively to treat patients with a poor prognosis can lead to prolonged disagreements among staff members (Lederberg 1989). Some settings, such as busy emergency rooms, have an inescapable and exhausting level of chaos and breed anonymity and alienation. Staff of overburdened psychiatric wards confront similar tensions, worsened by the subversive pull of psychological regression (Browner 1987; J. G. Jones et al. 1987).

The emotional responses of health workers working with patients who have acquired immunodeficiency syndrome (AIDS) have a unique intensity (Pasacreta and Jacobsen 1989). (Also, see Chapter 14.) For all these professionals, the usefulness of early and repeated opportunities to debrief, ventilate, and reinforce achievements in a team setting has been repeatedly stated (Berah et al. 1984; Durham et al. 1985; D. R. Jones 1985). It is of interest that Sanner and Wolcott (1983) observed true stress responses in disaster simulation exercises. Lastly, the training of medical personnel has always been viewed as stressful, albeit "character-building" (Ford and Wentz 1986; Smith et al. 1986; Walerstein et al. 1989; Weinstein 1983). However, in recent years, there has been a general awareness that the stresses are increasing and the rewards are decreasing.

Rewards and Effective Coping Strategies

Having outlined the stresses in some detail, it is equally important to look at the many rewards that come with doing such special work and to outline effective adaptations. To be sure, the data supporting these claims of positive rewards are empirical but persuasive. Well-adapted medical caregivers participate in basic and usually private human experiences, in which they may play a positive role. This can lead to an increased sense of competence, courage, and generosity, as well as a sense of being "initiates" of existential confrontations.

At a conscious level, caregivers are often proud of their intellectual capacities, their reliable emotional controls, their problem-solving stance, their ability to rise above superstition and fear, and their ability to function well under pressure. The acting out of positive identifications is a strong motivator, as is the desire to achieve mastery over feared events. Mature defenses such as altruism and humor are very useful.

Constructive sublimation is obviously commendable and need not be made conscious. However, it is almost universal for staff members to have varying intimations of their suppressed and unconscious reactions and beliefs, which they experience as shameful and incompatible with their professional self-image. They keep them secret, reinforcing their belief that they are alone in having them. This can lead to increasing isolation and decreasing self-esteem.

Special Advantages of Group Modalities

The special advantages of group modalities for helping personnel are seen at all psychological levels—from the overt and conscious levels to the unconscious ones. Note that this form of intervention differs from group therapy, but it offers many of the same advantages. These group modalities have long been recognized, as witnessed by the numerous reports of their use with nurses (Beardslee and DeMaso 1982; Cassem and Hackett 1979; Eisendrath, 1981; Gibbons and Boren 1985; Lederberg 1989; Mohl 1980a, 1980b; Moynihan and Outlaw 1984; Pasacreta and Jacobsen 1989; Rosini et al. 1974; Silberfarb and Levine 1980; Simon and Whiteley 1977; Weiner and Caldwell 1981, 1983;), hospice staff (Hover 1986; Larson 1986), medical students (Dashef et al. 1974; Plaut et al. 1982), house staff (Brashear 1987; Reuben et al. 1984; Siegel and Donnelly 1978; H. I. Swiller, Toward more humane medicine: group dynamics and medical education, unpublished manuscript, April 1989), and oncology fellows (Artiss and Levine 1973; Richards and Schmale 1974; Wise 1977).

A few reports included evaluations of the effects and showed mixed results in groups of nurses on intensive care units (Tyson et al. 1984; Weiner et al. 1983). The authors stated that support groups are more likely to succeed if they respond to a perceived need, if the leader has been previously experienced as useful, if early sessions are tightly structured, and if early discharge of highly negative feelings is avoided. Fawzy et al. (1983) suggested that psychiatric liaison activities, with staff support groups numbered among them, can play an important role in maintaining staff morale and decreasing turnover rate. Nursing educators generally regard nursing groups as very helpful (Scully 1981). A thoughtful dissenting note was sounded by Abrams and Sweeney (1982), who pointed out the dangers of too much self-involvement and possible acting out on the part of staff when there is not enough attention paid to work goals and clear boundaries during staff meetings on psychiatric units. These caveats can be extended to other types of units, and they are echoed in Collins and Grobman's emphasis (1983) on maintaining a firm structure and a clear work agenda in all staff groups in the general hospital setting. Lederberg (1989) took an intermediate view and suggested that the leader should be prepared with structure and contents as needed to keep group anxiety, overt hostility, and personal self-disclosure within tolerable limits, but also that the leader should allow unscheduled ventilation and exploration of feelings within the boundaries of the needs of the work setting.

The dynamics of staff support groups were discussed by Mohl (1980a, 1980b) and Eisendrath (1981). A schema for three stages of group development was developed by Lederberg (1982); this schema is described below.

Overall, successful support groups are an ideal place in which to ventilate and defuse pathological group behaviors such as displaced anger, scapegoating, and paranoid reactions. However, it also follows that without careful guidance, the power of these groups can be used in negative ways to reinforce scapegoating, cognitive distortions, and other destructive norms. They may dissolve under the anxiety of too much personal disclosure or inappropriate forays into psychotherapeutic material. That is why these groups, despite their origin in the self-help movements, need a strong leader.

Leadership of a Staff Support Group

Although staff support groups are becoming more common, they are often conducted by people without specific group training. Leaders must understand and manage the difference between therapy and support groups. In a therapy group, members agree to a contract dictating motivation for psychotherapy (presenting complaint), payment, attendance, personal disclosure, confidentiality, and tolerance of anxiety—all in the service of ultimately achieving individual goals.

In these staff support groups, the contract is usually inferred, if not absent; attendance is often irregular due to sudden work pressures; payment is usually absorbed by the institution; personal disclosure beyond a certain narrow range is to be discouraged; confidentiality is not available; and too much anxiety rapidly leads to dropouts or group dissolution. Staff members often have a wide range of misconceptions about the goals of support groups. Some are afraid that there will be a great deal of personal disclosure; a very few may look forward to the same. Others confuse the group with a personnel grievance proceeding in which they hope to redress their complaints. The leader must tolerate all of this comfortably and be ready to work with the group to define the goals and educate the group about its limitations.

Further, the group leader must make his or her own role clear to the group. For example, will he or she give any feedback to anyone outside the group? At first blush, this seems unthinkable, but in fact, many group leaders are employed in the institution and have complex and multiple roles. They must clarify these functions to themselves and to the group members. Does the group leader have an agenda? Will he or she work actively to implement change? In a therapy group, one might let the group struggle with these issues; in a support group, it is appropriate to clarify them promptly and free the group to focus on more fruitful work issues.

Theoretical Considerations

Historically, the canonical group model has been the long-term outpatient psychotherapy group, and it remains the teaching model used by most training programs. In recent years, the term "support group" has been used to describe a wide variety of endeavors that have in common only the lack of individual, insight-oriented psychodynamic goals. An unfortunate corollary has been a somewhat invidious comparison of the goals of therapy groups to those of support groups, which tends to minimize the complex dynamic issues operating in support groups.

In the case of high-stress staff support groups, the outpatient therapy model is the least helpful. Family therapy models are more useful, with their emphasis on a preexisting culture that has a life of its own, their strong homeostatic tendencies, and their well-honed capacity to exclude or co-opt the group leader (Lederberg 1982).

The dynamics of inpatient psychotherapy groups also bear reviewing, especially their emphasis on discontinuous time frames and complex boundary issues in an intense emotional climate that is often out of control (Klein 1977; Klein and Kugel 1981; Rice and Rutan 1981). Nothing prepares the inexperienced group leader for the distinguishing feature of these groups, namely, the sheer volume of human tragedy.

Starting a Staff Support Group

When a support group is requested, it is important to explore the accompanying agenda, looking at the overt and covert issues. Common requests include "coping with stress," "dealing with death," and "handling difficult patients or families." It is less often directly stated that a harried supervisor is hoping to lessen staff complaints about his or her leadership, or that the staff are hoping to create a forum in which they can combat their team leader or control and even ostracize difficult co-workers. These motivations do not invalidate the requests, but the group leader must explore and understand these covert agendas as fully as possible and attend to them in planning the group. They will influence whether or not the group will include the supervisor, head nurse, or attending physician, namely, the de facto team leader (as distinct from the group leader).

Groups in which the team leader participates are generally less frank and spontaneous, especially about issues of authority and discipline. An important benefit of team leader participation is role modeling for staff members and the demonstration of a positive attitude toward the group.

Whether or not team leaders attend, it is crucial to establish a supportive relationship with them and to earn their trust and genuine support. Mere lip service from them will not do, because group members will recognize it readily and will respond to the underlying message with disinterest and absenteeism. The group leader must always keep in mind that the team already has one or more de facto team leaders who have real power over the members' work lives and therefore are strongly (and appropriately) cathected with both real and transferential feelings. The leader who overlooks these feelings will not understand the group process. The leader who undermines them will lose the group to absenteeism or attrition. One must accept that the group's transference to the group leader will always be divided.

Early on, the leader needs to understand the group and system boundaries (see Chapter 6). Flexibility is the key. The group need not even be called a *group* if that term is experienced as too "psychiatric" by potential members who are leery of being "patients." It can be, for example, a workshop, psychosocial rounds, or an interdisciplinary meeting. Some leaders have found it necessary to literally feed the members, i.e., at a pizza lunch or a breakfast meeting. Although this is partly a reflection of leadership style, it also highlights the fact that in many situations, the staff feel so overworked and deprived that they will not readily attend extra meetings without some concrete gratification. Once that pattern is set, it is hard to change, even after the members become quite comfortable with the group format. The best setting is a private and, above all, convenient one, because by definition the members are working in stressful conditions and will not go much further out of their way.

Timing includes several issues. First, the actual time of day of the meeting can be quite critical in that it may favor attendance of particular members or shifts. The group leader should not be wedded to the open-ended weekly format characteristic of therapy groups. Much useful work can be done in bimonthly meetings with stable membership or in short-term groups that can range from 4 to 12 weekly meetings. The latter format is particularly helpful in crisis intervention or in focusing the attention of an ambivalent group. It also relieves the anxiety of members who fear too much exposure or intimacy.

Contents and Dynamics of Staff Support Groups

Staff support groups with stable membership, if not too rigidly structured, go through developmental stages that recur in a cyclical way (Lederberg 1982).

Early Stages of Group Dynamics

The topics of the early group usually involve predictable work complaints: overwork, hectic pacing, understaffing, a sense of being exploited, problems with authority (especially if the team leader is absent), problems with co-workers (intra- and intershift), and problems with other disciplines. One sees a preponderance of projection and externalization, along with a sense of passivity and helplessness. Ventilation of these issues is welcome by the group, but it is of limited usefulness if nothing more is done. However, one can usually help the group identify and label the various components of emotionally loaded issues. This usually defuses some of the negative affect and often uncovers component parts that are either acceptable or at least amenable to intervention. Focusing next on selected and achievable interventions mitigates the sense of passivity.

Doubts about treatment create guilt, as well as lower self-esteem if the staff member has internalized the problem. Groups are an excellent set ting in which to help some individuals absolve themselves and to help others to be more understanding of the professional and ethical beliefs that drive their co-workers.

Another common early topic is the difficult patient and/or family. Staff members relish the opportunity to complain and shed their usual mantle of discipline and courtesy. The group is a proper setting for this kind of release, for letting down and indulging in black humor. It also enables staff to remind themselves that such relaxation is inappropriate in less private settings. But the group work must not stop there. Difficult cases make it possible to discuss human behavior under stress. The universality of this behavior often helps staff to understand their own reactions. In any case, the discussion of their problem cases usually decreases their negative feelings and leads to better case management and an improved sense of mastery.

The group can function as an effective holding environment in which older staff members support and validate younger ones and each other around the grief, fear, and sense of inadequacy that can overwhelm all of them at unpredictable moments in their demanding work lives.

Middle Stage of Group Dynamics

If a group continues to meet with some regularity and some stability of membership, the dynamics change significantly, even while the topics remain the same. As more trust is developed, members may bring up the difficult "good" (as opposed to the "bad") cases, that is, the "special" ones to which they have become too attached. Sometimes a staff member associates to a crucial personal experience. The leader needs to modulate the disclosure and set a tone of respectful acceptance. The leader must stand ready to shield the member from overexposure. This is also the time when group members may do some cautious confronting. At this stage in a well-run group, members reflect on their professional identity and acknowledge their strengths and vulnerabilities. Interpersonal conflicts, when they come up, are less smothered in anger and blame, and protagonists begin to recognize and be more tolerant of characteristic coping patterns in themselves and others.

Late Stage of Group Dynamics

Many of the concerns and dynamics of the middle stage are on the boundary between work and personal issues. Many staff members rethink their professional attitude and their personal lives. At the very least, the individual caregivers usually feel less isolated and less anxious, and unit morale is higher.

In the support group, the sense of intimacy and trust may be quite heady; some members may begin to feel anxious, whereas others may want to blur even more the difference between a work and a therapy group. The group leader must not succumb to his or her own charisma and switch the contract, lest the ability of the staff to work together be compromised. Those members who resent the nonclinical focus may approach the leader privately and be referred for personal therapy.

Groups With Unstable Membership

The discussion of developmental group stages assumes a certain continuity of membership. However, this continuity is not present in an increasing number of medical settings. Twelve-hour shifts and a 3-day week for nurses means that a group leader may not see the same staff members for several weeks. At the same time, the shortening of work shifts for house staffs has also increased discontinuity on medical teams. Thus support groups may not develop beyond the early stages. Some leaders respond to this by becoming the group recorder and providing continuity through their summaries at the beginning of each group (M. Zimberg, personal communication, January 1989). This improves and enriches the group process and provides a model for good communication. It may play an even more important role outside the group because it combats the profound disruption that the 12-hour shift is felt to have caused in unit support and friendships, which influence staff morale.

The group leader could also think of each meeting as an entity, somewhat in the style described by Yalom (1983) for inpatient groups. The leader allows unstructured time for subjects to be brought up and then selects the ones that he or she feels are most fruitful and leads the group to discuss them; the leader also intervenes in the last 15 minutes with a wrap-up and a request for feedback and future agendas from the group.

Ad Hoc Groups

Another variant of unstable membership is the team that is gathered episodically for special tasks or unforeseen disasters. Recent work on posttraumatic stress disorders and other durable symptoms of stress in these caregivers has aroused interest in designing group interventions to meet their special needs (see Chapter 16).

If possible, preexposure groups with a strong practical and educational focus should be formed. These groups can be extremely useful because a sense of predictability and competence lowers the risk of later problems.

Postexposure debriefings are now quite generally recommended (Waeckerle 1991), and again, the group setting is felt to be an asset. Each worker should be given a leisurely opportunity to tell his or her story in the group. This in turn sets the stage for reviewing posttraumatic responses, such as unbidden visualizations, intrusive thoughts, dreams, nightmares, fears, and avoidant behaviors, which are known to occur in a significant percentage of personnel. Open discussion should be encouraged, and the experiences should be validated and normalized (L. Terr, personal communication, December 1991). The members can support each other and congratulate each other on their teamwork and their endurance, even while they forgive each other for their shared moments of panic. McFarlane (1988a) found a predominance of delayed over immediate posttraumatic symptoms in disaster personnel. Risk factors have variously been found to be extensive exposure to bodies and grotesque scenes of mutilation, youth, lack of experience, a field setting as opposed to a hospital or emergency room setting, and the usual psychiatric risk factors such as personality traits and preexisting psychiatric diagnoses and family history (D. R. Jones 1985; MacFarlane 1988b).

Conclusions

Support group leaders need to be strong and experienced. Leading these groups demands skill, tact, delicacy, and considerable maturity. It is also a privilege to lead one's peers and to participate in the healing aspects of a group that deals with universal human emotions.

References

Abrams RC, Sweeney JA: A critique of the process-oriented approach to ward staff meetings. Am J Psychiatry 139:769–773, 1982

Artiss KL, Levine AS: Doctor-patient relation in severe illness. N Engl J Med 288:1210–1214, 1973

Beardslee WR, DeMaso DR: Staff groups in a pediatric hospital: content and coping. Am J Orthopsychiatry 52:712–718, 1982

Berah EF, Jones HJ, Valent P: The experience of a mental health team involved in the early phases of a disaster. Aust N Z J Psychiatry 18:354–358, 1984

Brashear DB: Support groups and other supportive efforts in residency programs. J Med Educ 62:418–424, 1987

Browner CH: Job stress and health: the role of social support at work. Res Nurs Health 10:93–100, 1987

Campbell TW: Death anxiety on a coronary care unit. Psychosomatics 21:127–136, 1980

Cassem NH, Hackett TP: Stress in the nurse and therapist in the intensive-care unit and the coronary care unit. Heart Lung 4:252–259, 1975

Cassem NH, Hackett TP: Psychiatric medicine in intensive care settings, in Psychiatry Medicine Update: MGH Reviews for Physicians. Edited by Manschrek T. New York, Elsevier, 1979, pp 135–161

Collins AH, Grobman J: Group methods in the general hospital setting, in Comprehensive Group Psychotherapy, 2nd Edition. Edited by Kaplan HI, Sadock BJ. Baltimore, MD, Williams & Wilkins, 1983, pp 289–293

Dashef SS, Espey WM, Lazarus JA: Time-limited sensitivity groups for medical students. Am J Psychiatry 131:287–292, 1974

De-Nour AK, Czaczkes JW: Emotional problems and reactions of the medical team in a chronic haemodialysis unit. Lancet 2:987–991, 1968

Durham TW, McCammon SL, Allison EJ: The psychological impact of disaster on rescue personnel. Ann Emerg Med 14:664–668, 1985

Eisendrath SJ: Psychiatric liaison support groups for general hospital staffs. Psychosomatics 22:685–694, 1981

Fawzy IF, Wellisch DK, Pasnau RO, et al: Preventing nursing burnout: a challenge for liaison psychiatry. Gen Hosp Psychiatry 5:141–149, 1983

Ford CV, Wentz DK: Internship: what is stressful? South Med J 79:595–599, 1986

Fox RC: The Human Condition of Health Professionals (Distinguished Lecture Series, School of Health Studies, University of New Hampshire). Durham, NH, University of New Hampshire, 1980, pp 11–39

Freudenberger HJ: Staff burnout. Journal of Social Issues 30:159–165, 1974

Gibbons MB, Boren H: Stress reduction: a spectrum of strategies in pediatric oncology nursing. Nurs Clin North Am 20:83–103, 1985

Hover D: Development of a hospice staff support group. The American Journal of Hospice Care (September-October):39–41, 1986

Jones DR: Secondary disaster victims: the emotional effects of recovering and identifying human remains. Am J Psychiatry 142:303–307, 1985

Jones JG, Janman K, Payne RL, et al: Some determinants of stress in psychiatric nurses. Int J Nurs Stud 24:129–144, 1987

Klein RH: In-patient group psychotherapy: practical considerations and special problems. Int J Group Psychother 27:201–204, 1977

Klein RH, Kugel B: In-patient group psychotherapy from a systems perspective: reflections through a glass darkly. Int J Group Psychother 31: 311–328, 1981

Kubler-Ross E: On Death and Dying. New York, Macmillan, 1969

Larson DG: Developing effective hospice staff support groups: pilot test of an innovative program. The Hospice Journal 2:41–55, 1986

Lederberg MS: Stresses on cancer staff: the uses of group to mitigate them, in Current Concepts in Psychosocial Oncology. Edited by Holland JC. New York, Robert Gold Associates, 1982, pp 89–92

Lederberg MS: Psychological problems of staff and their management, in Handbook of Psychooncology. Edited by Holland JC, Rowland JH. New York, Oxford University Press, 1989, pp 631–646

Maslach C: Burned out. Human Behavior 5:16–22, 1976

Maslach C: The burn-out syndrome and patient care, in Stress and Survival: The Emotional Realities of Life-Threatening Illness. Edited by Garfield CA. St. Louis, MO, Mosby, 1979, pp 111–120

McFarlane AC: The Ash Wednesday bush fires in South Australia: implications for planning for future post-disaster services. Med J Aust 143:286–291, 1984

McFarlane AC: The longitudinal course of posttraumatic morbidity: the range of outcomes and their predictors. J Nerv Ment Dis 176:30–39, 1988a

McFarlane AC: The phenomenology of posttraumatic stress disorder following a natural disaster. J Nerv Ment Dis 176:22–29, 1988b

Mohl PC: A systems approach to liaison psychiatry. Psychosomatics 21:457–461, 1980a

Mohl PC: Group process interpretations in liaison psychiatry nurse groups. Gen Hosp Psychiatry 2:104–111, 1980b

Moynihan RT, Outlaw E: Nursing support groups in a cancer center. Journal of Psychosocial Oncology 2:33–47, 1984

Munley A: Sources of hospice staff stress and how to cope with it. Nurs Clin North Am 20:343–355, 1985

Pasacreta JV, Jacobsen PB: Addressing the need for staff support among nurses caring for the AIDS population. Oncology Nursing Forum 16:659–663, 1989

Plaut SM, Hunt GJ, Johnson FP, et al: Intensive medical student support groups: format, outcome and leadership guidelines. J Med Educ 57:778–786, 1982

Quinley S, Bernstein NR: Identity problems and the adaptation of nurses to severely burned children. Am J Psychiatry 128:90–95, 1971

Raphael B: Mental health responses in a decade of disasters: Australia, 1974–83. Hosp Community Psychiatry 38:1331–1337, 1987

Reuben DB, Novack DH, Wachtel TJ, et al: A comprehensive support system for reducing house staff distress. Psychosomatics 25:815–820, 1984

Rice CA, Rutan JS: Boundary maintenance in in-patient therapy groups. Int J Group Psychother 31:77–93, 1981

Richards AI, Schmale AH: Psychosocial conferences in medical oncology: role in a training program. Ann Intern Med 80:541–545, 1974

Rosini LA, Howell MC, Todres ID, et al: Group meetings in a pediatric intensive care unit. Pediatrics 53:371–374, 1974

Sanner PH, Wolcott BW: Stress reactions among participants in mass casualty simulation. Ann Emerg Med 12:426–428, 1983

Scully R: Staff support groups: helping nurses help themselves. J Nurs Adm 11 (March):48–51, 1981

Siegel B, Donnelly JC: Enriching personal and professional development: the experience of a support group for interns. J Med Educ 53:908–914, 1978

Silberfarb PM, Levine PM: Psychosocial aspects of neoplastic disease: group support for the oncology nurse. Gen Hosp Psychiatry 3:192–197, 1980

Simon N, Whiteley S: Psychiatric consultation with MICU nurses: the consultation conference as a working group. Heart Lung 6:497–504, 1977

Smith JW, Denney WF, Witzke DB: Emotional impairment in internal medicine housestaff. JAMA 255:1155–1158, 1986

Taylor AJ: A taxonomy of disasters and their victims. J Psychosom Res 31:535–544, 1987

Tyson J, Lasky R, Weiner M, et al: Effects of nursing-staff support groups on the quality of newborn intensive care. Crit Care Med 12:901–906, 1984

Vachon MLS: Motivation and stress experienced by staff working with the terminally ill. Death Education 2:113–122, 1978

Vachon MLS, Lyall WAL, Freeman SJJ: Measurement and management of stress in health professionals working with advanced cancer patients. Death Education 1:365–375, 1978

Waeckerle JF: Disaster planning and response. N Engl J Med 324:815–821, 1991

Walerstein SJ, Rosner F, Wallace EZ: House staff stress. N Y State J Med 89:454–457, 1989

Weiner MF, Caldwell T: Stresses and coping in ICU nursing, II: nurse support groups on intensive care units. Gen Hosp Psychiatry 3:129–134, 1981

Weiner MF, Caldwell T: The process and impact of an ICU nurse support group. Int J Psychiatry Med 13:47–55, 1983

Weiner MF, Caldwell T, Tyson J: Stresses and coping in ICU nursing: why support groups fail. Gen Hosp Psychiatry 5:179–183, 1983

Weinstein HM: A committee on the well-being of medical students and housestaff. J Med Educ 58:373–381, 1983

Wilkinson CB: Aftermath of a disaster: the collapse of the Hyatt Regency Hotel skywalks. Am J Psychiatry 140:1134–1139, 1983

Wise TN: Training oncology fellows in psychological aspects of their specialty. Cancer 39:2584–2587, 1977

Woolley H, Stein A, Forrest GC, et al: Staff stress and job satisfaction at a children's hospice. Arch Dis Child 64:114–118, 1989

Yalom ID: Inpatient Group Psychotherapy. New York, Basic Books, 1983

CHAPTER 10

Group Therapy With Medically Ill Patients

Melvin J. Stern, M.D.

Introduction

Group therapy with medically ill patients has a long history in modern psychiatry. The pioneer work was done by Joseph Henry Pratt, who together with his collaborator, the Reverend Elwood Worcester, held weekly classes for tuberculous patients beginning in July 1905 in the Protestant Episcopal Emmanuel Church in Boston, Massachusetts (Pinney 1978). The patients were taught what was then medically known about their disease and were encouraged to present progress reports to the group, which would then be commented on by Pratt, Worcester, and other class members. The major focus was to help the tuberculous patients cope with their worrisome thoughts and concerns and find renewed interest in life. Others have since used group techniques to treat patients with diseases affecting different organ systems, including the cardiovascular system (Adsett and Bruhn 1968; Bilodeau and Hackett 1971; Ibrahim et al. 1974; Mone 1970; Rahe et al. 1973; Stern et al. 1984), the pulmonary system (Forth and Jackson 1976; Groen and Pelser 1960; Pattison et al. 1971; Reckless 1971), the gastrointestinal system (Lammert and Ratner 1986; Lööf et al. 1987; Wise et al. 1982), and the neurological system (Bucker et al. 1984; Chafetz et al. 1955; D'Afflitti and Weitz 1974; Hartings et al. 1976; Oradel and Waite 1974). Patients with disease syndromes such as cancer (Baider et al. 1984; Spiegel and Glafkides 1983; Spiegel et al. 1981; Yalom and Greaves 1977), as well as those undergoing specific procedures such as transplants (Buchanan 1975) and ileostomy (Lennenberg 1954), have also participated in group therapy.

All medical therapy groups, independent of disease entity, tend to share common characteristics:

- They are usually homogeneous in composition (based on commonality of illness or symptomatology) and are generally short term (20 sessions or fewer).
- They emphasize education about the illness in question, including information about pathophysiology, etiology, and therapeutic alternatives.
- They support compliance with medical regimens.
- They teach patients how to obtain relief from anxiety by utilizing relaxation techniques and/or self-hypnosis.
- They focus on helping patients make changes in life-style, including diet, exercise, work, and recreation.
- They support patients in coping individually with the effects of their illness, allowing them the opportunity to ventilate feelings and helping them to relate more effectively to medical staff, family members, friends, and/or colleagues.

Medical patients differ from those with pure psychiatric conditions in that their focus of concern, at least initially, is on a target disease or procedure. As such, they are frequently symptom oriented and desire cognitive explanations. Many are also rigid, compulsive individuals who are unable to express negative feelings, particularly aggression. When presenting to a therapist, they are frequently seen as aloof and detached. They are reluctant to discuss emotional problems, which they view as a sign of weakness, and they consider any sharing of dependency needs as both frightening and shameful (Stein and Wiener 1978). Notwithstanding this characterization, medical patients are highly motivated to obtain effective rehabilitation and to form a positive alliance to work towards health. Providing a cognitive set with which to help the patient better understand his or her illness plus the use of stress and relaxation techniques to ease his or her tension is likely to encourage the patient's trust. If the patient feels adequately supported on this level, he or she may be willing to explore more emotionally laden issues, including those related to body image, sexuality, self-esteem, and existential factors (i.e., morbidity and dying). The therapist must always be prepared for the medical patient's tendency to revert to dealing with the facts of his or her illness, particularly if the patient is experiencing physical symptoms. The following case example illustrates a typical presentation of a medically ill patient and the therapeutic intervention needed to engage him in therapy:

Case 1

I saw Mr. A, a 45-year-old businessman, 4 months after he suffered the second of two heart attacks that had occurred in the space of a year. He had been referred by his cardiologist because of intermittent episodes of brief chest pain plus skipped beats. These were not associated with any (new) organic pathology. In our first session, Mr. A provided a detailed history of his physical problems. He said that after his initial hospitalization 9 months earlier he felt that his heart attack was a fluke. Although he gave up smoking two-and-a-half packs of cigarettes a day, exercised, and attempted to reduce his cholesterol level through dieting, he continued his frenetic pace at work. After his second heart attack he even attended a stress seminar but couldn't remember what he had heard other than that he needed to slow down and relax. As we talked, I was impressed with Mr. A's high level of anxiety, as manifested in the stiff way he held his body, the slight tremor in his hands, and the symptoms that had brought him to consult with me. Notwithstanding this anxiety and in direct contrast to it, he attempted to affect an air of denial and lack of concern—wondering out loud why he was coming for consultation. He was concerned enough about his symptoms, however, to agree to see me another time.

During the second session, Mr. A volunteered that he was highly impatient, couldn't bear waiting in line, and needed to be constantly active. When things didn't go his way, he could become verbally and physically explosive. He admitted that this manner of operating was quite stressful to his body and that stress was a major cause of his heart attack because he had been told that his myocardial infarction was probably secondary to vasospasm. This, he said, was most troubling to him because he didn't know what it would take for him to change his behavioral style and whether indeed he wished to put forth the effort to do so.

I saw Mr. A for five more individual sessions before referring him to a cardiac group that I led. During this time, he experienced two separate recurrences of anxiety-related cardiac symptoms. On each occasion he had not done his exercises or used the supplementary tranquilizers because he resented each as an infringement on his sense of control. On each occasion, he had been involved in some form of stressful activity (i.e., racing on the expressway to meet a friend for a golf game or playing poker at a gambling hall for high stakes). And on each occasion, he thought of leaving therapy because, in spite of our discussions, he was still symptomatic and vulnerable. We were able to surmount this near impasse by talking about his present need for control in life and his distrust of others in helping him regain the control he had lost. He traced his lack of trust in general to his early years, when he couldn't trust his passive father or his chronically dissatisfied mother to nurture or support him. Mr. A was very interested in working on this issue of trusting himself and others, and this became a major factor in his decision to enter group therapy.

Group therapy is especially helpful to medical patients such as Mr. A in that it provides a forum where they can talk about their fears and receive guidance about behaviors that they may adopt or avoid in coping with their illness. Just the act of acquiring knowledge often reduces the patients' anxiety. Additionally, group members can be confronted and challenged by their peers and encouraged to comply both with their medical regimen and with suggestions offered for dealing with life stresses. For many patients, the group experience offers a unique opportunity to share affects and emotions with peers; to be comforted by the knowledge that others, too, are struggling to cope with the same loss of control over bodily processes; and to be supported and valued.

Techniques of Leading Medical Group Therapy

Medical groups, independent of disease entity, tend to be homogeneous in composition based on commonality of illness or symptomatology. They are usually short term (20 or fewer sessions). In leading a medical group, the therapist must actively engage the patients and ensure that even silent patients participate. After the initial session in which the patients introduce themselves and describe what brought them to the group, the therapist, with the possible assistance of a nurse or medically oriented physician, should focus attention on providing knowledge about the disease in question and its medical management. After one or two sessions during which most questions about the physical illness are answered, the patients are ready to discuss the role their life-style has played in the etiology of their medical condition and/or in their rehabilitation. Self-hypnosis or deep muscle relaxation exercises are often taught to help reduce the general anxiety level of group members. The remaining sessions vary in focus based on the leader's therapeutic orientation and the needs of the specific medical group.

Behavioral Techniques

Behavioral or cognitive social learning therapists emphasize awareness of dysfunctional habits and cognitive distortions. They attempt to provide patients with an optimal mode of functioning and subsequently provide feedback to the patients as to how effectively they are changing their behaviors. Homework assignments are given in areas such as social skills and life-style. Patients record their behavioral observations in detail and report back to the group.

For example, in a cardiac group a behavioral-cognitive therapist would focus on modifying the patient's time urgency and free-floating hostility. Some behavioral therapists might also encourage substitution of acts of affection for acts of hostility and/or involvement in activity that is less goal directed (e.g., talking with old friends, leisurely reading, and attending concerts).

Psychodynamic Techniques

Psychodynamically oriented leaders actively elicit patients' psychological responses to their illness. They encourage ventilation about feelings of loss and rejection involving perceived changes in body image, professional identity, and family role. Group cohesiveness is cemented as members discuss concerns about feeling helpless and less lovable. Patients may talk about feeling responsible for their illness because of past transgressions. Therapeutic relief is obtained as patients develop a sense of communality with others and receive group-generated support for action in taking control of their lives. Reducing unhealthy reliance on inappropriate defense mechanisms, including denial, rationalization, and intellectualization, are major therapeutic goals.

For example, in a cardiac group, the psychodynamic therapist may encourage discussion of feelings about the difficulties of coping with the infarct itself, as well as concerns about its effect on work, family, and social relations and life-style. Problems in expressing affect, particularly love and hostility, are addressed as examples emerge in the here and now of the group. Existential issues, including facing the basic issue of life and death, are touched on to a greater or lesser extent depending on the group composition.

Other Techniques

Imagery can be used in both cognitive-behavioral and psychodynamically oriented groups. General healing images, such as having patients imagine lying on a beach absorbing the healing rays and warmth of the sun or floating on a lake surrounded by trees with a clear sky overhead, help facilitate the induction of a relaxed state and may be presented in the early phase of the group. Other general images can be used to promote activation of a specific healing system, such as the immune or circulatory system. Patients may be asked to imagine being in control of white cells killing cancer cells or driving a plow to widen a narrowed coronary artery. Still other self-derived images, elicited from patients in the latter phase of short-term therapy, may be used as a "waking dream" to explore feelings related to the medical illness and the unconscious dynamics that may be mediating these feelings.

Therapist Variables

Countertransference issues, although including the usual need for therapists to know themselves and be aware of their "blind spots," have unique manifestations in medical groups. Tyro therapists in particular express fear about pressing patients too hard to deal with cognitive-behavioral themes or underlying psychodynamic issues lest these patients experience acute physical symptoms (e.g., chest pains or paroxysmal respiratory difficulty) that may compromise their health. Although this is a real possibility, my experience is that the group itself serves as an adequate holding environment to shelter patients from exposing feelings too fast or too intensely. If, notwithstanding this caveat, patients experience distress, the leader may elect to use the next session of the group to deal with the problem. In more acute cases, holding a special individual session to help the patient gain perspective about his or her underlying feelings may be indicated.

Therapists often become discouraged by patients who choose to concentrate exclusively on physical symptoms and medical interventions, thereby avoiding dealing with underlying dynamics that may be contributing to their symptom complex. One way I have found to prevent this from happening is to impart knowledge to patients and answer their questions about the disease and its medical and/or surgical management in the initial sessions. This significantly reduces the patients' need to deal with strictly medically related issues in later sessions (Stern et al. 1984).

Acting out omnipotent fantasies to cure medically ill patients or to significantly relieve their disabling physical symptoms is a potential problem for all therapists who deal with these patients. Very often this idea is reflected in the medical patients' desperate wish for help after not having found succor in traditional medicine. Therapists who assume an omnipotent position are likely to become disheartened and depressed if their patients do not physically improve or if they become more physically incapacitated. The omnipotent therapist may then withdraw from or abandon their patients at a time when the patients may need more support in coping with the anxiety, disappointment, and despair associated with a worsening medical situation (Kaufman and Micha 1987).

The following case examples highlight therapeutic experiences within a psychodynamically oriented group for cardiac patients. In Case 2, members are learning of their mutual difficulty in dealing with hostile feelings.

Case 2

As had been the case recently, Mr. B opened the session and began talking about himself. Mr. C listened and then turned towards me with his back to Mr. B and asked whether the group had an organized format as to who was to speak and when. I said nothing. Mr. B spoke directly to Mr. C, whose back was still turned away, saying that he was being interrupted. Mr. C ignored him. Mr. B persisted in questioning Mr. C. Other group members then joined in, noting that Mr. C had intimated outside the group that he was annoyed with Mr. B for hogging the sessions and that he was dealing very indirectly with Mr. B about this. Mr. C was quiet (and remained so for the remainder of the session). Mr. D then talked about feeling empathy for Mr. C because he too tried to present himself to the outside world as a nice, quiet, calm guy while seething and in turmoil internally. During the next session, Mr. C talked about what had occurred in group the previous time. He apologized to Mr. B and commented on his knack for provoking anger in others and then stonewalling to avoid consequences.

In Case 3, members in the same group share a general feeling of isolation.

Case 3

Mr. E began the session by noting that whereas he had enjoyed the group initially, during recent group meetings he had felt that he was very much on the periphery—unable to get his own issues into discussion and feeling unattended to when he did talk. Several of the other members responded sympathetically, indicating that they had felt the same way—both in and out of the group. Mr. D said that with groups of people, he frequently had to push himself to talk versus just listening. Mr. F agreed, adding that when he was an adolescent someone had told him that he acted like he was in a barrel looking out. Mr. E sighed, nodding his assent to what had been said and clearly feeling more at one with the group.

In Case 4, which occurred several sessions after the preceding vignette, the group members share with one another their overall pessimism coupled with a sense that, no matter what they do, they are doomed.

Case 4

Mr. E said he wanted to talk about a recurring dream that had nagged him since childhood. In the dream, he was on the Cape Cod seashore. A big wave came up and the undertow dragged him out to sea. He was able, through hard swimming, to get back to land. He then walked to a higher place on the beach. Suddenly, yet another, bigger wave came and once again dragged him out to sea. He felt as if he were about to drown but used all his strength to negotiate his way back to shore. After this, he crawled to yet higher ground. Then, standing up, he surveyed his surroundings. Out of the corner of his eye, he became aware of a new disaster. A tidal wave was coming toward him at great speed and would surely engulf him. He then awakened. Members were mesmerized by Mr. E's presentation. Then, as if pressed by an inner force, they talked of their underlying paranoid feelings that they had heretofore carefully concealed. One member, a highly respected scientist, talked about feeling like an impostor at work. He feared he would someday be discovered and his career brought to an end. Another, a journalist, noted that no matter how many assignments she did well, she was always afraid she wouldn't be able to complete the next one satisfactorily and she would be ignominiously dismissed from her job. A third member felt he was rejected repeatedly by intimates and wondered whether his confidence in the group was misplaced and whether he'd be rejected in group as well.

Clearly, similar examples may be forthcoming in other kinds of groups. The difference with medically ill groups is that their homogeneity results in the members invariably vibrating as one in dealing with an issue. "It is as if," said one member, "you were me and you were telling my story."

In the second section of this chapter, I focus on specific medical populations. It highlights the major psychosocial problems that require attention in group to ensure that the therapeutic process is meaningful and effective for these patients.

Cardiac Patients

Cardiac patients are preoccupied with their heart's function, and they are fearful of dying or becoming disabled. Any activity that they consider to be stressful may be avoided because of these fears. Some patients avoid returning to previous work levels, whereas others do not engage in sexual relations or previous recreational pursuits in the belief that these activities will cause them to suffer another heart attack. Many are concerned that they will be seen as less worthwhile and will then be relegated to the sidelines. Approximately 25% of post-myocardial infarction patients experience anxiety and/or depression. These patients frequently have an excessive need for independence and control. Before the heart attack, they dealt with this need through intense devotion to work with little time left for human intimacy and recreational comfort. Without therapeutic intervention, these cardiac patients may regress into a state of brooding, depressive passivity or confused and purposeless agitation (Stern 1984). The same problems beset people who undergo bypass graft surgery, especially if they have not been prepared.

Short-term group intervention with coronary patients helps reduce their depression and anxiety, increases their sociability and friendliness, and concomitantly contributes to a reduction in friction in their interpersonal relationships (Stern et al. 1983). There is also some indication that patients participating in an educationally oriented group program have fewer deaths and reinfarctions and have a greater likelihood of remaining at work compared with control subjects in the years after the group therapy experience (Rahe et al. 1979).

Long-term, open-ended group therapy (longer than 6 months in duration) with coronary patients is designed to alter their underlying type A personality characteristics, most specifically their free-floating hostility and sense of time urgency, which left unchanged may contribute to their suffering a recurrent myocardial infarction. Either a cognitive-social restructuring or a psychodynamic model may be used. One large controlled study using the cognitive-social restructuring model showed that not only did group participants significantly modify their type A behavior but also that they had significantly fewer repeat infarctions over a 3-year follow-up period (Friedman et al. 1986).

Cancer Patients

Being diagnosed with cancer, even when it is removed in its early stages and a good prognosis is forecast, confronts the individual with life's fragility. Fears of death, recurrence, disability, and loss of functioning are common. Denial of the illness's impact is a frequent defense, but one that is fraught with danger, particularly if it leads the patient to avoid obtaining needed medical and emotional support. Some patients actively utilize their physicians and friends to gain information, receive support, and enjoy life in a planned, thoughtful manner. Still others ruminate about their illness, withdraw into themselves, and avoid socializing. These patients are prone to becoming anxious and/or depressed (Kaufman and Micha 1987).

A short-term group intervention can help these latter patients reduce their levels of anxiety, confusion, depression, and fatigue. Concomitantly, by helping the cancer patients to express their feelings and learn new coping methods, the group contributes to these patients' use of active behavioral and cognitive coping strategies and reduces their reliance on maladaptive avoidance (Fawzy et al. 1990).

For patients with metastatic carcinoma who have little or no hope for survival, effective coping involves mastering the stress of terminal illness. Group therapy is frequently open ended and long term. Patients remain in group as long as their physical condition permits. A major focus of the group is on dealing with the sense of isolation these patients experience. By expressing anger at their physicians, they are sometimes able to work through and separate the part that is justified—mostly associated with the impersonal and authoritarian stance of their surgeons and oncologists—from the part that is irrational. Finally, by dealing with the deaths of other group members, participants are better able to detoxify their own dying and look at it rather than avoid it (Yalom and Greaves 1977).

Patients with metastatic breast carcinoma who participated in a long-term psychodynamically oriented support group were found to experience less anxiety, fatigue, and confusion and to feel more vigorous than a control group of patients at a 1-year follow-up (Spiegel et al. 1981). Additionally, a 10-year follow-up of these patients revealed that their survival rate from the time they began treatment was nearly double that of a control group (Spiegel et al. 1989).

Patients With Gastrointestinal Conditions

Unlike patients with heart disease and cancer, who are reacting to a life-threatening and potentially disabling illness, patients with gastrointestinal conditions are distressed by their inability to obtain relief from chronic physical symptoms that have an impact on their ability to enjoy life. Abdominal pain, diarrhea, constipation, flatulence, nausea, and vomiting are but some of the symptoms with which these patients cope on a daily basis. Short-term group therapy usually has a strong educational and behavioral component (Lammert and Ratner 1986; Lööf et al. 1987; Wise et al. 1982). Physical symptoms are identified, and patients are instructed to keep diaries that document both food intake and putative life stressors to help identify those factors that make their symptoms worse. Utilizing this information to make life changes becomes a task for the individual and the group. In the process, members feel supported and less isolated. In the latter phase of the group, they may experience a greater sense of trust, resulting in their discussing personal issues, including problems with sexuality. Treatment results are variable, with only some studies reporting a reduction in physical symptoms after group participation. Wise et al. (1982) suggested that booster sessions might be necessary to maintain symptom improvement over time.

Patients With Other Conditions

Neurologically disordered patients (Bucker et al. 1984; Chafetz et al. 1955; D'Afflitti and Weitz 1974; Hartings et al 1976; Oradel and Waite 1974), diabetic patients (Aveline et al. 1985; Oehler-Giarratana and Fitzgerald 1980; White et al. 1986), vascular surgery amputees (Lipp and Malone 1976), and dialysis patients (Lubell 1976) are often anxious and depressed about their slow, painstaking, and often incomplete physical recoveries. They are concerned about further disability and are fearful of becoming a burden to others. When families also are involved in the group, communication between patient and family about accepting the disability and its limitations becomes a primary focus.

Patients with asthma (Forth and Jackson 1976; Groen and Pelser 1960; Reckless 1971) and chronic emphysema (Pattison et al. 1971) are frequently exquisitely sensitive to psychological stimuli, which alone or in combination with biological factors may precipitate paroxysmal respiratory difficulty. In a psychodynamically oriented group, these patients may develop asthmatic symptoms when affectively aroused. This can limit their group participation and may lead to their terminating further group involvement. Some studies have concluded that these patients would do better with a more educational and disease-focused model. One study (Reckless 1971) suggested that anxiety symptoms could be contained by focusing group attention on the patient experiencing an asthmatic attack in order to help him or her identify the emotional theme to which he or she might be responding. The patient was encouraged not to leave the room or reach for medication, but rather to make bodily contact with another group member, which eventually led to a decrease in anxiety and physical distress. Over time, these attacks occurred less frequently both in and out of the group in response to the themes that had originally triggered them.

Patients with hypertension (Patel and Marmot 1988) or low back conditions (Linssen and Zitman 1984) tend to be most responsive to a cognitive-behavioral approach. Anxiety is lessened through learning relaxation techniques. In addition, patients with low back conditions may be taught to identify antecedent situations and negative emotions related to pain and to combat these with adaptive, alternative thoughts.

Patients in multidiagnostic groups (Stuber et al. 1988) share common concerns, including feeling alienated from the "well" community, concern about ongoing disability, and conflicts over dependency. Group cohesiveness based on sharing a common set of symptoms is not present. This cohesiveness must develop as it does in a regular outpatient group through a gradual understanding among group members who share common concerns. Some groups tend to be established mainly to provide ongoing support, whereas in others, members are able to work through issues generated by their disabilities, feel increasingly comfortable, and then graduate from the group.

Conclusions

For many medically ill patients, participating in group therapy is a new and frightening experience. Talking with others in a group, when they have been emotionally isolated and instinctively distrustful of exposing themselves to any vulnerability, is something that these patients might not usually consider. Once they begin participating in a group, however, medical patients actively work in therapy. Their overcoming a sense of isolation and their developing an increased ability to cope with their illness are sources of gratification for all therapists who work with them.

References

Adsett CA, Bruhn JG: Short-term group psychotherapy for post-myocardial in-farction patients and their wives. Can Med Assoc J 89:577–584, 1968

Aveline MO, McCulloch DK, Tattersall RB: The practice of group psychotherapy with adult insulin-dependent diabetics. Diabetic Med 2:275–282, 1985

Baider L, Amikam JC, De-Nour AK: Time-limited thematic group with post-mastectomy patients. J Psychosom Res 4:323–330, 1984

Bilodeau C, Hackett TP: Issues raised in a group setting by patients recovering from myocardial infarction. Am J Psychiatry 128:73–78, 1971

Buchanan DC: Group therapy for kidney transplant patients. Int J Psychiatry Med 6:523–531, 1975

Bucker J, Smith E, Gillespie C: Short-term group therapy for stroke patients in a rehabilitation centre. Br J Med Psychol 57:283–290, 1984

Chafetz ME, Bernstein N, Sharpe W, et al: Short-term group therapy of patients with Parkinson's disease. N Engl J Med 253:961–964, 1955

D'Afflitti JG, Weitz GW: Rehabilitating the stroke patient through patient-family groups. Int J Group Psychother 24:323–332, 1974

Fawzy FI, Cousins N, Fawzy NW, et al: A structured psychiatric intervention for cancer patients, I: changes over time in methods of coping and affective disturbance. Arch Gen Psychiatry 47:720–735, 1990

Forth MW, Jackson M: Group psychotherapy in the management of bronchial asthma. Br J Med Psychol 49:257–260, 1976

Friedman M, Thoresen CE, Gill JJ, et al: Alteration of type A behavior and its effect on cardiac recurrences in post-myocardial infarction patients: summary results of the Recurrent Coronary Prevention Project. Am Heart J 112:653–665, 1986

Groen JJ, Pelser HE: Experiences with, and results of, group psychotherapy in patients with bronchial asthma. J Psychosom Res 4:191–205, 1960

Hartings MF, Pavlou MM, David FA: Group counseling of MS patients in a program of comprehensive care. J Chronic Dis 29:65–73, 1976

Ibrahim MA, Feldman JG, Sultz HA, et al: Management after myocardial infarction: a controlled trial of the effect of group psychotherapy. Int J Psychiatry Med 5:253–268, 1974

Kaufman E, Micha VG: A model for psychotherapy with the good-prognosis cancer patient. Psychosomatics 28:540–547, 1987

Lammert M, Ratner M: Group treatment of patients with irritable bowel syndrome. Soc Work Health Care 12:67–92, 1986

Lennenberg E: QT in Boston—ileostomy group. N Engl J Med 251:1008–1010, 1954

Linssen ACG, Zitman FG: Patient evaluation of a cognitive behavioral program for patients with chronic low back pain. Soc Sci Med 19:1361–1365, 1984

Lipp MR, Malone ST: Group rehabilitation of vascular surgery patients. Arch Phys Med Rehabil 57:180–183, 1976

Lööf L, Adami H, Bates S, et al: Psychological group counseling for the prevention of ulcer relapses: a controlled randomized trial in duodenal and prepyloric ulcer disease. J Clin Gastroenterol 9:400–407, 1987

Lubell D: Group work with patients on peritoneal dialysis. Health Soc Work 1:159–176, 1976

Mone L: Short-term group psychotherapy with post-cardiac patients. Int J Group Psychother 20:99–108, 1970

Oehler-Giarratana J, Fitzgerald RG: Group therapy with blind diabetics. Arch Gen Psychiatry 37:463–467, 1980

Oradel DM, Waite NS: Group psychotherapy with stroke patients during the immediate recovery phase. Am J Orthopsychiatry 44:386–395, 1974

Patel C, Marmot M: Can general practitioners use training in relaxation and management of stress to reduce mild hypertension? Br Med J 296:21–24, 1988

Pattison EM, Rhodes RJ, Dudley DL: Response to group treatment in patients with severe chronic lung disease. Int J Group Psychother 21:214–225, 1971

Pinney EL: The beginning of group psychotherapy: Joseph Henry Pratt, M.D. and the Reverend Dr. Elwood Worcester. Int J Group Psychother 28:109–114, 1978

Rahe RH, Tuffli CF, Suchor RJ, et al: Group therapy in the outpatient management of post-myocardial infarction patients. Psychiatr Med 4:77–88, 1973

Rahe RJ, Ward HW, Hayes V: Brief group therapy in myocardial infarction rehabilitation: three to four year follow-up of a controlled trial. Psychosom Med 41:229–242, 1979

Reckless JB: A behavioral treatment of bronchial asthma in modified group therapy. Psychosomatics 12:168–173, 1971

Spiegel D, Glafkides MC: Effects of group confrontation with death and dying. Int J Group Psychother 33:433–447, 1983

Spiegel D, Bloom JR, Yalom I: Group support for patients with metastatic cancer. A randomised prospective outcome study. Arch Gen Psychiatry 38:527–533, 1981

Spiegel D, Bloom JR, Kraemer HC, et al: Effect of psychosocial treatment on survival of patients with metastatic breast cancer. Lancet 2:888–891, 1989

Stein A, Wiener S: Group therapy with medically ill patients, in Psychotherapeutic Approaches in Medicine. Edited by Karasu TB, Steinmuller RI. New York, Grune & Stratton, 1978, pp 223–242

Stern MJ: Psychosocial rehabilitation following myocardial infarction and coronary artery bypass surgery, in Rehabilitation of the Coronary Patient, 2nd Edition. Edited by Wenger HK, Hellerstein HK. New York, John Wiley, 1984, pp 453–471

Stern MJ, Gorman PA, Kaslow L: The group counseling v. exercise therapy study: a controlled intervention with subjects following myocardial infarction. Arch Intern Med 143:1719–1725, 1983

Stern MJ, Plionis E, Kaslow L: Group process expectations and outcome with post-myocardial infarction patients. Gen Hosp Psychiatry 6:101–108, 1984

Stuber ML, Sullivan G, Kennon TL, et al: Group therapy for chronic medical illness: a multidiagnostic group. Gen Hosp Psychiatry 10:360–366, 1988

White N, Carnahan J, Nugent CA, et al: Management of obese patients with diabetes mellitus: comparison of advice education with group management. Diabetes Care 9:490–496, 1986

Wise TN, Cooper JN, Ahmed S: Group therapy of the irritable bowel syndrome: themes and process. Journal of Psychiatric Treatment and Evaluation 4:511–515, 1982

Yalom ID, Greaves C: Group therapy with the terminally ill. Am J Psychiatry 134:396–400, 1977

CHAPTER 11

Family Support Groups for Medically Ill Patients and Their Families

Kathleen Whiteman Carroll, M.S.W., L.C.S.W.

Introduction

In *The Village Voice* Paul Cowan (1988) spoke eloquently of his own experience of leukemia. Cowan learned there is a "land of the sick" with its own language, geography, and citizens, where normal life is changed forever. Regarding the impact of his leukemia on his family, Cowan initially felt guilty, saying, "Now the people I loved most would feel my illness as a constant weight" (p. 28). At first, he believed he was failing his loved ones. He worried that if he were sad or irritable he would alienate someone whose support he needed. "I had to let other people's love flow through me and nourish my self-esteem" (p. 31).

Cowan (1988) shared his concerns with his own family and also reached out to others who were similarly afflicted with serious illness. With their common language, they were able to discuss with each other the fears they could barely admit to themselves. He found that he was stronger than he realized and that "dreading death, I can still affirm life" (p. 33).

But what of Cowan's family? Surely his illness had a profound effect on every member. Family members tend to suffer from their own grief, anxiety, and helplessness in response to the patient's illness. However, they

The author is a psychotherapist at Kaiser Permanente, Department of Psychosocial Services, San Diego, California. She is also in private practice in San Diego. For 3 years, she was National Program Manager for the Leukemia Society of America, Inc.

also tend to deny or minimize their own emotional pain in their preoccupation with helping the one who is ill. This ability of family members to focus on the clearly more serious problems of the patient is a necessity for families to survive and function in ordinary life. However, this often adaptive ability to deny, neglect, or defer their own needs can be finally maladaptive for both family members and patient.

Serious illness is sudden and frightening for both patient and family. It forces a confrontation with one's helplessness and one's own mortality. The terror of a life-threatening illness can provoke an emotional withdrawal of patients and family members from each other at a time when communication is most essential. However, not all patients have Cowan's insight or honesty, so they may need the encouragement of other patients and their families to express their response to the illness and their needs.

The emotional impact of illness on the patient is addressed in Chapter 10 of this volume. This chapter focuses primarily on the efficacy of family support groups in helping patients and family members to maximize their ability to cope with the illness.

Addressing the Family's Response to Life-Threatening Illness

Life-threatening illness poses a threat to family homeostasis. The patient's response is naturally shaped by his or her earlier functioning, history of losses, and other concurrent stresses in his or her life. The family, too, brings to the illness its own history of losses, style of coping, and current stresses. Members of a family with a history of significant losses that were never adequately discussed or grieved for are more vulnerable. They may react to the diagnosis of a life-threatening illness with greater anxiety and poor inherent coping ability. Another family with numerous marital, parent-child, or financial problems could be a system already stressed to the breaking point. Add the diagnosis of a life-threatening illness and the whole system may founder as various individuals within the system cope in maladaptive ways.

Weisman (1979) defined coping as " . . . what one does about a problem in order to bring about relief, reward, quiescence, and equilibrium" (p. 27). According to Weisman, poor copers usually feel powerless and good copers tend to be resourceful in their approach to confronting a life-threatening illness, Weisman noted that coping is a skill that can be cultivated by following his "positive directives," including the need to confront reality, focus on solutions, consider alternatives, and *"maintain open, mutual communication with significant others."*.

Tringali (1986) surveyed the needs of family members of cancer patients, noting that the family, rather than the individual patient, is the client. Tringali noted that the family needs social support, factual medical information about the patient's condition and treatment, a belief that hospital staff care about the patient, and a feeling of hope.

Rolland (1989) described three major phases of an illness: the crisis, chronic, and terminal phases. The crisis phase includes events immediately preceding and succeeding the diagnosis. During this time, according to Rolland, the family needs to

- Create a meaning for the illness that maximizes a sense of mastery and competency
- Grieve the loss of the pre-illness family identity
- Begin to accept permanent change while maintaining a sense of continuity between past and future
- Pull together to achieve short-term crisis reorganization
- Develop a system with more flexibility with regard to future goals

The diagnosis affects the family in differing ways, depending on the phase of the family's life cycle and the stage of individual development of all the family members. When hospitalization removes the patient from the home and thus from the normal interrelationships within the family, the whole system must change to accommodate this event. If the patient is the head of the family, economically or emotionally, the shifts in the family dynamics are necessarily greater. Other family members must assume that person's responsibilities or the whole family system suffers a serious deprivation. Families can founder either temporarily or permanently under this stress, or they can rise to the challenge and adapt in surprising ways, including the acquisition of a new depth of intimacy.

Rolland stressed that the more the family can communicate about the illness, reallocate roles, problem-solve, and avail themselves of social support and community resources, the better they will handle the illness. If they can anticipate problems and devise solutions, many illness-related crises can be averted.

Optimal treatment for the patient, therefore, requires attention to the suffering of his or her family. A major treatment goal should be the facilitation of better communication between the patient and the medical team and between the patient and the family. This improved communication will increase family and social supports when they are most needed. Enhancing the family's ability to cope with the illness and related role changes, reducing their anxiety and helplessness, and helping them attain a sense of mastery will have an immediate positive effect on the patient. Appropriate support for the family also minimizes residual pain and dysfunction after the patient's death.

Busy medical staff tend to view family members as peripheral to the treatment of the patient. Therefore, the family becomes adept at keeping their concerns and emotional reactions to themselves. Lack of factual medical information often adds to their anxiety. If traditional supports are not in place (e.g., there is an absence of extended-family members, a loss of faith, or a need to travel to a distant city for treatment), the coping challenge for the family members becomes nearly unendurable.

When family members ask for medical information from hospital staff, they are often seeking attention and support, but staff time constraints make it difficult to respond to this need. On the other hand, members of other families who are in the same situation are uniquely qualified to provide this support. Their common experience with the illness enables family members of medical patients to help each other quickly and effectively.

During the chronic phase, families must adapt to the fluctuations of the illness as well as the uncertainty of its duration. The family's primary task during this phase is the maintenance of as normal a life as possible. The goal should be maximal autonomy for each member despite the necessary constraints imposed by the illness. In the terminal phase, death is seen as inevitable, forcing the family to begin mourning the loss of its ill member.

This section has focused on the various responses that the family may have to a life-threatening illness in one of its members. As noted, optimal treatment for the patient necessarily includes his or her family. Treatment for the family involves the following treatment goals:

• Learning more about the illness and the related role transformations in the family
• Reducing anxiety and helplessness and allowing emotions to be expressed and legitimated
• Improving communication between the patient and the family and between the family and the medical team
• Enhancing existing coping skills and acquiring new ones

- Increasing family and social supports
- Diminishing long-term negative sequelae

That groups are an effective treatment modality for medically ill patients has been shown in Chapter 10 of this volume, as well as by D'Afflitti and Weitz (1974), Johnson and Stark (1980), Silver and Lambert (1987), Spector and Conklin (1987), and Spiegel et al. (1981), among others.

Critical Components of a Family Support Group

Any discussion of medically related support groups requires that the model proposed here be distinguished from self-help groups and therapy groups. The literal definition of a "self-help" group is one in which similarly afflicted people meet to help themselves and each other without the leadership of a mental health professional. Although the group model proposed here is not a self-help group by this definition, it does have some of the same attributes of self-help groups. For example, groups offer a forum where members can share with each other the powerful emotions elicited by a life-threatening illness. Supporting and encouraging each other help members feel less alone, less helpless, more self-confident, and better able to cope. In addition, those group members who are perceived by the group to be handling the stress effectively become positive role models for the others.

The model proposed here is derived from that used by the Leukemia Society of America (1988). The Society has a unique national program of 34 professionally led family support groups of leukemia patients and their families. Eighteen of the Society's groups were included in a 3-year study, with data gathered at 1-year intervals. Whiteman (1987) found that hope, humor, anxiety, and anger were the feelings most often expressed in the group. Least often expressed was the feeling of hopelessness. Most community-based cancer support groups emphasize education rather than group interaction. In contrast, these groups focus on the interaction of the patients and family members with each other, offering support to one another, learning new coping skills, and expressing commitment to the group. Unlike traditional psychotherapy groups, extra-group contact was encouraged by the leaders, and provided additional support for the group members.

Parameters

For a family support group, meeting times, duration, and location should be a consistent as possible. Weekly meetings are best because of the rapid changes in the illness and the resultant differing needs for support among the group members. Ideally, the meetings should last 90 minutes. One hour is generally not sufficient time for all group members to talk. On the other hand, the last half hour of a 2-hour group session often has a number of early departures, suggesting that it is excessively long.

The location of the meetings in most cases will be determined by matters of convenience for the leaders and for the prospective group members. Generally, such groups meet at or near the medical center. A quiet conference room, preferably off the medical floor or away from the clinic waiting area, is ideal.

Patient Selection and Preparation

Patient selection and preparation are important aspects of starting a family support group. Although the norm in most medical centers is not to prescreen patients and family members for group, prescreening is strongly recommended. In a 15-minute interview either in person or on the phone, the leader can assess the medical patient or family member. He or she can also help them to decide whether the group might be suitable for their needs. Without some expectation that it will be helpful, patients and family members are reluctant to experience the inevitable anxiety of entering a new group. Although group is a highly therapeutic modality for many medical patients and their families, it is not beneficial for everyone. Patients with psychotic features or serious drug or alcohol problems, for example, should be excluded, which is discussed further in the section "Contraindications for Family Support Groups."

Family support groups are not therapy groups. It is unrealistic in such groups to expect family members to attempt significant characterological change. In addition, relatives of medically ill patients are not necessarily having interpersonal problems. Family members want support and concrete assistance with learning more about the illness, as well as specific behaviors they can utilize to cope more effectively.

The "contract" in a family support group is somewhat different than that in a therapy group. For a family group, the stated contract should be that members will share their thoughts and feelings honestly with each other. The goal is to help each other to cope more effectively with the illness and its treatment. Members need to be reassured that their continued attendance will be beneficial for them as well as the other group members. Working on their own problems either actively in the group or privately later becomes an established group norm rather quickly for most of the participants. However, the more anxious members may be quiet and participate less actively themselves. Instead, they learn from watching others work on their problems in the group.

Hope is a significant factor in both therapy groups and family support groups. In the former, the hope is that if the patient suffers or struggles through the process of therapeutic growth, he or she will get better. In the latter, however, hope may be even more important because these group members are in a greater, more immediate crisis. They are in urgent need of immediate relief from their emotional pain.

The conflict and rebellion noted by Yalom (1975) in the second stage of group development is not typical of family groups. These groups are not as intense as therapy groups because they do not work directly with transference or unconscious material. Therefore, the conflict expressed will be modulated by the norms of polite social behavior. For example, what is often talked about rather than expressed directly in the group is conflict between the patient and family members. Conflict between group members and the medical team is also a common topic. This hostility should be understood by the leaders as a natural and frequent form of displacement. The goal here should be to encourage more communication among patient, family, and medical team. If a modicum of communication with the physician is unattainable for the patient and family, they should be encouraged to seek a second medical opinion.

"Stability of membership is a necessary precondition for effective group therapy," according to Yalom (1975, p. 62). Yet for a family group, stability of membership is an unrealistic goal because of the constant disruptions caused by the illness and its treatment. Bailis et al. (1978) addressed the rapid and constant turnover in group membership in two groups for relatives of psychiatric inpatients. Their average group attendance was 1 to 10 members, and each member attended an average of two to three sessions. The group leaders, meeting time, and location remained constant, and there was always an overlap of at least 1 old member from week to week.

Bailis et al. (1978) also noted that the leader has a vital role in shaping therapeutic group norms and selectively reinforcing members for conforming to those norms. Their initial assumption was that a group with short-term membership and frequent entrances and departures would always be forming and would exhibit only the features of a beginning group. These features include "dependency to a great extent on the leader, lack of group cohesiveness, denial of problems, and use of cliches and formulas in seeking to aid other members . . . " (p. 405). What they found instead was a progression in the groups from the beginning to the more advanced stages of group development. They also noted "the subtle passage and evolution of group norms—the legacy of the group—from generation to generation of members" (p. 405). This "legacy" also operates in family support groups, enabling them to achieve more than the typical early-stage group.

According to Bailis et al. (1978), a group that is constantly reforming, like a family group, can develop a legacy of high cohesiveness. Although Yalom (1975) noted that the development of cohesiveness comes in the third stage, a family support group can become a highly cohesive group in the first meeting.

Spector and Conklin (1987) noted that cohesiveness developed quickly in their group for patients with acquired immunodeficiency syndrome (AIDS) and their partners. However, this cohesiveness broke down after 8 weeks when divisions developed between healthy and physically ill members. The authors attributed these divisions to patient denial and resistance and recommended that such that groups be composed of patients at similar stages of the disease.

Therapeutic Factors in Family Support Groups

Yalom (1975) cited several "curative factors" inherent in open-ended psychodynamic therapy groups. Several of these are useful therapeutic factors for the family groups proposed here. These include interpersonal input, imparting of information, universality, altruism, existential factors, catharsis, and the instillation of hope.

Interpersonal input.   Interpersonal input, which was ranked highly by Yalom's patients, includes learning how one is perceived by others and that self-disclosure leads to greater involvement in the group.

Imparting information.   Imparting information is a curative factor that includes didactic instruction such as the teaching used in patient preparation for group. Instruction about the illness and its treatment provides structure to the group, thereby reducing anxiety. Therefore, instruction should be a regular feature of a family group. Although Yalom found that members' advice to each other was usually not helpful, "the *process* (this author's emphasis) of advice-giving rather than the content of the advice may be beneficial since it implies and conveys a mutual interest and caring" (p. 12). The same is true of advice-giving in family support groups. Although information can be provided by the group leader, it has a greater impact when it comes from the group members. For example, a group member can validate the patient's or family member's concern about a particular physical or emotional reaction to the illness or treatment by reporting his or her own reactions. Members can also acquaint each other with the medical system and available community resources.

Naturally, the most frequent topics of discussion are those related to the patient's illness and symptoms, the impact of the diagnosis, the loss of functioning, and various strategies for maintaining as normal a life as possible. Communication is another frequent topic. This includes communication and its lapses between the patient and the medical team and between the patient and the adult as well as the child family members. Less often discussed are group members' relapses and deaths, which may be too emotionally laden for some groups or facilitators to handle. (This view was seconded by Hyland et al. [1984].)

Universality.   Universality is discussed in this chapter as an issue for seriously ill patients and their families. Most of them want to talk with their fellow sufferers, not their well-meaning friends who tell them, "I understand" when they cannot possibly know what the experience is like. As noted earlier, patients and family members are uniquely qualified to give and receive support by proving to each other that they do not face the stigma of a life-threatening illness alone. The feeling of universality is a powerful inducement to attend a family support group.

Altruism.   Altruism is an important part of the healing process for patients and family members alike. However, when they are first invited to join a family group, many cancer patients have suffered such a loss of self-esteem that they doubt that they have anything to offer the others. For some, their altruism has been superseded by their fear of seeing patients who are sicker and closer to death than they are. Patients soon learn that by helping each other, they feel better about themselves. This is perhaps the most powerful and therapeutic aspect of group participation and should be facilitated by the leader as often as possible.

Existential factors.   Another curative factor pertinent to medical groups is what Yalom called "existential factors." Learning that life involves suffering, pain, and existential isolation is inevitable for most seriously ill patients. Sharing this difficult learning experience with others makes it easier to bear. Patients' reactions to the group vary. One patient stated, "I delayed coming to this group because I thought it only consisted of people crying and feeling doomed. Yet I found the meeting very upbeat."

Catharsis.   Catharsis can be described as the emotionally climactic moments in a group when the members express powerful and often socially unacceptable feelings. It is experienced as a welcome release after the pressure of self-restraint necessary to confront the illness and treatment. Emotional reactions like anger, rage, and fear (especially of death) need to be expressed and validated. Catharsis is best facilitated by the support and acceptance that the leader models for the group. If there is a stigma attached to the disease, as with AIDS and sometimes with cancer, the value of the cathartic experience is greater.

Instillation of hope.   After catharsis, which can be quite frightening for the group, the group needs the resolution that comes with the reaffirmation of hope. Yalom stated that the "instillation of hope" is a factor that keeps the patient in treatment so that other curative factors may take effect. He defined the source of hope for patients as contact with others in the group who have improved. The operation of this factor is particularly evident in groups for postmastectomy patients who fear the loss of their sexual attractiveness. When they encounter other patients who are sexually active and whom the group members feel to be attractive, they feel more hopeful about their own situations.

In one group for bereaved parents, the instillation of hope was particularly difficult because of the enormity of their loss. Although the members initially wondered what there was left to hope for, they came up with the following answers: helping other parents, especially those more recently bereaved; raising money for cancer research; reading to the blind; donating blood for other pediatric cancer patients; and writing a story about their child's battle with the illness.

Contraindications for Family Support Groups

Psychotic members should be discouraged from attending family support groups for two reasons: 1) they can be highly disruptive to the group and thus prevent it from achieving its goals and 2) they require individual attention, and more effective therapeutic intervention is available elsewhere.

Obvious alcoholism or substance abuse is also highly detrimental to the group. Members who arrive at the group intoxicated should not be permitted to attend. This is an example of the gate-keeping function of the leader, who is responsible for protecting the group from extreme disruptions caused by an intoxicated or psychotic member.

Other types of dysfunctional members may also have to be excluded for the sake of the group. Although the extreme rage expressed by many patients with a borderline personality disorder may be treated effectively in psychotherapy groups, it is probably too damaging for this type of group to sustain. Similarly, some patients or family members may be too paralyzed by their own anxiety, shock, or denial to benefit from the support of the group. This is especially true of families struggling to cope with a recent diagnosis.

Generally, bereaved family members do not feel comfortable attending this type of group. However, some may wish to return to a group that knew their deceased relative. There are advantages and disadvantages to their attendance for the group as a whole. Some group members may feel threatened by the fact that the family in question failed to "conquer" the illness. Others see them as role models for having survived, illustrating for the group the final stage in the coping process. In any case, the leader should discuss with the family the advantages and disadvantages of returning to the group. The family should consider other options as well, such as a bereavement group in the community or a referral for psychotherapy.

Role of the Leader

A family support group, especially a new group, needs a consistent leader or two to help it accomplish its goals. A leader should maximize the group's curative factors by protecting its boundaries, reminding members of confidentiality, screening out disruptive patients, and adhering to consistency in meeting time and location. In short, the leader creates a safe environment in which the members can share their concerns with each other.

Although experience in group leadership is desirable for leading family groups, it is not required. Whatever the leader's experience, he or she should have compassion for the patients and family members and a commitment to helping them communicate honestly about the illness and its impact on their lives. Perhaps most important is the leader's humility. No matter how many years the leader has counseled patients with this particular disease, unless he or she has the disease herself, he or she is not the "expert." For example, the Leukemia Society of America (1988) carefully selects two volunteer group leaders called "facilitators." One is usually a mental health professional with experience in individual and group treatment, and the other is usually an oncology nurse, with technical knowledge of the illness, the treatments, and common patient reactions to both. This combination of leader expertise, utilized by Hyland et al. (1984) in a group for breast cancer patients, has also proven to be highly effective in the Leukemia Society's groups.

During the initial stage of group formation, the group tends to be very dependent on the leader. Family groups will always resemble beginning groups until the "legacy" cited by Bailis et al.(1978) is established. Yalom (1975) called the initial stage in group therapy one of "orientation, hesitant participation, search for meaning." This is a time of great dependency on the leader for structure, answers, approval, and acceptance. Often the leader of a family group will be seen by the group as the expert. His or her task is to help the members see that they have much more to teach and learn from each other than the leader can offer. Whenever a question about the illness or treatment is asked of a leader, the first response should be to redirect the question to the group. This gives members a sense of responsibility to and for each other for group cohesion to develop. In addition, the agent of change is the group itself, not the leader. A leader who accepts the title of "expert" that a nervous beginning group wishes to confer can create an overly dependent, leader-centered group.

The leader should therefore give ownership of the group to its members. This is done by teaching them that they are responsible for what transpires in each group meeting. From time to time the leader should elicit from the members their perception of the group and its purpose. He or she should also ask how they would like the group to be.

The family support group model proposed here is based on an interactional group in which communication flows toward and from every member and the leader. The leader is not a peer of the group members; rather, he or she has clear authority and tasks. These tasks include the establishment and maintenance of productive group norms that lead to the achievement of the goals stated above. The leader has to be active, consistent, and firm, especially with a new group. Members need to feel that the group is a safe environment where they can talk candidly with each other about the illness and its impact on the family. The leader should delineate commonalities and facilitate members' responses to each other, thereby enhancing their mutual support.

Postgroup follow-up is strongly recommended. Family support groups are often intensely emotional, which may frighten some members into dropping out. If possible, the leader should attempt to contact those who have left the group, eliciting reactions to the group and suggestions for improvement. This will also give the leader the opportunity to "debrief" the member and refer him or her for other professional help if indicated. Often this type of outreach will enable the member to feel supported enough to return to the group.

Another part of the leader's job is to communicate with hospital staff, because without their support, a family support group cannot succeed. Johnson and Stark (1980) noted that staff play an essential role in getting patients and families to attend. D'Afflitti and Weitz (1974) also found that they required the staff's compliance in having stroke patients bathed and fed in time for the group meeting. They explained that opposition to such a group is due to the fact that "the general medical ward atmosphere is often geared to the suppression of uncomfortable emotions" (p. 329).

Other issues include staff members' fear of patients' anger, fear that patients will become depressed by seeing others who are sicker than they are, and fear that patients will compare treatments and receive medical misinformation or change physicians.

The group leaders have primary responsibility for allaying staff concerns. These concerns diminish when staff are kept informed of the group from the beginning. Group themes can be relayed to staff without compromising the confidentiality of the individual members. The group leader(s) should stress that the staff as well as the patients and families will benefit from the group. Staff will be able to learn more about the patients and the families' reactions to the illness, and the group participants will be less anxious and make fewer demands on staff time. In addition, the group leader can help staff to have a greater belief in the inherent coping ability of patients and family members.

Conclusions

Most of the studies of the efficacy of groups for families of medically ill patients are retrospective and anecdotal. Although family groups appear to be therapeutic for families facing a variety of illnesses, further research is needed. Specific questions to be addressed include the following:

- Do family members obtain more support when they attend the same group as the identified patient?
- Should group leadership techniques vary with different medical diagnoses?
- How can one control for a possible negative effect of the group on the more vulnerable members?
- What are the best ways to encourage participation in a family group?
- Should groups be focused on a specific stage of the disease?

In addition, a model for training group leaders might be developed. Such a model would include a basic course in group dynamics for health care professionals who lack group experience.

Meanwhile, family groups are meeting in various medical settings around the country, and they are offering a unique and valuable form of support to their members. Coming together to talk with each other about the illness and its impact on their lives is tremendously helpful for most of the group members. And because such groups form naturally in hospital lounges and clinic waiting rooms, health personnel have a clear obligation to enhance their therapeutic effectiveness.

References

Bailis S, Lambert S, Bernstein S: The legacy of the group: a study of group therapy with transient membership. Soc Work Health Care 3:405–418, 1978

Cowan P: In the land of the sick: letter to a potential patient. The Village Voice, May 17, 1988, pp 27–33

D'Afflitti JG, Weitz GW: Rehabilitating the stroke patient through patient-family groups. Int J Group Psychother 24:323–332, 1974

Hyland J, Pruyser H, Novotny E, et al: The impact of the death of a group member in a group of breast cancer patients. Int J Group Psychother 34:617–626, 1984

Johnson EM, Stark DE: A group program for cancer patients and their family members in an acute care teaching hospital. Soc Work Health Care 5:335–349, 1980

Leukemia Society of America: Family Support Group Handbook. Alexandria, VA, Leukemia Society of America, 1980

Rolland J: Chronic illness and the family life cycle, in The Changing Family Life Cycle: A Framework for Family Therapy, 2nd Edition. Edited by Carter B, McGoldrick M. Boston, MA, Allyn & Bacon, 1989, pp 433–456

Silver D, Lambert A: The effect of a support group on the psychosocial well-being of brain tumor patients and their families (abstract). Oncol Nurs Forum 12 (suppl): 87, 1987

Spector IC, Conklin R: Brief reports: AIDS group psychotherapy. Int J Group Psychother 37:433–439, 1987

Spiegel D, Bloom JR, Yalom I: Group support for patients with metastatic cancer: a randomized outcome study. Arch Gen Psychiatry 38:527–533, 1981

Tringali CA: The needs of family members of cancer patients. Oncol Nurs Forum 34(4):65–70, 1986

Weisman AD: Coping With Cancer. New York, McGraw-Hill, 1979

Whiteman K: Unpublished paper presented at the meeting of the National Board of Trustees, Leukemia Society of America, Boston, MA, June 1987

Yalom ID: The Theory and Practice of Group Psychotherapy, 2nd Edition. New York, Basic Books, 1975

PART III

Special Populations in Group Therapy

CHAPTER 12

Creating the Adolescent Group Psychotherapy Experience

Albert E. Riester, Ed.D.

Introduction

Group psychotherapy provides the opportunity for an adolescent to explore, discover, learn, and communicate with others in a safe and nurturing therapeutic environment. It provides unique opportunities to develop age-appropriate interpersonal skills that are necessary to resolve conflict and frustration. The group enables the adolescent to experience and observe scapegoating phenomena, subgroup alliances, power and control dynamics, the development of trust, and the complex age, gender, and status issues that are present whenever people interact. The intense emotions associated with termination, absent leader, new member, authority, peer competition, and group confrontation motivate members to understand how their judgment and perceptions can be impaired in social encounters.

By working in the here and now, group members are able to recognize how their asocial and dysfunctional behaviors have made them captives of authority figures and obstructed the individuation process. As the group endures the stormy middle stage in group development, authority figures and peers emerge as resources in the adolescent's struggle for identity, respect, and autonomy. Furthermore, as problems are shared in the group, the adolescent recognizes that all people have similar needs, fears, and dreams for the future.

This powerful treatment modality provides a microcosm of adolescent society wherein the age-appropriate expression of anger, intimacy, and anxiety leads to group cohesiveness and emotional contact with others. The group's support enables the members to work through internal conflicts that have prevented them from functioning at their level of ability. As termination approaches and the expected regression occurs, the adolescent receives another confirmation that the group's acceptance, trust, and support is unconditional. Although rarely acknowledged by the adolescent, he or she leaves the treatment experience with a group-object that can be evoked in the future to cope with rejection, tragedy, disappointment, and joy. In brief, the group therapy experience serves as a laboratory to understand that nurturing and caring relationships and confrontation by others fuel rather than stall the individuation process and the attainment of one's goals.

The Purpose of Group Psychotherapy

Youths referred for outpatient and inpatient psychiatric services have one characteristic in common: Their behaviors have made them the unwanted teenagers of adolescent society. The unwanteds are at risk for moving into adulthood without the emotional and social maturity to cope and adapt well. These adolescents have not been able to function and respond to the basic expectations of their family, school, and peer group. Furthermore, they have been denied access to the socialization experiences necessary to develop in the cognitive, motor, and psychological domains. For many, severe language and learning disabilities, intellectual limitations, and perceptual motor delays have prevented mastery in school. For others, depression, anxiety, impulse regulation problems, and psychotic ideation have impaired their judgment. They have a poor capacity to form attachments with others. In brief, far too many young people will not make the passage through adolescence because their basic human needs will go unmet. These basic human needs include

> caring relationships with adults, guidance in facing sometimes overwhelming biological and psychological changes, the security of belonging to constructive peer groups, and the perception of future opportunity. (Carnegie Council on Adolescent Development 1989)

Because of a variety of political and socioeconomic factors, some fortunate unwanted or at-risk adolescents gain access to the health care and mental health system. Generally, a parent, school official, or law enforcement agent refers the adolescent for assessment and intervention to improve his or her level of functioning in the classroom, work team, peer group, clubs, and family. As the assessment reports document, these patients do not have the insight, social skills, self-esteem, and age-appropriate judgment necessary to interact with others according to their own expectations and the demands of society. For a high percentage, their neurological and psychological disorders and related behaviors have created tension and anguish. Simply stated, their "I" or self problems have resulted in rejection by small groups (family, peers) and large groups (schools, employers) and an inability to gain access to the opportunities in the community.

The adolescent patient's problem behaviors communicate his or her need for help; however, society responds by assigning adolescents low social status, where teaching, support, and love are often impossible to attain. This cycle of rejection or conflict becomes the central interpersonal experience for the unwanteds. Their problems are frequently manifested by dysfunctional and asocial behaviors. Others in their lives respond to these surface behaviors or symptoms with rejection, avoidance, and harassment, reinforcing the unwanted's negative self-image. In summary, access to socialization experiences is blocked, and these adolescents begin to drift aimlessly in a lonely search for ways to meet their psychosocial and biological needs.

Creation of the Therapeutic Group Climate

The group therapist is charged with the awesome responsibility of creating a therapeutic group climate that will enable unwanteds to become wanted. If the therapist understands and accepts the role of leader, the group can be a powerful modality to help youths who are depressed, hostile, anxious, confused, and unable to think or act in a logical manner. The following guidelines are presented to assist the group leader in developing a therapeutic milieu that will enable patients to attain their treatment goals.

1. The amount of group structure must be congruent with the developmental level of the patients in the group.
2. Goals for the group and patients must be formulated and utilized in the treatment process.

3. Nonverbal and verbal activities give the patients the opportunity to experience mastery.
4. The unwanteds will press the therapist to reject the group and thereby confirm their negative self-image while recreating a familiar emotional encounter with authority figures.
5. Knowing who does what with whom, as well as when, where, and how, will give the therapist a road map to understand group process.
6. Knowledge of the stages of group development will help the therapist to recognize and understand the patient's progress towards individuation.
7. The therapist's peer group history can be a resource in selecting verbal and nonverbal activities to establish a therapeutic alliance.
8. Supervision will help the therapist of unwanteds to draw on these adolescents' own resources to orchestrate the creation of a therapeutic milieu.
9. Termination must be dealt with throughout the process of treatment. The denial of "next" can prevent discussions of how the here and how can be utilized in the future.

These guidelines are discussed in more detail below to illustrate how they may be applied to group therapy with adolescents.

Developmental Level of the Group

Group therapy will be successful if the therapist provides the external structure and guidance to enable the adolescent patient to experience mastery in the group. Structure is defined as the degree to which the therapists initiate action that promotes the participant's cognitive, emotional, and social development. The amount of external structure needed to accomplish this task depends on the developmental level of the group. For example, severely emotionally disturbed, impulsive, and undersocialized adolescents need an auxiliary ego to enable them to benefit from the group experience. The therapists must be active in planning and conducting each session. For example, they must establish and enforce clear ground rules that correspond to community laws and the requirements of the office building, school, or clinic where the group meets. Also, the length of the group session, number of co-leaders, frequency of sessions, time allotted to a task, kind of furniture, activities, materials, and number of redirections and reminders are all elements related to developing the level of structure so patients can par-

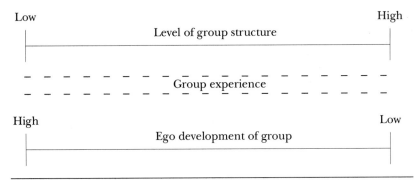

Figure 12–1. Level of group structure and stage of ego development.

ticipate in the group.

Figure 12–1 illustrates how the group's development level and amount of group structure orchestrated by the therapist must be congruent. For example, if the group structure and ego development are "low," chaos will emerge and patients will have pathological group experiences. It is imperative that group therapists orchestrate the appropriate level of structure to create a climate that is secure, caring, and supportive. If therapists permit social chaos, groups in general will be perceived as rejecting, overwhelming, and an "object" to avoid in the future.

Schamess (1986) and Scheidlinger (1960) both addressed the need for congruence between the amount of group structure and the level of ego development in group therapy of children. Because so many high-risk adolescents needing treatment are near the 3- or 4-year developmental level in the emotional and social domains, articles written for children offer a resource for the therapist in understanding the needs of the teenage population. Scheidlinger and Schamess endorsed the active role of the therapist in orchestrating the group so that positive socialization and therapeutic experiences will occur. Restating the goals, clarifying the established ground rules and consequences, and selecting appropriate verbal and nonverbal activities are examples of actions that the leader can initiate to create a therapeutic milieu.

Goals for the Group and Patient

A goal-oriented approach that corresponds to the therapist's theoretical orientation is suggested in planning for the adolescent group. The availability of group and patient goals enables the therapists to communicate

Group Psychotherapy Progress Notes

Patient: _____

Therapist: _____

Focus of Treatment in Group Therapy

Date	Session	Hours	CLUSTER I Peer behaviors				CLUSTER II Group skills				CLUSTER III Adult behaviors				Comments
			Interacts with peers	Accepts input/guidance from peers	Forms cohesive relationship with others	Communicates needs and feelings verbally	Demonstrates problem solving in the group	When frustrated, controls impulses in group	Utilizes group to gain insight and self-awareness	Communicates needs and feelings verbally	Accepts guidance and input from adults	Initiates request for assistance and clarification	Communicates with others about strengths as well as problems	Communicates needs and feelings verbally	

```
        1              2              3              4              5
   Impairs                     Within normal              Strength for
  functioning                     limits               social adaptation
```

Summary: _____
_____
_____
_____
_____

Figure 12–2. Group psychotherapy progress notes.

with parents, other clinicians, teachers, and prospective patients concerning the purpose of the therapeutic experience. It will also be easier to document and discuss how the group will contribute to reaching the goals and objectives of the patient's treatment plan.

Generally, goals address the reduction of dysfunctional behaviors and target the areas where the patient has significant developmental delays. I have successfully used goals that focus on peer-, group-, and adult-oriented behaviors. These three goal areas are outlined in Figure 12–2, and this format can be used by the clinician to document patient progress after each group session.

These three goal areas help the group to deal with a variety of psychosocial issues such as intimacy, identity, individuation, and interpersonal conflict resolution with adults and peers. Additional individualized goals that relate more specifically to the treatment plan can be included on this form.

Figure 12–3 illustrates how these three goal areas can be tabulated to document change in the total group (Jones 1989). Figures 12–4 and 12–5 are profiles of how two patients from the same group performed over a period of time as perceived by the therapist. David D (Figure 12–4) was diagnosed as having conduct disorder with depression and had a history of substance abuse. Frank (Figure 12–5) had a pervasive developmental disorder with schizoid tendencies.

Both patients had different rates of progress, but both reached similar levels of performance in the group before termination. Frank moved from weak interpersonal communication in the group to more active interaction with peers and adults. David quickly emerged as the leader in the initial session and had the opportunity in the group to apply these skills for constructive rather than antisocial purposes. In later sessions, he encouraged Frank as well as others to participate and verbalize their feelings and needs.

If we accept Wong's consensus (1983) that object relations theory will help guide psychotherapies in the future, the interpersonal goals shown in Figure 12–2 may be of interest to the practitioner. For the group represented in Figures 12–3, 12–4, and 12–5, patient progress could be documented. This convenient format gave the patients and therapists the opportunity to work toward goals in three critical interpersonal areas: peer, adult, and group as a whole. This graphic illustration of patient improvement also can assist parents and teachers in planning structured events where these social skills can be demonstrated in the community.

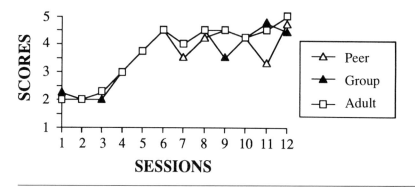

Figure 12–3. Group cluster comparisons.

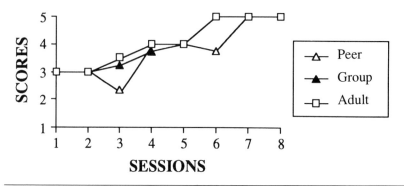

Figure 12–4. Individual cluster comparisons: (David).

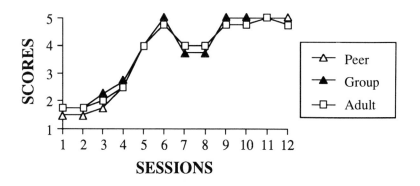

Figure 12–5. Individual cluster comparisons: (Frank).

Activities: Nonverbal and Verbal

The debate over verbal versus nonverbal activities in conducting child and adolescent groups occurs in every clinic, hospital, and private practice setting. In planning for the group, the therapist must understand that verbal discussion and a project involving fine and gross motor skills are both examples of a kind of "activity." Both verbal interaction and project participation facilitate group development, participation, interpersonal communication, and cohesiveness.

The degree to which the activity is based on the verbal versus motoric mode of communication is related to the developmental level and competencies of the group members. In other words, a group with high language development can participate successfully in verbal discussion with less need for activities requiring gross and fine motor skills. In contrast, groups with poor language sophistication generally experience greater mastery and inclusion in groups where there are projects that utilize their fine and gross motor skills. Figure 12–6 presents a model designed to ensure that the group experience contains the appropriate blend of verbal and nonverbal activities.

It is crucial to be flexible and creative in blending verbal and nonverbal activities that represent the interests, abilities, and developmental readiness of the group. The therapists, because of their developmental level and language sophistication, will be more comfortable with verbal activities (discussion) because they feel that through these skills they have mastery and control. The nonverbal activities (gross and fine motor expression) frequently pull the therapists into a domain where they have less skill, interest, and knowledge than their patients. However, as long as there is open and direct discussion and awareness of what is occurring in the here and now, nonverbal and verbal activities can be blended to fit the situation. For example, snack time can become a common ground to enable group cohesiveness to develop, stimulate interaction, and give members a positive social experience.

In a residential facility, the early-adolescent group voted to build a race car for a derby. The race car became a symbol for the group and was used to discuss the patients' journey on the road to progress so they could be discharged from the hospital. Several group members with poor language skills were able to teach highly verbal therapists with poor motor and carpentry skills how to follow directions and create a symbolic representation of their group. The derby race car was a catalyst for here-and-now activation, whereby interpersonal skills, fun, and environmental

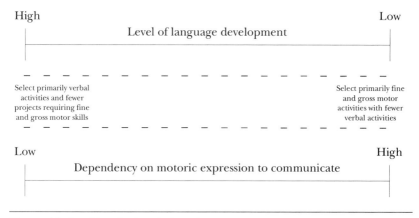

Figure 12–6. Blend of verbal and motoric activity by developmental level of group.

mastery were experienced for the first time. When the therapists were unable to perform a task, they modeled how to seek and accept help from others. Most importantly, the activity enabled patients to experience mastery in their relationship with the group therapists and peers.

The Therapist Will Be Pressed to Reject the Group

Frequently, adolescent unwanteds have experienced family and peer group rejection, and the therapy group evokes intense feelings associated with past experiences. In the initial stage of the therapy group's development, even the most ego-deprived adolescents demonstrate some control of their feelings. For this reason, therapists begin to develop initial confidence in their ability to manage impulsive and provocative patients. However, as the adolescents begin to feel accepted and protected from humiliation, they begin to express anxiety, hostility, and frustration originating from past encounters.

During the middle stage of the group's development, these feelings are communicated verbally and nonverbally to the group, resulting in confrontations that are paranoid and hostile in nature. If structure, support, reassurance, and careful planning are provided by the therapists, this stormy middle stage can become the occasion to recognize that the group is the accepting and nurturing "mother" object. During this stage, therapists frequently are consumed by their subjective perceptions and begin to psychologically abandon the group. Negative countertransference is manifested by coming late for the group session, focusing on the adolescents' hostile behaviors, ignoring patient progress in participation and commitment, and permitting scapegoating to occur. The experience could reconfirm the adolescents' low self-image and paranoid perception of groups and authority figures in general. The group will confront the therapists' authority, challenge their values and beliefs, and reject their suggestions and interpretations during the conflict stage. Ambivalence about being a group member dominates the discussions as the therapists struggle to save the group that they may be rejecting at an unconscious level.

There is no easy way to survive the conflict stage without some supervision and time to debrief the sessions. The supervision and collaboration process enables the therapist to understand emotionally that this is how the unwanteds recreate the chaotic and rejecting family and peer groups from their painful past. Primitive behaviors emerge, representing the participant's unsocialized expression of his or her need for greater autonomy from the mother group. With this insight, leaders can plan and structure positive here-and-now experiences. This attitude will enable the group to ride out the stormy stage and learn age-appropriate ways to facilitate the individuation process.

Group Process Illumination

Group process commentary can be a powerful intervention to assist adolescents in gaining insight and learning how to communicate more effectively in a group. Therapists must recognize the patterns of interaction that occur in the life of the group because they may reveal unconscious issues that interfere with interpersonal communication. When content statements provoke others, recognition of the process will help the group understand why the statements or themes elicit intense emotion. Also, the pattern of who does what with whom, as well as when, where, and how, is helpful in unraveling some of the processes that impair the group's forward progress. In one group, Austin, age 17 years, began the session with a description of how a recent fist fight caused his obvious eye injury. The group responded by discussing alternative ways to deal with conflict, which Austin accepted. By looking at the process, the leader reminded the group that every week Austin would open the discussion with a "then and there" problem for the group session to solve. By illuminating how the group was operating as a system, the members discussed their own difficulty in discussing their problems and how Austin's style enabled them to be participant observers. By dealing directly with a group process, members began to encourage each other to interact.

By observing where group members sit, and identifying the group's sociometric pattern, the leader can point to the unconscious concerns of the group. Process illumination enables the adolescents to discuss how their interaction patterns in the group are related to their personality dynamics. The following case example illustrates how group process illumination facilitates the working through of internal emotional conflicts:

Case 1

> In a recent group, Susan always sat next to the male cotherapist but directed all of her comments and eye contact to the female cotherapist who was seated across from her. One week, the cotherapists intentionally sat next to each other. The members' initial discussion focused on marital conflict, divorce, and abandonment themes. When the therapists asked if the new seating pattern had an impact on the content of their discussion, Susan began to share her ambivalent feelings about the male therapist. She perceived him as a temporary group member who was not concerned about her problems. She quickly learned that this subjective perception was based on her history where her father abandoned the family when she was three. The here-and-now discussion of transference dynamics was activated by group process illumination.

Individuation and Stages in Group Development

Initially, the adolescents' press to be separate and autonomous from the therapists' values and views is evident at every turn. The conflict stage of group development is the best time to witness the adolescents' march towards individuation from the symbolic mother group. At this time, therapists may conclude that the adolescents in their group are uncooperative, rebellious, egocentric, poorly motivated, and oppositional. This attitude will block the creation of a therapeutic alliance, and group members will begin to respond to the leaders from a paranoid world view. This oppositional behavior should be recognized by the therapists as "reaching out for individuation" and understood as a means to become independent (Fried 1970). The unwanteds, however, express their innate need for autonomy in ways that result in greater dependency on the group. In other words, they communicate their ambivalence about achieving greater autonomy by behaving in ways that will create a hostile, dependent relationship on therapists, parents, teachers, and friends. We know that emotionally disturbed adolescents are not able to achieve greater autonomy because society has excluded them from opportunities to learn how to communicate frustration and gain self-knowledge. Through understanding of the developmental process and by riding out the stormy conflict stage, therapists can form the group bond that facilitates individuation.

A discussion of how asocial and developmentally inappropriate behaviors guarantee dependent relationships with authority figures always gains the group's attention. When the therapists side with the innate need for autonomy, the group will be motivated to explore ways to change hostile, dependent relationships. For example, poor grades and discipline problems in school can be discussed in the context of how these behaviors elicit more frequent interactions with teachers, family, and school authorities. These confrontations provide the unwanteds with the emotional contact with parental objects that they cannot obtain through activity that our culture accepts and values. Through discussion, the group will come up with new ways to gain parental object recognition that do not thwart the attainment of autonomy. The group will identify the cultural requirements for greater independence (e.g., good grades for college or skills needed for employment) and present new ways to meet their emotional needs. By bringing the discussion into the here-and-now life of the group, the adolescents will experience greater emotional independence as they respond to the responsibilities of group membership. For example, resolving conflict through group problem-solving and following through on commitments will enable the group to engage in "fun" activities.

Therapist's Peer Group History

The therapists' own peer group history has a powerful influence over their values, leadership style, understanding of peer group dynamics, selection of activities, and ability to focus on a group-as-a-whole issue. Group leaders will recall that their own adolescent society was a mosaic of informal social subgroups with contrasting and often hostile attitudes and leisure time patterns (Riester 1968). However, we often forget that each clique has its counterpart in adult society. For example, the leading crowd in high school has comparable adult subgroups in the community who recall that in high school they were from the popular group. The delinquent, asocial, and disruptive teenage subgroups have adult counterparts who have a history of rejecting society's rules, mores, and values.

The teenager's membership in a clique begins to make a statement concerning his or her identity and role in society that is likely to continue into adulthood. The assumption that clique membership is a phase and is unique only to adolescent society may be the reason it is rarely addressed in psychiatric assessments. Perhaps the adolescents who become core members of the preppies, jocks, kickers, freaks, socials, intellectuals, hoods, or greasers will internalize their subcultural mores and join corresponding adult subgroups as they grow older. We can accept that adolescence is a time for exploration. However, the freedom to move in and out of different cliques may not be an option for the unwanteds. Membership in certain cliques may be physically unsafe because of their drug use, sexual mores, and asocial activities. Perhaps the option of joining an unconventional subculture for an interim period during adolescence is riskier in a highly competitive and unsafe world.

When therapists are leading a group of 14-year-old adolescents, it is important for them to be in touch with their own 14-year-old group history. For example, were the therapists members of the popular or leading crowd in high school, or were they members of the "intellectual" crowd where they experienced rejection from "in crowd" social activities? Some therapists may not have experienced membership in a cohesive peer subgroup and may have had only peripheral membership in a teenage clique. Was the therapist's life at 14 more adult centered, with leisure time spent with family and teachers (music lessons, athletics), or was it peer group oriented?

A group discussion of high school cliques, including clothing styles, beliefs, values, and leisure time activities, is a comfortable way to deal with identity and inclusion issues. Therapists must recognize the difficulty that emotionally disturbed students have in gaining access to the peer groups that may support the mores and life-styles familiar to the therapists. For example, if they leave an asocial clique (hoods), can they become a member of another subgroup that provides the cohesiveness and support that they crave emotionally? How can they leave the asocial subgroup where they occupy a leadership role and become a peripheral member of the subgroup that represents the values of the therapists? What skills are needed to join the subgroups that more closely approximate the subgroup where the therapists held leadership roles? Are the therapists suggesting that clique membership is not necessary because it evokes painful memories of group rejection when they were 14? The answers to these fascinating questions will emerge in the life of the group if therapists begin to share their own peer group history.

Supervision: A Necessity for Survival

Adolescents desperately need adult wisdom, guidance, support, and encouragement. However, the need to be autonomous and establish their own identity is so strong that they seem to dismiss adult viewpoints. At times, the group therapists feel isolated, alone, unloved, and rejected. Without supervision, therapists may be blind to the group's metaphorical and nonverbal communication that acknowledges the therapists' caring and wisdom. Even as treatment progresses, adolescents seem egocentric and insensitive to the needs and concerns of adults.

Supervision helps to translate the patients' presence in the group into a statement that they are motivated to change. The adolescents' confrontation is now understood as a need for autonomy, and expressions of hostility now convey a growing trust for others. When group cohesiveness develops, supervision helps the therapists to recognize that the group must also deal with sexual fantasies and intimacy issues. The following case example illustrates how supervision can help the therapist stay with the group process and become aware of countertransference:

Case 2

In one session, several group members confronted the therapists concerning their opinions about illegal drug use. The latter expressed their strong opposition to drug use and were able to control their feelings when several group members promoted the use of drugs. In supervision the therapists had a feeling of hopelessness about the future of some group members. However, the supervisory process gave them the encouragement to remain as the positive and caring parental objects. A few months later, one group member who was adamantly pushing drug use for everyone wrote the following in English class:

It takes a long process of therapy and willpower to break an addiction. But first an addict, just like an alcoholic, must admit there's a problem. There's the common addict's line "I can stop any time I want."

It sounds easy, but is it? I think a good question for someone currently on drugs is "Can I really stop?" If so "I dare you!!!" Another question you should ask if you're thinking about taking drugs is— "Do you want to find out how hard it is to stop?"

Termination

As the group develops cohesiveness, communication is more direct, open, and constructive, and the denial of group death dominates. Here-and-now issues are handled with less anxiety, and the historical roots of feeling and perceptions dominate the discussions. A focus on "next" is avoided, and termination rituals are not planned to help deal with separation anxiety.

Adolescent patients generally will not be in treatment for more than 10 sessions because of funding realities and the logistics of gaining access to services in a rapidly changing health care system. For this reason, termination issues must be addressed in the beginning and not at the end of treatment.

A discussion of the number of sessions and the ways that members can terminate must be presented early in treatment. During group therapy, unwanteds have learned some social skills but do not have the experience of obtaining membership in prosocial peer groups in adolescent society. They may quietly drift away without attention to the departure and to how group therapy has prepared them for the community.

Dealing with the anxiety of termination and teaching termination rituals must be major goals in all therapy groups. Adolescent patients experience a society that does not often have reunions, and their groups abruptly disband when their purpose has been accomplished.

Planning the termination "party," accompanied by discussions about "next," must be on the agenda in every therapeutic group. The denial of termination occurs as a countertransferential phenomenon that is a topic for discussion in supervision and cotherapist debriefings. For example, when the therapists have succeeded in achieving cohesiveness and harmony, there is awareness of how the group becomes an externalization of their values and beliefs. Dealing with group death may remind the therapists of their own mortality, which is a countertransferential phenomenon that should be discussed in supervision.

It may be easier to deal with termination when the therapists accept that adolescents will internalize the group object and draw on it for life. As termination approaches, therapists find it difficult to accept this and believe they must continue to be present to ensure that treatment is successful. In a few sessions on a hospital unit or outpatient facility, patients are able to incorporate the group object and develop new ways to cope with conflict with others. However, the therapists' feelings of abandonment and lack of control over the treatment planning result in avoidance of the termination issue. Perhaps awareness of the therapists' own termination history and approach to separation from their teenage groups is the first step in recognizing why this issue is frequently avoided. Again, the supervision session can be used to discuss this emotionally charged issue. The here-and-now discussion of the group's denial of its own imminent death and the therapists' termination history will provide a powerful learning experience. During the last session, regression to the choppy conflict stage is common as the discussion focuses on "next" and termination. Confrontations that conceal separation anxiety and sadness will occur. Case 3 illustrates how leaders can respond to denial and model how to say goodbye:

Case 3

In a recent group, the special snack of breakfast tacos furnished by the therapists was the symbolic reminder of the reality that the time together was ending. As the group avoided the topic, the therapists dealt with the termination of their own long relationship. This gave the adolescents a moment to observe two adults who were able to reflect on the past, say goodbye in the present, and cherish their relationship, which built a foundation to meet the new challenges of tomorrow. The cohesiveness and bonds that emerged from this emotional experience enabled the members to internalize the group object, which will help them to become accepted and wanted by others and cope in our uncertain society.

The magnitude of the challenge to help this high-risk population is overwhelming. The change and progress that adolescents demonstrate in group psychotherapy enable the therapists to view life with the caring perspective of the boy in the starfish story:

As an old man walked the beach at dawn, he noticed a boy ahead of him picking up starfish and flinging them into the sea. Finally catching up with the youth, he asked him why he was doing so. The answer was that the stranded starfish would die if left until the morning sun.

"But the beach goes on for miles, and there are millions of starfish," countered the old man. "How can your effort make any difference?"

The boy looked at the starfish in his hands and threw it to safety in the waves. He said, "It makes a difference to this one."

References

Carnegie Council on Adolescent Development: Turning Points: Preparing American Youth for the 21st Century. New York, Carnegie Corporation of New York, 1989

Fried E: Individuation through group psychotherapy. Int J Group Psychother 20:450–459, 1970

Jones JH: The Holmgreen study: group psychotherapy with emotionally disturbed adolescents and changes in interpersonal behaviors (Unpublished M.A. thesis). San Antonio, TX, Trinity University, 1989

Riester A, Zucker R: Adolescents' social structure and drinking behavior. Pers Guid J 47:304–312, 1968

Schamess G: Differential diagnosis and group structure in the outpatient treatment of latency age children, in Child Group Psychotherapy: Future Tense. Edited by Kraft IA, Riester AE. Madison, CT: International Universities Press, 1986, pp 29–68

Scheidlinger S: Experimental group treatment of severely deprived latency-age children. Am J Orthopsychiatry 30:356–368, 1960

Wong N: Fundamental psychoanalytic concepts: past and present understanding of their applicability to group psychotherapy. Int J Group Psychother 33:171–189, 1983

CHAPTER 13

Group Psychotherapy for Elderly Patients

Beryce W. MacLennan, Ph.D.

Problems of the Elderly

People of all ages must make major changes in their lives. They lose their spouse or other intimates, are forced out of jobs, become physically or mentally disabled, or become dependent and terminally ill. However, the problems of the elderly involve special stresses. The elderly need attention that is focused thoughtfully on their particular life circumstance and their particular dilemmas.

The average elderly person over 65 years of age has at least one physical disability. Losses are much more frequent, and there is less time and hope for regeneration. Because loss and reduction of resources and capacities are almost universal aspects of becoming old, the tasks of the elderly are to readjust their lives, to maintain hope, and come to terms with an aging image of themselves in a society that does not value old age as a source of wisdom or authority. Old people do not abandon earlier ways of adjusting to change. Some are wonderful survivors. Some have never been very competent. Others find that old ways of overcoming difficulty and fending off anger, anxiety, and depression are no longer available to them. Persons who have bolstered their self-esteem through success at work, physical prowess, or sexual admiration may find these defenses no longer viable. Some who have depended on parents and spouses for their very identity may now find themselves alone.

In this chapter I explore how group therapy can be useful to the elderly in reorganizing their lives to best advantage, overcoming losses and disabilities, and coming to terms with death. Groups for the elderly range across the spectrum of group therapy: elderly patients may be placed in heterogeneous therapy groups or groups designed exclusively for them. Some are treated in psychodynamic groups; others are treated in cognitive restructuring groups; and still others are treated in supportive groups. The latter may have special foci, such as coping with retirement, bereavement, or alcoholism. Groups also are designed for more infirm patients in community and institutional settings; these groups are focused around activities combined with discussion. Tross and Blum (1988) have undertaken a comprehensive review of the literature.

Deciding on the Appropriate Group

To decide on the most appropriate group for the elderly patient, the therapist needs to take several factors into consideration:

- The patient's self-image
- The age specificity of the presenting problem
- The theoretical focus and group goals
- Practical options

The Patient's Self-Image

Although some old people have truly become "senior citizens" and live in the world of the elderly, other elderly people do not identify themselves as old and still see themselves as part of the regular adult world. Knowing how patients view themselves is crucial for making the decision about where to place them; people who do not see themselves as old prefer to work in mixed therapy groups rather than in groups specifically designed for the old.

Benitez-Benz (1988) regularly works with older patients in her mixed groups and finds that they do very well. Selection for them is similar to that for any other adult patient. However, therapists have to cope with the attitude and expectations of some other patients about older people. For instance, in one group, an attractive, intelligent woman in her early 60s was struggling to separate from her mother, with whom she had had a dependent, contentious, argumentative but all-consuming relationship throughout her life. Even after her mother's death this dialogue continued in her mind. Finally, with the help of the group she was able to break free, look around, and consider other possible relationships. She then found herself joined by the other group members, all much younger then herself, in despair because she had wasted her life, never married, never had children, and could never hope, they thought, at the age of 62 to have any new satisfying relationships. The younger members could not conceive of "an old woman" of 62 being desirable and able to develop an intimate and satisfying relationship with a man. There were no role models in the group to help them. It was left to the therapist to challenge this assumption and to encourage the patient and the other members to explore what was happening to other older people in the world around them and to speculate about what this woman could hope for. The experience was ultimately useful, both for the woman herself and the other group members.

Age Specificity of the Presenting Problem

Older and younger adults do have some different issues. Because those over 60 have probably lived at least two-thirds of their lives, the past may be more significant to them than the future. Becoming independent is a major issue for the young. Combating increased dependence is a concern for the elderly. Developing a career and advancement are likely to be important for the younger adult, whereas older people may have already given up the world of work. Many younger adults are very concerned with childrearing, whereas older people are more concerned about their adult children or their even more aged relatives.

In a study of groups composed of old and young members, Lakin (1988) found significant differences between the groups in how they related to the leader and their attitude toward the group. In particular, the older group members related more to the leader and relied more on him for leadership, whereas the young group members took more initiative. The elderly were also more likely to be supportive and reassuring.

Cohorts of elderly patients differ from each other. Older cohorts have more women, and the older the women are, the more likely they are to have been full-time mothers and wives for a considerable part of their lives. Fewer older women will have had careers or will drink or smoke, and more will have religious backgrounds and affiliations.

Theoretical Focus and Group Goals

Three categories of groups are available to the elderly: psychodynamic group therapy, cognitive-behavioral group therapy, and supportive group therapy.

Psychodynamic group therapy.   When the choice is made in favor of insight therapy, some therapists have formed traditional psychodynamic groups for the elderly. Because of the narcissistic injuries accompanying old age, self psychology groups have been considered particularly useful in treating the elderly (Lothstein and Zimet 1988; Weiner and White 1988). The therapist aims to develop a supportive group climate that serves as a warm, accepting family, with the therapist as a loving parent. The group members deal with the narcissistic injuries and relationship problems that have been present throughout life and rework these issues within the context of current problems.

Weiner and White (1988) wrote that the analyst becomes a selfobject for the patient through two types of transference, one mirroring and the other idealizing. They stated, "In the mirroring transference the patient maintains self cohesion through the mirroring of his/her archaic omnipotent wishful self, while in the idealizing transference it is maintained through merger with the analyst as an idealized parent image." They described a group in which the members presented with different problems, all of which affected their perception of themselves and their object relationships. Lothstein and Zimet (1988) described a similar group in which one woman experienced the death of her mother, who was her sole object. Another had to retire and lose her social world. One male patient felt a sense of emptiness because his wife had developed a special friendship with another woman and his children had moved away. Phyllis, the woman whose mother had died, believed she could never love again but began to feel differently about herself as group members accepted and admired her. Harry and Phyllis developed a "twinship" relationship. Their pairing and mutual admiration were helpful to both in repairing their damaged self-esteem.

Cognitive-behavioral groups.   In addition to psychodynamic group therapy, other models have proven to be successful with this population. In recent times, cognitive-behavioral techniques, developed by Beck and Rush (1978), have been adapted for the treatment of depression in the elderly. Cognitive-behavioral therapy tackles the distortions of thinking that underlie the behaviors and helps the patients recognize that they are creating their depression and can overcome it. This form of treatment adapts well to groups in that patients help each other recognize their distortions and work out ways to deal with them through task assignments, role-playing, and assertiveness training.

A recent development emerging from health psychology has been the formation of life-style enhancement and habit control groups for the elderly, aimed to ward off chronic illness and maintain health. These groups deal with diet control focused on calorie control and low-fat and low-cholesterol diets or on compliance with specific diets such as for late-onset diabetes. They also encourage the maintenance of a moderate regimen of exercise, sufficient sleep, socialization, and stress management and the minimal use of alcohol and tobacco. The importance of finding ways to obtain life satisfaction and to avoid situations that will provoke relapses are also emphasized. Most such groups for the elderly have been age specific.

Support groups.   Support groups for the elderly are often symptom focused and short term. They are formed to deal with acute mental breakdown or special life crises such as bereavement and retirement. These groups may be organized as closed, time-limited groups, in that the selected members are invited to commit themselves for a limited number of sessions and after the second or third meeting no new members are admitted. However, other groups that are short term for the individual members are, in fact, conducted long term as open-ended groups. Some examples of such groups are in-hospital groups for short-stay acute psychogeriatric patients or older patients who are recuperating from a heart attack (Weiner 1988). Sometimes bereavement groups are conducted as open-ended groups, and the members gain courage from other persons who have already resolved the worst of their grief and are beginning to remake their lives successfully.

Groups in institutional settings with more disabled patients very frequently start out as short-term activity and discussion groups without any rigorous selection of members. In these groups, there may be a second stage in which the members are more carefully selected, and a short-term activity group may be converted into a long-term, closed psychotherapy or mutually supportive group with the agreement of the members.

Even problem-specific groups that are short term take on a different character for the elderly. Elderly bereaved individuals do not have to cope with the same practical problems during bereavement that younger individuals have, nor do they have quite the same options, even though the grief work is similar. Late-onset alcoholism may take on a different character, and retirement is not usually an option for the young. Most individuals in long-term-care settings are elderly, so the age of a group may be predetermined.

Practical Considerations

Sometimes the choice is a pragmatic one. There may be no groups exclusively for the elderly. However, when a choice is available, the decision is generally based on the focus of the group and the attitude of the older person.

Examples of Special Focus Groups

Many supportive groups, particularly those for the active elderly, are focused around specific life crises or problems such as retirement, remaking their lives after 60, bereavement, or the management of depression or substance abuse. In this chapter, I describe retirement and bereavement groups and groups for the elderly who have problems with alcohol. These three types of groups illustrate most of the dilemmas associated with treating the elderly in group therapy.

Group Psychotherapy After Retirement

A National Institute of Mental Health study of retirement (Sheldon et al. 1975) identified five factors as potentially problematic for individuals after retirement: loss of function, loss of self-esteem, loss of role, loss of colleagues, and a change in the balance of the relationship between couples living together. In spite of their anticipation of freedom from obligation and routine, some people miss the structure of going to work every day and of completing assigned tasks. Many retirees begin to feel worthless and useless after they give up their life's work. Their self-esteem and sense of status were bound up in their work, and they no longer know exactly who they are. In their work, they occupied a particular position, and at home they may well have been the chief breadwinner. Both of these roles may be eliminated after retirement. Others find that their social life and friendships were bound up in their work and that after retirement they are excluded. They no longer have common interests, and they become lonely and depressed. Still others are suddenly forced into early retirement by ill health or are edged out by younger employees and suffer both narcissistic and financial damage. Some grieve for the competencies they are no longer allowed to exercise and for a sense of achievement they will never experience again. Some people find that they not only have work loss but also losses from developing disabilities, reduced sight or hearing, arthritic pain, and impaired mobility, all of which add to their anxiety and depression.

Many programs are conducted today to prepare those who are nearing retirement. These programs generally deal not only with the psychological elements of retirement but also with the financial, social, recreational, and health care aspects. However, many retirees are not able to deal with their losses in an anticipatory way and do so only after they are retired. Short-term groups have been developed for them in areas where there are many retirees. Salvendy (1989), for instance, described 12-week groups for those who had been retired for a short time and were experiencing difficulties. These were held at the Retirement Clinic, Toronto Psychiatric Hospital, Toronto, Canada, and were led by a male and a female therapist team. Those selected were interested in working out their psychological problems and were not psychotic, uncontrollably alcoholic, or severely clinically depressed or confused. The therapists encouraged the members to feel hopeful about the future and to examine their problems and options realistically. Salvendy cited examples of pessimistic distortions that were challenged by the group; these included a man who thought that everyone looked down on him because his bank manager no longer spent as much time with him as before; another member was reminded that his excellent negotiating skills, no longer used at work, proved useful in the group.

The aims of such groups are to help the members view themselves realistically and to consider how they wish to spend the next period of their lives. How do they want to occupy their time? How will they remake their social life? How can they develop new roles for themselves? How can they have fun?

A major problem for many who retire is how they will relate to their spouse. A common situation in times past has been the husband who retires and tries to take over and reorganize the wife, who has stayed home all her life. Today, a second situation frequently occurs: one spouse is still at the height of his or her career while the other is ready to retire. The ways in which they want to spend their time are very different. For instance, one university professor retired and felt very depressed because he was no longer able to do research or teach. His wife was a very busy member of a consulting firm and often worked long hours and on weekends. He wanted her around to do things with him, and also he wanted her to give up her work and travel with him, which she was not willing to do. The couple attended several weekend group meetings for recently retired couples who were encountering similar problems. As a result, they reaffirmed their love for each other and made some compromises. He managed to develop some interesting volunteer and paid projects, whereas she modified her schedule so that they were able to spend more time together and do some of the travelling that he wanted. In the group there were many identifications across couples and exclamations of "I understand, I feel just like you do." They realized that their problems were not unique but were an inevitable part of adjusting to retirement in the modern world. If they wanted to stay together, they had to work out a life-style that was acceptable to both.

Bereavement Groups for the Widowed

Bereavement groups for the widowed are sometimes open to widowed people of all ages and sometimes only to the elderly. Although the processes of grieving are similar for young, middle-aged, and old people, the life tasks and expectations are different. Young widowed people may have children, and their prospects for remarriage and for careers are greater. Elderly people, who have often been married for many years and who may also have lost a number of their close friends and relatives, can become particularly desolate and distressed by the loss of a spouse. Ginsburg (1987), herself a widow, identified a number of reactions to the loss: initial shock and denial, confusion, emotional release, anger, guilt, depression, and self-isolation and ultimately acceptance of the death, reintegration of the self, and the beginning of making a new life. Not all widowed persons react in the same way or in the same sequence. However, there is a tendency immediately after the death for many widowed people to keep tight control and to operate as if they were conducting "business as usual." They experience an emotional numbing. After the first shock wears off, they begin to feel the pain.

In their demonstration of widow-to-widow programs, Silverman et al. (1974) used widowed persons whom they had trained as outreach workers. They found that after a few weeks family and friends tended to give less support and the widowed were in need of one-to-one and then group support. They ran groups for persons who had been widowed between 6 months and 1 year and who were in the process of working through their grief. These groups were led as mutual support groups by trained widow leaders.

Yalom and Vinogradov (1988) are among the few who described the process of therapy groups they led for widows of spouses who had died of cancer. They worked with 36 spouses in four therapy groups over 8-week periods. The therapists ran these groups as semistructured with interpersonal interaction and some structured exercises. For example, in addressing the theme of identity, they used one of two exercises that explored with the members how they saw themselves. These exercises were centered on the question "Who am I?" Toward the end of each group, they asked members to bring in photographs of their families and spouses.

Other familiar themes surfaced in these groups. Members noted a change in their social status. At first they continued to be invited to their old "couples" society. However, gradually, these invitations fell off. As a woman in a different project noted, "I became a Thursday rather than a Saturday night guest." They found out that if they wanted a social life they must enter the world of "singles." They had to make the adjustment of role and identity from that of a "married person," one of a couple, to that of a "widowed person" on their own. They experienced the urges to remarry and reconstitute the familiar married state; alternatively, they were tempted to give up their home and flee from the environment that they had shared with their spouse. They were encouraged not to make hasty major changes until they had worked through some of their emotional turmoil. Loneliness was a universal theme. Anger at fate and guilt about things they might have done differently were common. Members faced the transitory nature of life and the potential imminence of their own death. They were encouraged to take responsibility for themselves in remaking their lives and rebuilding their futures. Some began to enjoy the freedom of being on their own—the freedom to grow and take on new tasks. The therapists found themselves concentrating on "growth, self knowledge, and existential responsibility." They judged these groups to be successful in that they were cohesive, the members attended regularly, and the meetings dealt with relevant and emotionally charged content.

Horowitz et al. (1984) analyzed published reports of group therapy for the bereaved. In particular they described a study of 52 patients who received brief group psychotherapy. They concluded that highly motivated patients responded better to exploratory therapy, particularly when they had previously been well adjusted, whereas those patients who were poorly motivated and who had previously been less stable were better able to use a more supportive form of intervention. Paradoxically, a criterion for the differential use of mutual support or professionally led therapy groups may be that better-adjusted patients respond better to the latter.

The focus of the interventions can also be related to the stage of bereavement. Lieberman and Videka-Sherman (1986) evaluated self-help groups for widowed and divorced persons (mainly widowed) 3 to 4 years after their loss and found that those groups that fostered active social networking appeared to be most helpful. This confirms the need for individuals at this stage of recovery to actively make new roles for themselves and new intimate relationships.

Group Therapy With Elderly Patients Who Have Problems with Alcohol

The exact numbers of elderly people who have problems with alcohol are not known, but evidence has begun to surface. Researchers and clinicians such as Wood and Elias (1982) and Rathbone-McCuan (1988) clustered the elderly into early-onset and late-onset alcoholics. Early-onset alcoholics are individuals who have had problems with alcoholism throughout their lives. They are the survivors of the general population of alcoholics who neither have been able to give up alcohol nor have died from it. These elderly people range from public inebriates who are living in deteriorated and sometimes homeless conditions to those who occasionally have binges but in between are able to live relatively normal lives and who have developed a way of coping with their addiction.

Communities have tended to refer early-onset older alcoholic people to structured 12-step group programs and then to social service agencies for help with their multiple problems of living.

Late-onset alcohol problems are both more complex and often more treatable. Rathbone-McCuan (1988) pointed out that it is now known that reactions to alcohol can vary for individuals over their life span, so that some elderly people react more negatively to the same amounts of alcohol as they age. A second subset of elderly people experience dangerous reactions to the combination of alcohol with some of the drugs that many of them have to take for chronic medical problems. A third subset are those elderly people who use alcohol to self-medicate for the problems and pains experienced in aging, such as the many physical and psychosocial losses they experience.

As with other substance abusers, denial of alcohol problems is a major coping mechanism among elderly alcoholics, and it is often necessary to work with family, physicians, and other service providers in order to confront the elderly person and to bring him or her into treatment.

Multiple family groups can be very helpful for those elderly people who fail to recognize their problems. For instance, in one such group (led by myself) a family member described how his mother was always falling over and appeared to have slurred speech by the middle of the afternoon.

They had found empty sherry bottles all over her apartment. The mother, a rather prim woman of 78, said that she had a middle-ear problem and this affected her balance so that she often fell down. One of the other elderly women, who also had an alcohol problem, exclaimed, "Oh come on dear, we all know that you start drinking sherry at 10 in the morning and never give up until you pass out. Don't we all know how that bottle gets to us and prevents us from thinking about a lot of unhappy things?" Another elderly woman said, "Aren't you lonely living in that house by yourself knowing no one in the neighborhood?" The mother replied that she wished her son and daughter-in-law would come and see her more often. One of the men in the group exclaimed, "You can't expect to have your children take care of all your needs. They have their own life to live. Why don't you move somewhere where you can have some companionship of people your own age?" Although she was not required to admit to her alcohol problem at this point, her problem was tacitly recognized in the group and the members began to help her confront some of her needs that were leading her to drink. She eventually moved into a graduated health care setting where she could have her own apartment and still live independently but where there was both companionship and a 24-hour emergency health care system.

Some widowed individuals take to drinking excessively after their spouse dies. The first need is for help in getting sober. They can then often enter a regular bereavement group to deal with their grief while attending alcohol education and Alcoholics Anonymous groups for their alcoholism. Some of those who use alcohol to cope with psychological problems, such as loneliness or grief, may well be able to return to controlled drinking because they do not have true physiological craving for alcohol.

Many elderly people who are retired start the habit of attending "happy hours" in the late afternoon and do not recognize that they can no longer drink even two or three drinks as they had done in the past. Some of these elderly people drive home after drinking and get into alcohol-related accidents. Alcohol education groups dealing with the adverse effects of alcohol on the aging brain and some planning about other ways to socialize can often take care of the problem. Rathbone-McCuan (1988) emphasized that whatever the nature of the problem and the form of treatment, "it is essential that an emphasis on conscious material be maintained" (p. 145). This thinking is based on the assumption that arousing affect-laden unconscious material frequently may set off further drinking bouts as a defense against painful feelings.

Group Therapy in Institutions

Therapists who work with the frail elderly must reach out to wherever they are to be found: in mental hospitals, retirement homes, nursing homes, day treatment programs, or acute-care psychiatric units in general hospitals. Most groups for this population are supportive and often combine activity and discussion; some use reminiscence (Poulton and Strasberg 1986) or remotivation therapy (Dennis 1978).

In retirement homes and nursing homes, consultants from outside the home may be brought in to lead the groups. When this occurs, it is important that the consultants build good relationships with the staff and make sure that the latter understand what is being planned.

In teaching hospitals, turnover of student leaders, particularly residents who stay only a few months at a time, may create some difficulty in maintaining the continuity of the group. To some extent this can be ameliorated by the use of a permanent staff member as the primary therapist. More importantly, age contrasts can be very painful; the young trainees are forever going off to happier options, leaving the elderly to note the contrast this presents to their own lives.

Reintegration Groups

Elderly patients who have been in a hospital or nursing home for a long time may need special retraining to be able to return to a less-confined setting.

As part of a deinstitutionalization program, staff at the Ypsilanti State Hospital in Michigan developed a program for very regressed elderly mental patients who had lived for 15 or more years in a back ward in the hospital. They created a concentrated program, using different kinds of group activities for rehabilitative purposes. Members played name games to revive their sense of identity, for many were so disoriented that they did not know who or where they were. They had to relearn the skills necessary for self-care, such as tying shoe laces and dressing themselves. They learned to do exercises, to dance, and to sing. As they progressed, the group went on trips to relearn what life was like outside the hospital and to reacquire skills such as how to use buses, shop, and manage their money. A film of this program, called *To Live With Dignity* (Ypsilanti State Hospital 1974), shows how several of the patients were able to make remarkable progress over a 3-month period. The film culminates with a

Christmas party organized by the patients. Although the program was conceived and directed by a mental health professional, many of the group leaders were ward staff trained in group management.

Bienenfeld (1988) described group therapy with geriatric patients in a state hospital. These patients were less regressed than the Ypsilanti patients, although they also might have lived for a number of years at the hospital. Unlike the Ypsilanti program, Bienenfeld excluded patients who "have an organic incapacity to understand or participate, who are unmanageably disruptive and who are unworkably lacking in motivation" (p. 179). Like Linden (1954), who was a pioneer in working with institutionalized elderly patients, Bienenfeld worked with a female cotherapist and found a partner useful in clarifying and refining interventions. The goals for these groups included promoting discharge and diminishing management difficulties. As in all institutional settings, problems of personal autonomy and responsibility, power, and authority were found as themes in his groups. Reality was clarified in the group, and the patients were better able to make their own decisions.

Goodman (1988) formed groups for elderly patients in a psychiatric program in a teaching hospital when she found that the small number of elderly patients, about 19%, were complaining that they felt out of place and had no one to talk to among the many young acutely ill patients. Goodman, a social worker, ran the groups variously with a psychiatric nurse and with an occupational therapist experienced in leading activity groups. Many of these patients were very depressed, and activities were helpful in stimulating interaction.

Activity Groups in Nursing and Boarding Homes

In visiting large boarding homes, intermediate-care facilities, and nursing homes for the elderly, one is frequently confronted with numbers of residents lining the walls, staring into space, apparently uninterested in anyone. They often do not know the names of other residents in the house, even if they have lived alongside them for several years. Sometimes they have lost count of time and may no longer know their own age or even their names. Several authors (e.g., Johnson 1985) have described the use of activities and the arts to prevent such deterioration. For example, Stern (1988) worked with the residents in developing improvisational drama. In one group she had the members imagine that they were an acting troupe preparing for their tour. They each had to say their name and state an object that they would take with them; the next person repeated what had been said before and added their name and object, and so on. It was challenging, fun, and helped stimulate their memories and get them to know each other better.

Morrin (1988) sometimes combined art and music therapy and had her group members paint associations to the music. Sometimes the art led to very personal discussions, as when one member tried to draw a picture of her son, her favorite child, and others talked also about their favorites. This, in turn, led them to their husbands and to their feelings about their losses.

Losses are continuous. Some patients die; others become severely physically ill and must be moved elsewhere. Staff may leave or transfer to another unit. Bienenfeld (1988) maintained that it is most useful to recognize the ubiquity of these losses and to help the patients with their mixed feelings about the losses, their feelings about making any commitment to others, and their fears of their own vulnerability. Shura Saul (1988) helped her patients in a nursing home group grieve through poetry. Sidney Saul (1983) described how the elderly talk of death.

Groups for Alzheimer's and Other Confused Patients

Many elderly patients in long-term-care settings suffer from temporary or progressive confusion. Sidney Saul (1988), working in nursing homes and day treatment settings, ran groups for such patients, either alone or in conjunction with families and other caregivers. He found that working with these patients in groups led to improved socialization among members, modification of dysfunctional behavior, and reduction of depression. The groups were also used to help the families clarify the problems they were having in caring for their spouse or parent and to find acceptable solutions.

In one group, a wife reported that her husband refused to allow her to bathe him. Another patient suggested that the husband did not recognize his wife anymore and was embarrassed at having a strange woman care for him so intimately. She decided to hire a male aide to bathe him and this problem was solved. In another session, the therapists brought two mangos to the group, and the members spent time working out what kind of fruit they were and afterwards sharing them. Saul believed that fun, humor, and laughter are very important in lightening the spirits of confused patients.

Role of the Leader

The particular tensions facing the leader of groups composed of elderly patients emerge from a number of factors:

- Age bias and the limitations of empathy
- Maintaining hope
- Countertransference related to unresolved conflicts with their own parents
- Fear of their own aging

Taken as a group, these factors generate tension in the clinician, who is probably considerably younger than the patients being treated in the group. An age difference of 20 or more years may stretch the empathic limits of even the most dedicated clinician. How does he or she enter into the internal experience of a patient who has lost a job, a spouse, a child, or a critical body function? The capacity to maintain hope beyond such loss is usually hard won and constitutes an important aspect of maturity. Especially for the younger group therapist besieged by the pain of eight or more such patients, perspective may be difficult to maintain.

An additional countertransferential difficulty may present itself in the reemergence of past or present conflicts with the therapist's own parents.

Although the barrage of such feelings may stretch the empathic capacity of the clinician, the benefits to his or her clinical and personal development are impressive. Once the clinician has seen a few apparently hopeless elderly patients emerge with new zest and an array of previously unrecognized options, his or her despair around loss and reconstitution is permanently confronted and reduced—to the benefit of the patients but also as a ray of hope and optimism for one's own inevitable future.

Summary

In this chapter I have examined a range of groups that have been found to be useful in helping the aged face their problems, improve their functioning, and feel happier about themselves. Just as the elderly are a varied population with many different needs, so do the groups vary from support to insight, use activities or discussion, and take place in many different settings, wherever the elderly are to be found. Although some groups have a general orientation, many deal with special issues such as retirement, bereavement, and alcoholism. Common themes that run through these groups are the ubiquity of loss, the acceptance of death, and the value of humor in lightening the mood of the elderly. Finally, the healing power of human communities is clearly seen throughout the life span, and it generates hope while life lasts.

References

Beck AT, Rush AJ: Cognitive approaches to depression and suicide, in Cognitive Deficits in the Development of Mental Illness. Edited by Serban C. New York, Brunner/Mazel, 1978, pp 235–258

Benitez-Benz R: Including the active elderly in group psychotherapy, in Group Psychotherapies for the Elderly. Edited by MacLennan BW, Saul S, Weiner MB. Madison, CT, International Universities Press, 1988, pp 33–42

Bienenfeld D: Group psychotherapy with the elderly in the state hospital, in Group Psychotherapies for the Elderly. Edited by MacLennan BW, Saul S, Weiner MB. Madison, CT, International Universities Press, 1988, pp 77–166

Dennis H: Remotivation therapy, in Working with the Elderly. Edited by Burnside IM. New York, Duxbury, 1978, p. 219

Ginsburg GD: To Live Again: Rebuilding Your Life After You've Become a Widow. Los Angeles, CA, Tarcher, 1987

Goodman RK: A geriatric group in an acute care psychiatric teaching hospital: pride and prejudice, in Group Psychotherapies for the Elderly. Edited by MacLennan BW, Saul S, Weiner MB. Madison, CT, International Universities Press, 1988, pp 151–164

Horowitz MJ, Marmar C, Weiss D, et al: Brief psychotherapy of bereavement reactions. Arch Gen Psychiatry 41:438–448, 1984

Johnson DR: Expressive group psychotherapy with the elderly: a drama approach. Int J Group Psychother 35:109–128, 1985

Lakin M: Group therapies with the elderly: issues and prospects, in Group Psychotherapies for the Elderly. Edited by MacLennan BW, Saul S, Weiner MB. Madison, CT, International Universities Press, 1988, pp 43–56

Lieberman MA, Videka-Sherman L: The impact of self help groups on the mental health of widows. Am J Orthopsychiatry 561:435–449, 1986

Linden ME: The significance of dual leadership in gerontologic groups. Int J Group Psychother 4:262–273, 1954

Lothstein L, Zimet G: Twinship and alterego selfobject transferences in group therapy with the elderly. Int J Group Psychother 38:303–318, 1988

Morrin J: Art therapy groups in a geriatric institutional setting, in Group Psychotherapies for the Elderly. Edited by MacLennan BW, Saul S, Weiner MB. Madison, CT, International Universities Press, 1988, pp 245–256

Poulton JL, Strasberg DS: The therapeutic use of reminiscence. Int J Group Psychother 36:381–398, 1986

Rathbone-McCuan E: Group intervention for alcohol-related problems among the elderly and their families, in Group Psychotherapies for the Elderly. Edited by MacLennan BW, Saul S, Weiner MB. Madison, CT, International Universities Press, 1988, pp 139–150

Salvendy J: Brief group psychotherapy at retirement. Group 13:43–57, 1989

Saul, Shura: The arts as psychotherapeutic modalities with groups of older people, in Group Psychotherapies for the Elderly. Edited by MacLennan BW, Saul S, Weiner MB. Madison, CT, International Universities Press, 1988, pp 211–222

Saul, Sidney: Old people talk about death, in Aging: An Album of People Growing Old. Edited by Saul S. New York, Wiley, 1983, pp 61–67

Saul, Sidney: Group therapy with confused and demented elderly people, in Group Psychotherapies for the Elderly. Edited by MacLennan BW, Saul S, Weiner MB. Madison, CT, International Universities Press, 1988, pp 199–221

Sheldon S, McEwan PJM, Ryser CP: Retirement: Patterns and Predictions. Rockville, MD, National Institute of Mental Health, 1975

Silverman P, Mackenzie D, Peltipas M, et al: Helping Each Other in Widowhood. New York, Health Sciences, 1974

Stern R: Drama gerontology, in Group Psychotherapies for the Elderly. Edited by MacLennan BW, Saul S, Weiner MB. Madison, CT, International Universities Press, 1988, pp 257–268

Tross S, Blum JE: A review of group therapy with the older adult: practice and research, in Group Psychotherapies for the Elderly. Edited by MacLennan BW, Saul S, Weiner MB. Madison, CT, International Universities Press, 1988, pp 3–32

Weiner W: Groups for the terminally ill cardiac patient, in Group Psychotherapies for the Elderly. Edited by MacLennan BW, Saul S, Weiner MB. Madison, CT, International Universities Press, 1988, pp 165–176

Weiner MB, White MT: The third chance, in Group Psychotherapies for the Elderly. Edited by MacLennan BW, Saul S, Weiner MB. Madison, CT, International Universities Press, 1988, pp 57–61

Wood WG, Elias M (eds): Alcoholism and Aging: Advances in Research. Boca Raton, FL, CRC Press, 1982

Yalom ID, Vinogradov S: Bereavement groups: techniques and themes. Int J Group Psychother 38:416–436, 1988

Ypsilanti State Hospital: To Live With Dignity (videotape). Ann Arbor, MI, Ann Arbor Audio-Visual Center, 1974

CHAPTER 14

Group Psychotherapy With HIV-Positive and AIDS Patients

Joel C. Frost, Ed.D.

Introduction

Acquired immunodeficiency syndrome (AIDS) was first described by the Centers for Disease Control (CDC) in 1981 (1981a, 1981b). Human immunodeficiency virus (HIV) is the retrovirus that causes AIDS. The growing body of both clinical and lay material provides additional information about both the disease and its victims. (For an introduction, see Batchelor 1984, Backer et al. 1988, and Simon 1988, as well as E. K. Nichols 1986, Barrows and Halgin 1988, Kelly and St. Lawrence 1988, Ostrow 1990, and Morrison 1989.) Many clinicians have not yet had the experience within their general practice of working with people with AIDS or people who are HIV positive. Even fewer clinicians have worked with these patients within their therapy groups. The complexity of AIDS and the issues specific to this disease present many problems for group members, as well as for group therapists. This chapter addresses the rationale for treating AIDS patients in groups.

The first populations affected by the virus in the United States were predominantly gay men and intravenous drug abusers. Therefore, AIDS has been colored by a moral stigma because of the early associations with these minority target groups in general and with sexual and intravenous drug use behaviors in particular. People do not react to AIDS as just another disease. Knowledge about both the stigma and the beliefs surrounding AIDS is important for clinical management, as well as for an empathic understanding of the people infected and those around them, including other group members. (For a review of the psychosocial experiences of people with AIDS, see Chimiel et al. 1987, Forstein 1984, Lùpez and Getzel 1984, Morin et al. 1984, and Tross and Hirsch 1988).

Because ignorance about AIDS transmission persists, people with AIDS often feel unsafe when others are able to perceive that they have AIDS (e.g., when people know their diagnosis or can see a Kaposi sarcoma [KS] lesion visible on their exposed skin). Their fear of public exposure affects both their sense of safety and anonymity and their sense of their health (Lander 1989). Consistent with the impact of stigma, people with AIDS have been blamed and scapegoated by many people for contracting the disease. Many even blame themselves, wondering about having done anything that would warrant such a disease. At the time of diagnosis, many people with AIDS report losing their lovers, friends, families, co-workers, jobs, and homes. There is an ever-present aura of shame and lowered self-esteem that results in isolation and is particularly appropriate for group interventions.

Disease Stages

HIV-positive people pass through three phases. The first occurs at diagnosis. The second is a relatively healthy phase, and the third is the phase of chronic illness. On diagnosis, many people initially feel confused, frightened, out of control, and suicidal. Early clinical intervention often follows a crisis intervention model. Groups particularly help alleviate the stigma and psychosocial complications. Initial clinical intervention with someone who learns he or she is HIV positive is aimed at stabilizing the person emotionally, focusing on risk reduction for the person and others, and helping the person build a supportive network that will sustain him or her throughout the course of the illness (Grant 1988; Kelly and St. Lawrence 1988; Lenihan 1985; Newmark 1985).

Although the initial phase is often short lived, the second phase can last for years. It is a time when the person lives with all of his or her personality conflicts from before diagnosis, as well as with the problems that surface because of the diagnosis. During this second phase, long-term psychotherapy groups can be very helpful. The third phase, that of chronic illness, is a complex period that can last for a relatively long time. It can also be seen as the end stage of the disease, and therefore of the person's life. This last phase requires special attention and management. It is this third phase that raises the most concerns about whether to mainstream AIDS patients into heterogeneous therapy groups or to segregate them into homogeneous AIDS therapy groups.

Types of Groups

Crisis management groups (psychoeducational or activity groups), support groups, and psychotherapy groups are appropriate for people with AIDS. In practice, the distinctions among these groups are not always clear, and there can be some shifting back and forth among the models. Crisis management groups are often run like support groups, but they are time limited and generally only include people who have recently been diagnosed as HIV-positive. The format is structured and psychoeducational (e.g., 12 weeks, with a set topic for each week that includes teaching and discussion sections). Topics generally include safer sexual practices, stress management, reality testing about AIDS, suicide management, risk reduction, and network building (Kelly and St. Lawrence 1988).

Activity groups allow a newly diagnosed person to interact with other people with AIDS in a minimally threatening way. This type of intervention is helpful as the individual gets over the initial shock of the diagnosis and begins to employ denial (S. E. Nichols 1984).

Crisis management often means helping the patient understand his or her anxiety, focus his or her attention on coping skills, develop a support structure, manage suicidal thoughts, and put himself or herself back into a position of control. After the patient is stabilized, he or she is often referred to a support group for long-term needs. In large urban cities, there is often a network of crisis groups and support groups for people with AIDS. The idea of including people with AIDS in therapy groups is somewhat new, although as people who are HIV positive or who have AIDS live longer, the idea of a long-term therapy group is becoming more viable.

Support groups and therapy groups differ with regard to the role of the leader, contract of the group, and group goals. Each of these three categories is addressed separately.

Role of the Leader

The demand on the leader in an AIDS support group is to be active and directive in giving advice and in role-modeling; to be highly involved and yet noninterpretive; and to contain, redirect, and build defenses around affect. Intrapsychic exploration is kept to a minimum. The leader is often called on to provide medical knowledge about AIDS and various treatments; therefore, at times it is recommended that either the leader or one of the coleaders be a physician (Beckett and Rutan 1990). It is also recommended that the leader work with a coleader for mutual support (Child and Getzel 1990).

In a support group the leader works to contain regression rather than to foster it, as would occur in a therapy group. In a support group the leader is often asked to take an active stand and directly give advice and prohibitions, in contrast to the neutral stance of the leader of a therapy group. Not unlike members of any therapy group, people with AIDS often have very high expectations of the group leader. The following case example illustrates both the poignancy and the scope of the expectations that people with AIDS can hold for the therapist:

Case 1

On the initial interview, Mr. A, who had been diagnosed as having AIDS 3.5 years before, said that his goal for the therapy was to make it be 1975 again so that he could take away the disease. His denial was beginning to break down as his body began to be covered by KS lesions. Hope had begun to fail, and he actively needed the therapist to bring either new or more powerful hope to bear. The therapist wanted very much to be able to do this for Mr. A. Mr. A said in a half-joking way: "Please make it 1975 again, please make all this go away, I want to go back to the spontaneity and joy that I had back then." His wish was to be put into a group comprising long-term survivors. The therapist felt that hidden in this request was a wish on Mr. A's part to find a way to compound the "magic" that was keeping them alive separately.

This set of expectations can have a profound impact on the therapist, who often brings to his or her work an unconscious wish to be all-powerful and all-healing. In psychotherapy, the therapist attempts to analyze and break through denial to help patients live happier and more productive lives. With people who have AIDS, the therapist may experience the breaking down of denial as a process of encouraging the patient to give up hope and face death. The bind is that hope is often all that a person with AIDS has to keep going. This hope can take on a magical quality, with blind faith in the omnipotence of the therapist. The pull is for the therapist to imagine that he or she can and must fulfill this wish.

Renneker (1957) found that health care workers whose specialty was cancer patients suffered from their experiences with these dying patients. The deaths were experienced as treatment failures and blows to the workers' unconscious narcissistic and omnipotence needs. Their loss of hope was also felt as "injurious" to the cancer patient. Having believed in their own omnipotence, the health care workers had unconsciously "promised" to cure the patient.

The Role of Hope

The maintenance of hope is critical and raises many transference and countertransference dilemmas within clinical work. People with AIDS are predominantly young people who are developmentally closer in age to the time of total dependency on their parents. Thus the transference pull is for the therapist to be the omnipotent, omnipresent parental figure, the remembered and idealized "fantasy mother," who will make everything well again. The countertransference pull for the therapist who has gone into health care to "cure disease and illness" is to fulfill that wish. The therapist's own wish is often to live up to the AIDS patients' intense set of expectations that the therapist will be the all-powerful and magical parental figure who will take care of them, make this disease go away, and make them live.

In addition to hope, people with AIDS often feel that their attitude has a direct effect on their health and longevity. HIV-positive patients do not all follow the same course of illness; some live years longer than others. This fact can result in a conscious belief that attitude and feelings are determining factors in the patient's allotted amount of life.

This set of expectations pulls for the group therapist to be very active and openly encouraging, which may be one of the reasons that clinicians often use behavioral, cognitive, and guided imagery approaches. The support group contract allows for and encourages acting on one's feelings within the group session (promoting hugging and touching) or outside of the group (dinner dates, supportive telephone calls, or visits to the hospital to see sick group members). The focus is here and now, with active problem-solving and sharing of experiences. Indeed, recent research reported that support groups prolong the life expectancy of cancer patients by encouraging the group members to take a more active role in their medical treatment. (See Chapter 10 in this volume.)

The role of a leader in a support group for people with AIDS can be very different from that in a psychotherapy group. The position calls for a proactive stance and may involve active community and agency outreach and intervention into health care systems and funding agencies

(Child and Getzel 1990; Rounds et al. 1991). Childs and Getzel (1990) went so far as to list one of the four functions of the leader as follows: "They are members of the group, expressing their own emotional response and becoming involved in the supporting process, thereby lessening the patient's fear of the medical or social work institution and lessening the patient's sense of stigmatization" (p. 79). This stance may feel too exposing for group therapists who generally work at a greater objective distance from their patients.

It is important for the leader to have some conceptual framework for group work with people with AIDS, so that he or she can be realistic in his or her efforts. Spector and Conklin (1987) found Weisman's psychosocial stages of dying (1980) useful for this work. Getzel (Getzel 1991; Getzel and Mahoney 1990) found it helpful, for both therapist and patient, to focus on the existential needs of people with AIDS. Therapists need to be aware of what they are doing and why this can help as they continuously struggle with how close and distant and how self-revealing and withholding they should be with the group. A withholding stance on the part of the therapist can lead to the empowering of an individual or group. However, group members who feel their death to be imminent may feel disempowered by a withholding stance.

The Group Contract

The contract in an AIDS support group calls for the leader to encourage and foster connections among members both inside and outside the group. The focus is on active problem solving and network building that extends beyond the group. In contrast, the leader of a therapy group tries to foster the connections within the group, with a contract that often asks members not to have, or to limit, outside group contact (Rutan and Stone 1984; Yalom 1975). The duration of the support group contract is usually short, ranging from 12–15 weeks. Some groups allow for self-renewing commitments. This feature can allow members to move from a short-term commitment to a long-term commitment if feasible.

There is also often a provision in the contract that the therapist may choose to move a member to a different group as his or her medical or clinical condition changes. For example, a patient's ability to participate in the group may change due to AIDS dementia (Buckingham and Van Gorp 1988) or severe medical illness. The decision to move a person with

AIDS to another group as his or her medical condition deteriorates is often based on two premises: 1) his or her condition may make management in the group more demanding (as with AIDS dementia) and 2) as a person with AIDS gets more ill, medically healthier group members with AIDS may begin to lose hope as their denial is broken down. The counter approach is that when intergroup connections are made, they should not be broken. One person with AIDS remarked: "And in God's love, if you drop me when I'm like that, I'll kill you all because if I think you're all I got now, you'll really be all that I got then" (Child and Getzel 1990, p. 72). This issue of group membership is a complex one, and it is not easily resolved. It may well depend on how much the therapist feels that he or she can tolerate.

Because the role of the therapist and the contract of a therapy group are very different from those of a support group, discord can be experienced by HIV-positive persons or people with AIDS who simultaneously participate in both modalities. The following case example illustrates how difficult it can be for a person with AIDS to balance the styles of two therapists working in very different modalities:

Case 2

Mr. B, an HIV-positive member of a psychotherapy group, talked about how cold and unsupportive he felt the group leader to be. The leader was not active the way his support group leader was; he also forbade Mr. B to touch other members or to call them outside the group. Mr. B had always relied on physical contact, especially sex, for making contact with other men. Without this he felt very alone. He had a difficult time understanding why having to sit with these feelings was good for him; it certainly did not feel good. He saw it as a punishment. The group therapist struggled with how to make interpretations that would be helpful to Mr. B, while he was aware of his own thoughts that this man's inability not to touch had played a role in his having contracted the AIDS virus. The therapist was also aware of wanting to "protect" the other group members from Mr. B. The therapist had to remind himself of the patient's psychopathology, separate from his seropositivity.

Group Goals

The goals of an AIDS support group are to help the members feel better, lessen loneliness and isolation through fostering attachments to other group members, reestablish a sense of control in members' lives, bolster their sense of self-esteem, and develop and foster hope. The goal of group patients is ultimately to feel better, but the HIV-positive patient's ability to wait for this is limited. The person with AIDS often experiences difficulty with delay of gratification, whereas some non-HIV-positive group members can wait, as their future seems limitless. HIV-positive patients differ in that they often have limited goals for therapy, not unlimited goals like non-HIV-positive group members. The heterogeneous group may benefit by the inclusion of an HIV-positive group member when the reality sets in that any of us could die tomorrow. The non-HIV-positive group member's resistance to change that is aided by the sense of living forever may be punctured. Appreciation of this need for denial may help us to anticipate and better understand the non-HIV-positive group members' resistance to the inclusion of such patients. Limitless time and hope often go together, as do limitless time and resistance.

Hope is a critical variable with people who have AIDS, as this is still considered a fatal disease, with no cure as yet. We too must maintain the hope that our supportive interventions do make a difference in the quality and duration of the lives of these people. Indeed, some research with cancer patients reaffirms this hope (Spiegel et al. 1989). Perhaps some denial is healthy, so that relatively healthy people with AIDS can continue living. Medical personnel and therapists must struggle with how to titrate denial versus facing reality or, in other words, hope versus despair. Caregivers can experience a sense of guilt if they feel they have "taken the patient's hope away."

The Changing Picture of AIDS

Initially, people who become seropositive do not see themselves as living very long. As part of the expected initial reaction, the newly diagnosed person often attempts quickly to change everything in his or her life. This can be understood clinically as relating to feelings of hopelessness (Boris 1976). Once the person is able to slow down and stabilize, the focus shifts to health, safety at work and home, and preparing for death. As more people with AIDS live longer and relatively healthy lives, their needs shift from crisis management and support to more long-term goals. They have to manage their illness status, but they also have to continue to manage the same life issues they struggled with before their diagnosis. Indeed, often it is the task and goal of the therapist to refocus a person with AIDS back toward living rather than dying. Getzel (1991) turned to the insights of Rank (see Menacher 1982): people not only fear death, they fear living as well.

The impact of HIV and AIDS complicates and intensifies emotional reactions of the group leader as well as the group. A dramatic difference exists between a support group's goals of feeling better and of being more actively involved with people and the goals of a psychotherapy group (i.e., the goal of character change). In the latter, members face painful realities such as their sense of aloneness, hopelessness, despair, loss, grief, and mortality. Members are encouraged to dredge up the painful events of their life experiences and present relationships. Regression is promoted. Including a person with AIDS in a therapy group intensifies affects in ways often not anticipated. The directness and intensity of anger and rage, the propensity for blaming and scapegoating the victim, the emergence of homophobia (Weinberg 1972), and the fear of contagion often blind-side the leader.

The therapist's capacity to manage his or her homophobia and to find a gay life-style acceptable, the ability of the group members to accept a gay member, and the stage of development of the gay identity of the patient are all important factors regarding group placement of a gay patient (Frost 1990). Historically, gay men have had negative experiences in mixed groups, and as a result have often sought out gay-affirmative therapy groups and therapists. With greater acceptance of gay life-styles in many areas, clinicians regularly include gay men and lesbians in heterogeneous groups.

As mentioned earlier, the stigma around AIDS raises the level of shame beyond just the shame about being gay. Thus part of the rationale concerning support groups has been that they are a homogeneous and therefore "safe" environment for gay HIV-positive members. Yet many people confront death with new courage to look deeply into the self and restructure their world view. There is strong reason to include these patients in traditional long-term group therapy. With the changing picture of AIDS, more nongay people are being infected. These people are frequently black or Hispanic men and women who do not want to be considered gay and often are not willing to be in the all-gay support groups. Shame also has to do with people surviving on disability or Medicare payments, losing their home, and being unable to work yet having periods of time when they are healthy. When everyone in the group feels ostracized, the group can support a wide diversity of ethnic, sexual orientation, and socioeconomic backgrounds (Child and Getzel 1990). One creative way to offer help in rural areas was to use a telephone group (Rounds et al. 1991).

Impact on Other Group Members

Scapegoating is a problem in psychotherapy groups with members who are seen as significantly different or unacceptable (e.g., lesbians, gays, blacks, Hispanics, blue-collar workers, and intravenous drug abusers), but it is especially salient in the context of AIDS. Adding people with AIDS to an existing group can often create problems.

At a workshop entitled "Group Psychotherapy With Gay Men" held at the 1986 American Group Psychotherapy Association national convention, a group therapist talked about the difficulty she was having managing her group:

Case 3

> The therapist had brought Mr. C, a patient she knew to be gay, into one of her long-term groups. Mr. C developed AIDS, rapidly became ill, and died. The group was furious at her. They felt that she should have protected them better and that she had no right to expose them to such a horrible experience. Their anger was intense and blaming. The leader felt completely unprepared for such an attack. She wondered whether she had made a mistake.
>
> Indeed, the group had a powerful unconscious reason to be enraged at her; much about the situation was not fair. It was not fair that a young man whom they had begun to like and accept into their lives was so horribly treated by a disease. Mr. C's disfigurement, loss of function, and death at such an early age were all unfair. However, the members responded to the stigma that surrounds AIDS and blamed the leader as the bearer of the disease, rather than the disease itself. She, not AIDS, was seen as the beast. The leader, feeling blamed and unprepared, was unable to redirect the rage toward the disease or to help the group acknowledge the unfairness of life and sit with their sadness and grief at Mr. C's death.

The introduction of an HIV-positive member into an ongoing group greatly raises the anxiety of the other members and breaks through denial that anyone could be at risk. The risk also includes having to face the affects connected to the reality of the disease.

The reality of another member's having progressed to a later stage of illness is a major consideration, because it breaks down the denial of healthier members who are HIV positive or who have AIDS. For this reason, Spector and Conklin (1987) recommended that groups be composed of patients at similar stages of the disease. Beckett and Rutan (1990) cited many reasons why HIV-positive people and people with AIDS should be treated only in homogeneous groups. This issue is not easily resolved, and it may have something to do with whether the group therapists are themselves gay, lesbian, or heterosexual. Beckett and Rutan's experience was based on four homogeneous (all members having AIDS-related complex or AIDS) psychodynamic groups over a 2-year span. The issue of sexual orientation was not mentioned, as was true in Spector and Conklin (1987). The group leader's anxiety around working with these men who were gay and had AIDS-related complex or AIDS was also not addressed.

AIDS is a reality in the gay community, and thus resistance is more easily interpreted (Tavares and Lùpez 1984). The gay community now has had enough years of being surrounded by AIDS so that a heterogeneous group, at least mixed HIV-positive and HIV-negative, is more possible. But AIDS is not an accepted part of heterosexual or ethnic minority communities. Therefore, resistance by heterosexual group members and by heterosexual group therapists may not be so easily understood or addressed. The following case example illustrates how a specific community (primarily heterosexual hemophiliac patients) needed to actively deny and reject the intrusion of the reality of AIDS:

Case 4

Ms. D, a member in a parent's support group at a hemophilia clinic, angrily told the leader that he had made a bad decision to include the parent of an HIV-positive child in the group. She said that when the child got sick and died, the other parents would have no choice but to bond together and reject this parent. The level of the denial that these parents had to live with was too great; they felt unprepared to face the reality that their children with hemophilia could also get ill with AIDS and die. They would have to save themselves by expelling the enemy, here the bearer of the unacceptable reality.

The inability to predict accurately the intensity of the reactions of the other group members can lead to problems within a mixed group, as the following case example illustrates:

Case 5

Another clinician introduced Mr. E, an HIV-positive gay man, into a mixed gay and nongay psychotherapy group. After a few months of hinting, Mr. E announced his HIV status. Mr. F, another gay man, became frightened and overwhelmed with anticipated loss. He angrily demanded to know why Mr. E had not done a better job of protecting himself from AIDS. He said that he was furious that Mr. E was now going to die quickly, although Mr. E tried to point out that he was only HIV-positive and in good health. The other group members were horrified by Mr. F's reaction. They attacked Mr. F, telling him that he should be ashamed of himself. Mr. F became very defensive and humiliated. An impasse developed in which the other group members would not acknowledge their negative feelings toward Mr. E, nor would they forgive Mr. F for his comments. Mr. F could not regain his footing, and left the group 4 weeks later.

In retrospect, the therapist saw that he had not anticipated the intensity of the group reaction, nor had he anticipated the possibility of blaming the victim. He had failed to normalize Mr. F's anger and redirect it toward the disease itself and the anticipated loss. The therapist also knew that Mr. E had a long history both of promiscuity and suicidal intent. Dynamically, Mr. F had been partly correct in his assessment of Mr. E. The group and therapist were caught in a bind of trying not to "blame the victim" and the need to look at Mr. E's unexpressed suicidal intent and his sexual practices.

Special Group Problems
Evoked by People With AIDS

AIDS adds an intensity to the affect experienced within the group and in so doing promotes regression. This regression both allows and forces the reworking of character issues. People who are not normally hostile or bigoted find themselves feeling and saying things that they could not have anticipated. The therapist, an individual group member, or the group as a whole may experience guilt at having survived after the death of an HIV-positive group member. This is especially true when there has been a strong sense of identification with the HIV-positive patient.

The leader must be aware of his or her own history of possible exposure and HIV status, especially if he or she is gay or may otherwise identify with the person with AIDS.

Empathy can be difficult at times as the person with AIDS makes constant internal emotional and physical adjustments to the disease. The leader and other group members are often much slower in their ability to assimilate these adjustments. It is sometimes difficult for people who are not HIV positive to perceive themselves adjusting as quickly or as well to dramatic changes such as wearing diapers, using a cane, vomiting continuously for short periods of time, periodically losing all energy, taking medications at all hours of the day and night, or losing vision. This empathic break can occur as the therapist or group members attempt to adapt while the person with AIDS changes. During this lapse the person with AIDS may feel isolated. This can be especially true if caregivers and group members distance themselves as the person with AIDS nears death.

Suicidality is always present with HIV-positive patients, whether they talk about it or not. Initially after the HIV diagnosis, suicidality often focuses around the sense of crisis, felt lack of control, and inability to predict the future. Later, often after the diagnosis of AIDS is made, the individual may focus on the fear of pain and suffering versus an actual wish to die. Addressing the option of suicide can often help people with AIDS regain a sense of control. When encouraged to talk about their suicidality, people with AIDS need help in differentiating their fears of pain and suffering from a wish to die; most people with AIDS are concerned about the former. Often, in the very last stages of the illness most people with AIDS begin actively to want to die.

Suicidality is obviously not alien to people who are HIV negative. Discussing the matter directly can benefit all group members as they decide how to live life to its fullest. However, the leader may have a fear of suicidality contagion and be concerned for the other patients in the group.

It is difficult for the therapist to balance the HIV-positive patient's need for hope and denial with the therapist's own need to set aside denial in order to help a patient prepare for death. Generally, a therapy group's goal is not to help a member prepare for death, but this may arise in a group with a person who has AIDS. It is critical for the group therapist to make accurate clinical assessments of the needs of the person with AIDS and not act on the inevitable countertransference resistances.

The end stage of AIDS presents an additional problem for therapy groups with a traditional group contract that prohibits out-of-group contact. As a group member with AIDS becomes increasingly incapacitated, his or her ability to attend the group will be seriously compromised. Other group members may want to contact this member or visit him or her at home or in the hospital. After the person with AIDS dies, the group will have to decide whether to attend the wake or funeral together. These issues should be raised and explored. Beckett and Rutan (1990) held the position that leaders should notify each group member immediately on the death of another member.

The numbers of people who are HIV positive are steadily increasing. It is inevitable that more HIV-positive people and people with AIDS will be in heterogeneous therapy groups. Bisexual and closeted men and women within mixed groups often come to terms with or act on their bisexual or gay orientation. Group members with a history of unsafe sexual relations with someone who later comes down with AIDS will become seropositive during the course of the group. Adolescent and college-age men and women often experiment with both sexes as they search out their sexual identities and orientation (Melton 1988). Intravenous drug abusers, their spouses and sexual partners, and people with hemophilia all comprise present or potential group members.

Most of this chapter has been written with gay males in mind. Gay men make up the largest segment of the AIDS population, although there is an increasing shift toward intravenous drug abusers. To date, gay men have been more likely to seek out and use support groups or therapy groups because of class issues, financial ability, familiarity with service systems, and a sense of belonging to a clear community and set of organizations. It is hoped that women, especially poor women of color, will avail themselves of this opportunity to struggle with the agony that cuts across gender, class, or sexual orientation to find healing in the common bond (Cochran and Mays 1989). Groups are by nature empowering vehicles and therefore can play an important role in social change.

References

Backer TE, Batchelor WF, Jones, et al (eds): Special issue: psychology and AIDS. Am Psychol 43:835–987, 1988

Barrows PA, Halgin RP: Current issues in psychotherapy with gay men: impact of the AIDS phenomenon. Professional Psychology: Research and Practice 194:395–402, 1988

Batchelor WF: Psychology in the public forum (editorial). Am Psychol 39:1277–1314, 1984

Beckett A, Rutan JS: Treating persons with ARC and AIDS in group psychotherapy. Int J Group Psychother 40:19–29, 1990

Boris HN: On hope: its nature and psychotherapy. Int Rev Psychoanal 3:139–150, 1976

Buckingham SL, Van Gorp WG: Essential knowledge about AIDS dementia. Social Work 112–115, 1988

Centers for Disease Control: Pneumocystis pneumonia—Los Angeles. MMWR 30:250–252, 1981a

Centers for Disease Control: Kaposi's sarcoma and pneumocystis pneumonia among homosexual men—New York City and California. MMWR 30:305–308, 1981b

Child R, Getzel GS: Group work with inner city persons with AIDS. Social Work with Groups 12:65–80, 1990

Chimiel JS, Detels R, Kaslow RA, et al: Factors associated with prevalent human immunodeficiency virus (HIV) infection in the multicenter AIDS cohort study. Am J Epidemiol 126:568–577, 1987

Cochran SD, Mays VM: Women and AIDS-related concerns. Am Psychol 44:529–535, 1989

Forstein M: The psychosocial impact of the acquired immunodeficiency syndrome. Semin Oncol 11:77–82, 1984

Frost JC: A developmentally keyed scheme for the placement of gay men in psychotherapy groups. Int J Group Psychother 40:155–167, 1990

Getzel GS: Survival modes for people with AIDS in groups. Social Work 36:7–11, 1991

Getzel GS, Mahoney KF: Confronting human finitude: group work with people with AIDS (PWA's). Journal of Gay and Lesbian Psychotherapy 1:105–119, 1990

Grant D: Support groups for youth with the AIDS virus. Int J Group Psychother 38:237–251, 1988

Kelly JA, St. Lawrence JS: The AIDS Health Crisis: Psychological and Social Interventions. New York, Plenum, 1988

Lander S: Practitioners and AIDS: face-to-face with pain. APA Monitor 19(1):14–15, 1989

Lenihan GO: The therapeutic gay support group: a call for professional involvement. Psychotherapy 22:729–739, 1985

Lùpez DJ, Getzel GS: Helping gay AIDS patients in crisis. Soc Casework 387–394, 1984

Melton GB: Adolescents and prevention of AIDS. Professional Psychology: Research and Practice. 19:403–408, 1988

Morin SF, Charles KA, Malyon AK: The impact of AIDS on gay men. Am Psychol 39:1288–1293, 1984

Morrison CF: AIDS: ethical implications for psychological intervention. Professional Psychology: Research and Practice, 20(3):166–171, 1989

Newmark DA: Review of a support group for patients with AIDS. Top Clin Nurs 38–44, 1985

Nichols EK: Mobilizing Against AIDS: The Unfinished Story of a Virus (Institute of Medicine, National Academy of Sciences). Cambridge, MA, Harvard University Press, 1986

Nichols SE: Social and support groups for patients with acquired immune deficiency syndrome, in Psychiatric Implications of Acquired Immune Deficiency Syndrome. Edited by Nichols SE, Ostrow DG. Washington, DC, American Psychiatric Press, 1984, pp 77–82

Ostrow DG (ed): Behavioral Aspects of AIDS. New York, Plenum, 1990

Renneker RE: Countertransference reactions to cancer. Psychosom Med 19:409–418, 1957

Rounds KA, Galinsky MJ, Stevens LS: Linking people with AIDS in rural communities: the telephone group. Social Work 36:13–18, 1991

Rutan JS, Stone WN: Psychodynamic Group Psychotherapy. Lexington, MA, Collamore Press, 1984

Simon R: Confronting the spector of AIDS: what do therapists have to offer? (editorial). Family Networker 12:20–51, 1988

Spector IC, Conklin R: Brief reports: AIDS group psychotherapy. Int J Group Psychother 37:433–439, 1987

Spiegel D, Bloom JR, Kraemer HC, et al: Effect of psychosocial treatment on survival of patients with metastatic breast cancer. Lancet 2:888–891, 1989

Tavares R, Lùpez DJ: Responses of the gay community to acquired immune deficiency syndrome, in Psychiatric Implications of Acquired Immune Deficiency Syndrome. Edited by Nichols SE, Ostrow DG. Washington, DC, American Psychiatric Press, 1984, pp 105–110

Tross S, Hirsch DA: Psychological distress and neuropsychological complications of HIV infection and AIDS. Am Psychol 43:929–934, 1988

Weinberg G: Society and the Healthy Homosexual. New York, St. Martin's Press, 1972

Weisman AD: Thanatology, in Comprehensive Textbook of Psychiatry, 3rd Edition. Edited by Kaplan HI, Greedman AN, Sadock BJ. Baltimore, MD, Williams & Wilkins, 1980, pp 2042–2065

Yalom ID: The Theory and Practice of Group Psychotherapy, 2nd Edition. New York, Basic Books, 1975

CHAPTER 15

Dynamic Group Therapy for Substance Abuse Patients: A Reconceptualization

Sarah Golden, Ph.D.
Kurt Halliday, Ph.D.
Edward J. Khantzian, M.D.
William E. McAuliffe, Ph.D.

Introduction: Groups and Substance Abuse

As substance dependency has emerged as a compelling problem in our society over the past three decades, it is striking that the most widely recognized and accepted solution is the group approach. Regardless of whether the explanation for the addiction is seen as intrapsychic and psychodynamic, biological and hereditary, or social and environmental, our response to the growing numbers suffering the physical, psychological, and social ravages of alcoholism and other addictions is in this way significantly different from the individual, client-centered clinical approaches we customarily adopt for medical and psychiatric problems.

Given the changing, controversial, though often simultaneously held views of addiction as a problem of morality, of disease, or of psychosocial development, it is not surprising that self-help groups such as Alcoholics Anonymous (AA) that could "fuse the disease and the moral perspectives" (Orford 1985, p. 309) were the first to gain attention and to enjoy wide acceptance and popularity. Established in 1935 by two alcoholics, Bill Wilson and Dr. Bob, and modeled on the idea of a Christian fellowship, AA is a self-help group that involves sharing "one's life story" and "acknowledgement of character defects," often in a public meeting (Orford 1985, pp. 301–302). Change occurs within the group setting, in which elements of support, surrender, spirituality, and altruism prove ultimately to be "therapeutic" and transformational (Khantzian and Mack 1989). The success of AA has led to the application of the same model for other addictions and compulsions involving cocaine, narcotics, overeating, gambling, and sexuality.

Therapeutic communities such as Synanon, established in the 1960s in response to the emerging "heroin epidemic," similarly used the group as the context for change, but more radically and aggressively (Cherkas 1965), by combining elements of confinement, structure, regimented living and work assignments, and heavy confrontation. Changing attitudes is a cornerstone of this approach. As Orford points out, beyond the support inherent in AA and the therapeutic community, they also provide "a new set of attitudes and values, and it is to the group's ideology or 'will' that the novice must submit if he or she is to become a successful member" (1985, p. 303). Although this "total" group approach is not for every addict, therapeutic communities such as Daytop and Phoenix House continue to flourish.

In addition to the self-help group approach, several other major group models more recently have emerged in the treatment of addictions: the psychoeducational approach, which draws on cognitive-behavioral and social learning theory; and various psychodynamic approaches, which draw on the psychoanalytic tradition. The psychoeducative group seeks to inform addicts factually about the behavioral, medical, and psychological consequences of their use of substances. Such group experiences are now considered a standard component of most rehabilitation programs (Nace 1987). Similarly, McAuliffe and Ch'ien (1986) developed relapse prevention techniques that use a curriculum in a highly structured and didactic group format to highlight cognitive and behavioral factors, such as recognizing the social and environmental cues that lead to relapse. In the psychoanalytic tradition, the work of Yalom (1974) and Brown and Yalom (1977) articulated a psychodynamic, interpersonal application of group interactional principles for the group therapy of alcoholic individuals. This work, further developed by Vannicelli (1982, 1989), has been the mainstay in guiding psychodynamic therapists who treat substance abusers in groups.

It may be that the proliferation and popularity of group approaches to substance abuse and other addictions reflect what Orford (1985) called the essentially "social nature" of the change or recovery process, with the group offering a social context that has certain advantages for facilitating this change. Groups, regardless of a broad range of theoretical orientations, respond to the basic needs and vulnerabilities of addicts and alcoholics through the common elements of support, understanding, shared experiences, information, and opportunities for self-observation and confrontation that can make available and modify the psychological vulnerabilities associated with addictive behavior. But although the group is at the heart of each approach, its form and method vary according to its particular theoretical explanation of addiction. Even the question, "why a group?" may be answered differently depending on the type of group treatment offered.

A Psychodynamic Model

In this chapter we draw on a contemporary psychoanalytic perspective on substance dependence to provide a basis to understand and actively treat the vulnerabilities of addicts in group therapy. We describe a new group approach, modified dynamic group therapy (MDGT), first developed to treat cocaine addiction in the Harvard Cocaine Recovery Project, a program sponsored by the National Institute on Drug Abuse. Although developed specifically for cocaine addicts, MDGT is suited for treatment of most substance abusers with few, if any, changes. MDGT builds on the interpersonal model of group therapy described by Yalom (1974) and Brown and Yalom (1977) and the supportive-expressive approach for individual psychotherapy described by Luborsky (1984) and Luborsky et al. (1981) for substance abusers. The MDGT approach is designed to avoid the ambiguity of unstructured conventional dynamic groups, to go beyond the strictly interpersonal focus of interpersonal groups, and to actively provide understanding and treatment for the psychological vulnerabilities and related characterological problems that precipitate and perpetuate dependence on substances.

Theories of Addiction

Theory and Practice

The assumptions we hold regarding the etiology and nature of psychological disorders guide our clinical practice. Currently, in the field of addictions, the clinical implications of our assumptions about addiction are underdeveloped; there is even a tendency to use the assumptions themselves as excuses not to offer an adequate and appropriate treatment to substance abusers. Current theories of addiction, both psychodynamic and nonanalytic, reflect both conceptual disagreement about the needs of addicts and the inability to develop practical methods that follow adequately from theoretical considerations.

In the first half of this century, American psychiatry was informed by Freudian psychoanalytic thinking. As a consequence, we view psychological problems as originating in a person's childhood as a result of frustrated instinctual strivings and inadequate parenting. More recently, the advancing technology that enables us to measure the biological workings of the brain has produced new information about how the brain and biochemical processes regulate or determine emotions, behavior, and psychopathological conditions. Given these developments, a growing number of modern-day clinicians more often concern themselves with targeting an individual's dopamine or serotonin neurotransmitter systems rather than exploring an unhappy childhood in an effort to alleviate the patient's distress.

These apparently mutually exclusive explanations, the psychological and the biological, continue to be invoked in the ongoing controversies about cause-consequence, nature-nurture, and psyche-soma in medicine and psychiatry. These debates have been extreme and often counterproductive in the field of substance abuse. Although most agree that the etiology of alcoholism or addiction involves no single pathway, there is still a tendency to consider a particular perspective or element of the biopsychosocial equation to the exclusion of the others. In this review our perspective derives from the psychodynamic, psychoanalytic tradition as distinguished from biological and social models. We focus on what we believe to be some of the important psychological vulnerabilities that can lead to substance abuse problems. In order to clarify our model and to place it in the context of other current theoretical models, we first briefly discuss these other prevalent theories of addiction.

Biological Theories

There is clear evidence that heredity plays an important role in the etiology of alcoholism. The role of genetic-hereditary influences in the development of drug dependence is less clear. Family, twin, and adoptive studies indicate that genetic factors are involved in the high coincidence of alcoholism among male family members (Cotton 1979; Goodwin 1979; Schuckit 1985). However, the role of genetics has not been as clearly identified in the development of alcoholism in women. A series of further studies indicates that family drinking patterns, behavioral problems, and environmental factors interact with genetic factors to influence how or whether alcoholism develops (Cadoret et al. 1985; Cloninger et al. 1981; Frances et al. 1980). Along similar lines, the search for biological markers for alcoholism has revealed that individuals who are genetically at high risk for alcoholism display a decreased intensity of reaction to alcohol (e.g., less intoxication or body sway), as well as differences in evoked brain potentials, electroencephalographic alpha-wave activity, and acetaldehyde levels (Schuckit 1985). Tarter et al. (1984, 1985) proposed that genetic influences for alcoholism mainly manifest themselves through temperament and behavior and cause individuals so affected to behave and react to alcohol in ways that make the development of alcoholism more likely.

Cultural Factors and the Longitudinal Perspective

Vaillant (1983) traced the influence of culture and societal attitudes on drinking behavior and the development of alcoholism. He contended that such influences interacting with genetic factors are more important than personality factors or family environment in the etiology of alcoholism. Critics of Vaillant's findings and conclusions have argued that his longitudinal studies did not adequately discover or evaluate childhood environmental influences, which thus were minimized in his conclusions (Donovan 1986). In contrast, Shedler and Block (1990) recently presented longitudinal findings with a sample of 18-year-old subjects and their families following from the time they were 3 years old. They found formal significant correlations between emotional and behavioral maturity and patterns of substance abuse (marijuana and alcohol). Individuals who were immature and who came from dysfunctional families displayed more extremes in their patterns of use and dependence on substances.

Psychodynamic Theories of Addiction

The psychodynamic theory of addiction holds that early experiences and development predispose certain individuals to become substance dependent and implicates particular psychological vulnerabilities in this dependency. Our modified psychodynamic group treatment seeks to identify and address these psychological vulnerabilities.

Psychoanalytic theory since Freud has addressed the problem of addiction, conceptualizing the addiction to drugs as symptomatic of a psychological problem. Early views foreshadowed the self-regulating, self-medicating conception of compulsive drug use. Freud (1930) wrote in *Civilization and Its Discontents* that "the service rendered by intoxicating media in the struggle for happiness and keeping misery at a distance is so highly prized as a benefit that individuals and people alike have given them an established place in the economics of the libido" (p. 78). Theorists such as Rado (1933) and, later, Fenichel (1945) specifically described drug addiction as an attempt to self-medicate dysphoric affects, which stem from preexisting psychopathology within the individual.

These earlier views are still at the heart of the current psychoanalytic theory of compulsive drug use. Psychoanalytic theory over the past 20 years has largely elaborated on the nature of the defects of self, both intrapsychic and characterological, that can lead to addiction. Weider and Kaplan (1969) described addictive drug use as a "prothesis" that temporarily improves the adaptation of an individual with characterological vulnerabilities. Krystal and Raskin (1970) ascribed these vulnerabilities to childhood psychic trauma and pointed to the addict's inadequate affect development, particularly the inability to tolerate affect, as the cause of addiction. Contemporary psychoanalytic theory targets the structural and narcissistic nature of the vulnerability. For Kohut (1977), this was a "defect in the self," the inability to supply oneself "with self-approval or with a sense of strength through [one's] own inner resources . . . " (pp. vii–viii). The drug supplies, however fleetingly, the self-esteem, the feeling of acceptance, and the self-confidence that are missing within. Wurmser (1978) and Meissner (1986) described a narcissistic depression or crisis in which the painful affects associated with narcissistic wounding of the fragile self—anxiety, anger, depression, shame, emptiness, and doubt—emerge overwhelmingly. Again, the drug offers temporary, illusory "resolution" of the crisis by soothing, restoring, and strengthening.

Khantzian's work (1974, 1978, 1985) further elaborated on the psychological and narcissistic vulnerabilities of the potential addict: his "self-medication hypothesis" holds that addictions result when a person seeks to relieve the painful affects and suffering deriving from defects in ego capacities, in the sense of self, and in object relations. The drug is used to "medicate" poor self-esteem, intolerable affects, interpersonal problems, and lack of self-care. This model demonstrates how the individual's narcissistic and ego deficits play themselves out in the various dimensions of everyday life, which together produce an experience of ongoing narcissistic crisis. For example, a cocaine addict may use the drug to experience "a sense of empowerment that can enhance a state of self-sufficiency or [to] make contact and involvement with others exhilarating and exciting. Sexually, the user, short term, may also feel increased arousal and potency, and a sense of being glamorous and appealing" (Khantzian 1988, pp. 9–10). In another dimension—that of affective experience—cocaine may be used to overcome the fatigue, low energy, and boredom associated with depression.

Reconceptualization of Theory and Practice

Psychodynamic conceptualizations of addiction hold that although environmental, interpersonal, and physiological variables are important, the central problem remains the individual's own structural and developmental vulnerability. It is this often-severe vulnerability that treatment must address to effect lasting change in recovery. Although psychoanalytic theory offers a powerful explanation of substance dependence, at the same time addicts have been seen as unsuitable for psychodynamic treatment because of the very defects that contribute to their addiction: they are too disturbed, too intolerant of affect, and too prone to acting out. Both the negative view of the addict and a constricted view of what constitutes dynamic therapy can be used as rationalizations for not offering psychodynamic treatment to addicts.

If the therapy is seen mainly as an evocation of deep conflicts and affects, with a therapist whose role is to make transference interpretations, the addict (especially the newly recovering one) will not be able to stay in and benefit from treatment. In our group psychodynamic model, the focus remains on the intrapsychic and characterological vulnerabilities of the individual, but the method of working with the addict is modified to provide support, maximize safety, and address the potential for drug and psychological relapse, even as the characteristically self-defeating ways of experiencing oneself and acting with others are activated and emerge in the group setting.

Some of the adaptations or modifications in our model are related to the development of nonanalytic techniques for working with the substance abuser. Many nonanalytic approaches to addiction hold that the primary emphasis must be on abstinence, relapse prevention, and managing the cravings stirred by the pitfalls of an unsafe external world and the dangerous properties of the drug itself (McAuliffe and Ch'ien 1986; Milkman and Shaffer 1985). These approaches recognize the fragility of the addict in early recovery, and a treatment environment of safety and containment is established—one where the atmosphere is not too vigorously confrontational and where the addict is not expected to relinquish needed defenses too readily (Bean 1981; Zweben 1987). This is an important contribution to the specialized treatment of addiction. However, with their focus on external threat and extreme internal vulnerability, these methods underestimate the individual's strengths and the restorative capacity of exploring and understanding one's own suffering beginning in early recovery. In fact, some counsel that psychodynamic treatment may be indicated only after as much as 2 years of sobriety (Bean 1984). We question whether this is throwing out the baby with the bath water.

Other valuable adaptations of traditional approaches are also offered by practitioners of psychoanalytic treatment with a strongly interpersonal focus. This school of therapy conceptualizes the addict's difficulties as primarily interpersonal or relational (Brown and Yalom 1977; Luborsky 1984, 1989; Rounsaville et al. 1985; Vannicelli 1982, 1989; Yalom 1974). The treatment is supportive-expressive and most often takes place in a group as the natural medium of interpersonal experience and reenactment. Although interpersonal understanding and experience comprise a key dimension of our modified psychodynamic approach, we emphasize understanding of the individual's dysfunctional characterological patterns and intrapsychic structure as they become apparent in a group setting and the supportive emergence of the group members' commonalities as they help the individual to face these patterns and structures.

Focus of Modified Dynamic Group Therapy

Our reconceptualization of the therapy of addiction holds that the treatment must address the needs and difficulties of addicts as we understand them psychodynamically in a safe way that promotes recovery from addiction. These are seen as vulnerabilities in four dimensions: 1) tolerating and regulating affect, 2) problems with relationships, 3) failures of self-care, and 4) deficits in self-esteem.

These dimensions focus on "how character structure manifests itself in everyday life for everyone—intrapsychically, interpersonally, and in the larger world" (Khantzian et al. 1990, p. 16). MDGT is a supportive-expressive group psychotherapy that is designed to address the underlying vulnerabilities and characterological difficulties that lead to the addict's susceptibility to using drugs.

MDGT was developed as a group treatment for the Harvard Cocaine Recovery Project, a study of cocaine addiction funded by the National Institute on Drug Abuse and carried out at the Cambridge Hospital, a teaching hospital for Harvard Medical School (Khantzian et al. 1990). This study, in progress since 1987, is designed to compare two group treatments with each other and with a no-group control treatment with respect to their effect on outcome, including drug use and psychological functioning. The Harvard study explores both the effectiveness of group treatment versus a no-group treatment and also the relative efficacy of a supportive-expressive psychodynamic model and a cognitive-behavioral social conditioning one. It should be emphasized that the 214 addicted individuals who participated in the study were recruited through television and newspaper advertisements, radio announcement, and agency referrals and constitute a highly motivated, voluntary sample. Although they often suffered from severe, long-term addiction to cocaine, they were able to go through a rigorous intake process and make a strong commitment to a 6-month treatment. Our modified dynamic group therapy was developed for them and further tailored to address their specific needs as the project progressed.

The first modification offered by our approach is that even though we seek to use psychodynamic group therapy to address character disorder, we have an ongoing concern for the addicts' abstinence and prevention of relapse. Without abstinence, the characterological difficulties can be obscured and fueled by continuing crisis. With abstinence, these same difficulties become readily apparent in the group setting. MDGT is designed to "evoke salient themes of psychological vulnerability and characteristic defensive styles" (Khantzian et al. 1990, p. 20) but also to provide a context in which they can be understood and change can begin.

This context is one of safety and support, which is established in several ways. Safety and support are provided by an active, directive, and friendly group leader who begins by explaining the nature and expectations of psychodynamic therapy, distinguishing it from other addiction treatments (such as 12-step programs) with which group members may be more familiar. The anxieties common to joining a group are also directly acknowledged and the issues of abstinence and relapse prevention addressed as needed. A group leader may need to intervene directly (as in any "difficult" group), for example, by reminding the group to speak one at a time or to reestablish order by making sure disruptions are talked about (Rice and Rutan 1987). At the same time, group members as well as the leader are encouraged to take an active role in observing, reaching out to each other, and offering their insight and understanding.

The principles of interpersonal group therapy described by Brown and Yalom (1977) are employed in the MDGT model to promote the rapid development of cohesiveness, to maintain a focus on the here and now, and to create an interpersonal milieu in which group members can best "overcome feelings of self-contempt, loneliness, alienation and disengagement . . . " (p. 428). However, the MDGT focus is on how each individual's character style and structure play themselves out in the group, rather than on the interpersonal interactions themselves. We ask the group members to look at how they are in the group, how they experience themselves and others, and how their interpersonal behavior relates to inner experience and vulnerabilities. In this sense, the comfortable "interpersonal milieu" is necessary but not sufficient for the goals of MDGT. If all goes well, the MDGT group member will learn about himself or herself in all four dimensions: regulation of affect, relationships, self-care, and self-esteem. The focus of the work shifts between the interpersonal and the intrapersonal (i.e., between the experience of others and the experience of the self).

The discovery and understanding of character are more likely to occur once the group members feel they are on some "common ground" (Khantzian et al. 1990). Common ground is similar to the curative factor of "universality" described by Yalom (1985). It is perhaps more specific (and sometimes problematic) in a group that comes together because of common problems with substance abuse. It has been our usual experience that group members first seek to bond around their addiction. An important early transition they must make in an MDGT group is to realize that this is not the only common ground they share, but that the shame, the feelings of inadequacy, and the overwhelming nature of certain affects are also commonly felt by others. They realize that such things as accumulating parking tickets, never seeing the dentist, having frequent accidents, and getting deeply into debt are ways of not caring for themselves or not attending to possible dangers around them. They begin to see a pattern of such lack of self-care in others in the group and find a new common ground on which to meet. They see that they are not alone in their desire to find love, recognition, and security but that their characteristic means of attempting to do so may be grandiose, self-defeating, or in others ways familiar to others in the group who avoid the "middle ground" of ordinary, everyday life ("I showered gifts on my first wife; I really put her on a pedestal—then she left me suddenly"; "I always felt better if I was carrying a large amount of cash at all times"; "I worked out until I collapsed on the floor"). The common theme of never finding satisfaction with the middle ground may be greeted with knowing laughter and bring forth more stories in a similar vein from the group.

The shift from drug abuse as common ground to problems of living and of self as common ground is what distinguishes MDGT from other treatments for addiction. Part of the process of understanding one's own characterological patterns is to see how they can make one more susceptible to drug use as a temporary "solution," but this is not the main focus of the discussion. Often, especially early in the development of the group, members resist any view of their problems beyond the explanation that drugs are responsible. ("I'm here for one reason only—to deal with my drug addiction"; "My disease is very devious"; "This is what brings us together, you know what I'm talking about.") The necessary shift from thinking about drugs to thinking psychologically is addressed from the inception of the group. Self-understanding beyond the narrow focus on drug-taking is promoted, thereby also shifting from an emphasis on reaction to an external threat to a more active, autonomous experience. The goal is the same as that of all insight-oriented psychoanalytic psychotherapy, that of "restoring the integration of the individual and, in fact, of enlarging, through some kind of selfknowledge, the realm of self-direction or personal autonomy" (Shapiro 1989, p. 118).

MDGT In Action

In the following case example from an MDGT group, the effort was to focus on the characteristic way that one group member, Mr. A, participated in the group and to help him become more aware of how he denied his need for others and the depth of his own feelings. Mr. A's apparently "good" behavior—always being helpful to others while never troubling the group with his problems, playing the peacemaker, and in general keeping a very low profile—led in this particular group meeting to a keen disappointment in his fellow group members.

Case 1

Mr. A, a quietly friendly, appealing young man who worked in a mental health clinic for schizophrenic patients, had been a steady group member for several months. He was always on time and never missed a group meeting. His participation in the group usually involved a somewhat unemotional report on the progress of his separation from the woman with whom he had been living for some time, his frequent statements that he never experienced "cravings" for cocaine since becoming abstinent (and that he knew he'd never use the drug again), and great attention to the problems of others in the group. Although he often seemed to hold back initially before joining in, his expression betrayed a strong emotional response as he listened, and he seemed to feel most comfortable asking others about themselves and offering advice and support. His stance in the group exemplified his conflicting desire for empathy and his fear of it (the dilemma of the narcissistic group member that Liebenberg [1990] described).

One evening, as the group got under way, with much joking and talking at once, another group member, Mr. B, noticed Mr. A's increasingly uncomfortable silence: "[Mr. A], you look like you have something on your mind." Mr. A replied, "Well, I just think it's hard to say this, but . . . I've been thinking that there's too much competition to speak. Everyone talks at once . . . we need to reach out to each other more."

At this point, the other group members, somewhat chastened, hastily agreed, saying they liked it when "everyone participates" and everyone "gets a chance." They then seemed somewhat at a loss as to how to proceed. The leader asked Mr. A whether he had something he wanted to bring up about himself. Mr. A said, "Well, it's my birthday today, and I'm kind of disappointed . . . you know, kind of let down, that no one I know remembered." The others responded, "Hey! Happy birthday, man! We could have had a party!" But Mr. A continued, "I don't know, I always remember other people's birthdays, and at least get them a card or something."

Mr. A obviously felt sorry for himself, and several group members responded by telling their own stories of being neglected and disregarded. Ms. C spoke of coming from "a large, negligent family," too disorganized to recognize each individual child. Mr. D said that because his parents were both gone, holidays and birthdays were especially painful for him. Mr. E said his parents had always treated him as "an adult," and this meant never celebrating his birthday ("I don't think they remembered when it was!").

Although these other group members were able to respond empathically to Mr. A's distress, their own references were all to parents and their childhood experiences and not to the present realities of their lives. In their own poignant renditions of unhappiness, they both overshadowed Mr. A's concern about his birthday and seemed to accept his presentation of himself as the hapless victim of others' disregard. Perhaps Mr. A's leading off with a criticism of the group process, his history in the group of avoiding anything emotionally revealing about himself and denying problems, and his consistent focus on others contributed to this lack of response to him.

In fact, he seemed quite content to listen to the others' stories. His mild expression of dissatisfaction with the competition to speak in the group and his assertion that he never forgot a birthday himself were his only attempts to get some attention—and he got very little.

Finally, the group leader, acknowledging that the group seemed to understand and identify with Mr. A's emotional experience, wondered aloud whether they would let themselves get in the same spot as he had, as adults, and asked Mr. A how it had happened that such a caring, attentive person couldn't get anyone else to remember him. The sharing of common, related experience was not enough to address Mr. A's passivity and inability to ask for something, which so often had left him feeling disenchanted, alone, and angry at others—feeling that he gives so much and gets nothing in return. In merely serving as the catalyst for a discussion of neglect, Mr. A was again left alone. The group needed to move on to directly address the "protective shield" Mr. A characteristically used to deny his own vulnerability and his limited view of himself as the "only one who gets along with everyone," the self-sacrificing peacemaker, the "quiet" one who is forgotten.

At this point Mr. A himself became quite animated, describing his own family and his role within it for the first time. He described the tension he felt at having to mediate between his parents, who divorced when he was a teenager, the sense of responsibility for his younger brothers, and the pressure of being "the only one in the family who talks to everyone else." Within this delicate balance, he felt he could not even experience, let alone give voice to, his own feelings, for fear of upsetting the balance. Isolated, going through a painful separation himself, he was disappointed and angry that no one responded as he himself would have—his forgotten birthday was only the tip of the iceberg.

The group was much more able to respond to Mr. A's revelations about his experience than to his sulky, victimized, and self-righteous facade. He was able in this meeting to receive some of the support he desperately wanted and hoped would come to him if he was "good" and waited patiently. The group meeting ended with a discussion of "letting oneself be reached" and known, as well as "reaching out" to each other. Past experiences were explored in the context of present difficulties, and ongoing, characteristic patterns of protecting the vulnerable self were identified.

It is important to note that in this meeting the group's "common ground" was established around life problems other than the compulsive use of drugs. Identifying how the self-defeating solutions to these life problems leave one more susceptible to drug use is always an important dimension of the group process, because drug use is the ultimate "solution" for the substance abuser's narcissistically compromised position.

Advantages of Group Therapy

In MDGT the group functions not only to elicit the characteristic ways of interacting and experiencing but also to effectively demonstrate the "cost of character defenses" (Alonso 1989). Even as the defenses exact their price, the cohesion of the group provides safety, and the active presence of other group members gives rise to new possibilities for action. Fried (1985) saw the insight of the group members as resulting from this encounter with others, not from interpretation alone. Thus the group modality provides the fertile common ground for character-ological patterns to grow, the milieu in which the self-defeating, self-destructive, or ineffective nature of these patterns can be appreciated, the safety and containment for the acknowledgment of these patterns and their "cost," and the encounter that can motivate change.

The group modifications necessary for working with the newly recovering addict were developed in groups for "acting-out" patients who come into treatment in crisis, such as those described by Borriello (1979), and in groups geared to the needs of the borderline or narcissistic patient, as described by Stone and Gustafson (1982). The focus is on the "uniqueness" of the group member and on addressing the characteristic "action" defense by which the addict attempts to avoid feeling (Khantzian et al. 1990, p. 49). Confrontation can occur only in an atmosphere of support and acceptance, one in which the vulnerability and traumatic histories of many of the group members are appreciated. The advantages of group treatment for the characterologically disordered patient are to provide a medium for self-observation and interaction that avoids the "narcissistically injurious or accusatory interpretations" and the angry impasses that can arise in the intensity of the individual therapy situation (Tuttman 1990, p. 23) and to promote the growth of a sense of self and self-esteem without overwhelming someone who both yearns for and resists empathy. The group provides strength and containment for the lonely, isolated, vulnerable, and action-prone substance abuser so that reflection and development can occur.

Conclusions

MDGT is based on specific modifications of psychoanalytic, psychodynamic practice for substance abusers who have often been excluded from more traditional therapies or who have been relegated to nonpsychodynamic programs stressing education; a more exclusive focus on relapse prevention; and a concern for external threat. Safety, an active group leader, a cohesive interpersonal milieu (without an exclusively interpersonal focus), a development of common ground, an enlargement of psychological understanding beyond the presenting problem, and the supportive use of the group to promote individual insight and growth into characterological patterns—all these are "modifications" of psychodynamic therapy that can be relevant for other patients who are not seen as "appropriate" for traditional group or individual therapy. Character-disordered, acting-out, or traumatized individuals—who are usually not considered good candidates for insight-oriented, psychodynamic, or group therapy—may benefit from this approach.

References

Alonso A: Character change in group therapy. Paper presented at Psychiatric Grand Rounds, The Cambridge Hospital, Cambridge, MA, September 1989

Bean M: Denial and the psychological complications of alcoholism, in Dynamic Approaches to the Understanding and Treatment of Alcoholism. Edited by Bean MH, Zinberg NE. New York, The Free Press, 1981, pp 55–96

Bean M: Clinical implications of models for recovery from alcoholism, in The Addictive Behaviors. Edited by Shaffer HJ, Stimmel B. New York, Haworth, 1984, pp 91–104

Borriello JF: Group psychotherapy with acting-out patients: specific problems and technique. Am J Psychother 33:521–530, 1979

Brown S, Yalom ID: Interactional group therapy with alcoholics. J Stud Alcohol 38:426–456, 1977

Cadoret RJ, O'Gorman TW, Troughton E, et al: Alcoholism and antisocial personality: interrelationships, genetic and environment factors. Arch Gen Psychiatry 42:161–167, 1985

Cherkas MS: Synanon foundation—a radical approach to the problem of addiction (editorial). Am J Psychiatry 121:1065, 1965

Cloninger CR, Bohman M, Sigvardsson S: Inheritance of alcohol abuse. Arch Gen Psychiatry 38:861–868, 1981

Cotton NS: The familial incidence of alcoholism: a review. J Stud Alcohol 40:89–116, 1979

Donovan JM: An etiologic model of alcoholism. Am J Psychiatry 143:1–11, 1986

Fenichel O: The Psychoanalytic Theory of Neurosis. New York, WW Norton, 1945

Frances RJ, Timm S, Bucky S: Studies of familial and nonfamilial alcoholism. Arch Gen Psychiatry 37:564–566, 1980

Fried E: The process of change in group psychotherapy. Group 3:3–13, 1985

Freud S: Civilization and Its Discontents (1930), in The Standard Edition of the Complete Psychological Works of Sigmund Freud, Vol 21. Translated and edited by Strachey J. London, Hogarth Press, 1961, pp 64–145

Goodwin DW: Alcoholism and heredity: a review and hypothesis. Arch Gen Psychiatry 36:57–61, 1979

Khantzian EJ: Opiate addiction: a critique of theory and some implications for treatment. Am J Psychother 131:160–164, 1974

Khantzian EJ: The ego, the self and opiate addiction: theoretical and treatment considerations. International Review of Psychoanalysis 5:189–198, 1978

Khantzian EJ: The self-medication hypothesis of addictive disorders: focus on heroin and cocaine dependence. Am J Psychiatry 142:1259–1264, 1985

Khantzian EJ: The primary care therapist and patient needs in substance abuse treatment. Am J Drug Alcohol Abuse 14:159–167, 1988

Khantzian EJ, Mack JE: Alcoholics anonymous and contemporary psychodynamic theory, in Recent Developments in Alcoholism, Vol 7. Edited by Galanter M. New York, Plenum, 1989, pp 67–89

Khantzian EJ, Halliday J, McAuliffe W: Addiction and the Vulnerable Self. New York, Guilford, 1990

Kohut H: Preface, in Psychodynamics of Drug Dependence (NIDA Research Monograph No 12: DHEW Pub No ADM 77-270. Edited by Blaine JD, Julius DA. Washington, DC, National Institute of Drug Abuse, 1977

Krystal H, Raskin HA: Drug Dependence: Aspects of Ego Function. Detroit, MI, Wayne State University Press, 1970

Liebenberg B: The unwanted and unwanting patient: problems in group psychotherapy of the narcissistic patient, in The Difficult Patient in Group. Edited by Roth B, Stone W, Kibel H. Madison, WI, International Universities Press, 1990, pp 311–322

Luborsky L: Principles of Psychoanalytic Psychotherapy: A Manual for Supportive-Expressive Treatment. New York, Basic Books, 1984

Luborsky L, Woody GE, Hole A, et al: A Treatment Manual for Supportive-Expressive Psychoanalytically Oriented Psychotherapy: Special Adaptation for Treatment of Drug Dependence, 4th Edition (unpublished manual). Philadelphia, PA, VA Medical Center, 1981

McAuliffe WE, Ch'ien JMN: Recovery training and self help: relapse prevention program for treated opiate addicts. J Subst Abuse Treat 3:9–20, 1986

Meissner WW: Psychotherapy and the Paranoid Process. New York, Jason Aronson, 1986

Milkman HB, Shaffer HJ (eds): The Addictions. Lexington, MA, DC Heath, 1985

Nace E: The Treatment of Alcoholism. New York, Brunner/Mazel, 1987

Orford J: Excessive Appetites: A Psychological View of Addictions. New York, John Wiley, 1985

Rado S: The psychoanalysis of pharmocothymia (1933), in Classic Contributions in the Addictions. Edited by Shaffer H, Burglass ME. New York, Brunner/Mazel, 1981, pp 77–94

Rice CA, Rutan JS: Inpatient Group Psychotherapy. New York, Macmillan, 1987

Rounsaville BJ, Gawin F, Kleber H: Interpersonal psychotherapy adapted for ambulatory cocaine abusers. Am J Drug Alcohol Abuse 11(3–4):171–191, 1985

Schuckit M: Genetics and the risk for alcoholism. JAMA 254:2614–2617, 1985

Shapiro D: Psychotherapy of the Neurotic Character. New York, Basic Books, 1989

Shedler J, Block J: Adolescent drug use and psychological health: a longitudinal inquiry. Am Psychol 45:612–630, 1990

Stone W, Gustafson JP: Technique in group psychotherapy of narcissistic and borderline patients. Int J Group Psychother 32:29–47, 1982

Tarter RE, Alterman AI, Edwards KL: Alcoholic denial: a biopsychological interpretation. J Stud Alcohol 45:214–218, 1984

Tarter RE, Alterman AI, Edwards KL: Vulnerabilities to alcoholism in men: a behaivor-genetic perspective. J Stud Alcohol 46:329–356, 1985

Tuttman S: Principles of psychoanalytic group therapy applied to the treatment of borderline and narcissistic disorders, in The Difficult Patient in Group. Edited by Roth B, Stone W, Kibel H. Madison, WI, International Universities Press, 1990, pp 7–29

Vaillant GE: The Natural History of Alcoholism. Cambridge, MA, Harvard University Press, 1983

Vannicelli M: Group psychotherapy with alcoholics. J Stud Alcohol 43:17–37, 1982

Vannicelli M: Group Psychotherapy with Adult Children of Alcoholics. New York, Guilford, 1989

Weider H, Kaplan EH: Drug use in adolescents: psychodynamic meaning and pharmacogenic effect. Psychoanal Study Child 24:399–431, 1969

Wurmser L: The Hidden Dimension: Psychodynamics of Compulsive Drug Use. New York, Jason Aronson, 1978

Yalom ID: Group psychotherapy and alcoholism. Ann N Y Acad Sci 233:85–103, 1974

Yalom ID: The Theory and Practice of Group Psychotherapy, 3rd Edition. New York, Basic Books, 1985

Zweben J: Recovery-oriented psychotherapy: Facilitating the use of 12-step programs. Psychotherapy 19:243–251, 1987

CHAPTER 16

Groups for Patients With Histories of Catastrophic Trauma

Bessel A. van der Kolk, M.D.

Posttraumatic Stress Disorder

Experiences that overwhelm a person's ability to cope and that destroy one's sense of safety and predictability have long-term effects on psychological and social functioning. Posttraumatic stress disorder (PTSD), the syndrome of involuntarily reliving elements of the trauma in feelings, images, or actions, alternating with numbness and lack of positive emotions, often follows overwhelming stressors such as intrafamilial violence, war trauma, incest and rape, muggings, shootings, explosions, accidents, and other physical and sexual assaults. The helplessness and rage accompanying these experiences alter a person's sense of safety and trust and inevitably affect his or her ability to pursue and enjoy mutually satisfying relationships.

In PTSD, the overpowering nature of the experience causes trauma-related images and feelings to intrude, consciously and unconsciously, through reactions and emotions that were appropriate responses at the time of the trauma but are not relevant now. When exposed to situations of intimacy, trust, dependency, and aggression, which unconsciously remind them of the previous violation, PTSD patients often react as if they were being traumatized all over again. They blow up or withdraw, fight or flee. Unaware of the origins of these reactions, but conscious of their effects, they become ashamed, angry, and frightened. While attempting to negotiate their emotions, they become prone to sensation-seeking, overwork, and alcohol and drug abuse (van der Kolk 1987).

Effects on Interpersonal Functioning

It is difficult to recognize that the long-term psychological responses to traumatization—dissociation ("spacing out"), sensation-seeking, emotional constriction, and drug and alcohol abuse—are in fact ways of coping with trauma-related memories. The psychological consequences of such unresolved trauma encompass a variety of psychiatric problems (van der Kolk 1989). The most common are

- *Distortions in affect regulation.* These cause extreme reactivity to internal and external stimulation, depression, self-mutilation, anxious dependency, and passivity to control affect states.
- *Distorted concepts of self.* These lead to self-blame for uncontrollable circumstances, volunteering for the scapegoat role, dissociative phenomena and amnesias, and confused intermingling of pleasure and pain.
- *Distorted interpersonal relations that tend to have an all-or-none quality.* In other words, aggression, sexuality, and intimacy are either excessive or inhibited. Careless self-disclosure alternates with paranoid watchfulness, and the other's needs are approached with extraordinary sensitivity or insensitivity.
- *Fear of stable long-term interpersonal commitments* and a lack of confidence that conflicts can be peacefully resolved.

Attachment as Protection Against Traumatization

The essence of psychological trauma is the loss of a sense of safety and predictability. Trauma results when one loses the feeling of having a secure retreat, either within or without oneself, where frightening emotions and experiences can be confronted. Emotional attachments are a person's primary protection against helplessness and meaninglessness. They are essential for biological survival in children and existential meaning in adults. In all people, children or adults, severe stress dramatically increases the need for attachment and protection. Pain, fear, fatigue, and inaccessibility of familiar caregivers all elicit efforts to attract increased care. The availability of a caregiver who can be blindly trusted when one's own resources are inadequate is, in fact, the most powerful protection against overwhelming experiences. Thus the etiology and the cure of trauma-related psychological disturbance depend fundamentally on the security of interpersonal attachments (van der Kolk 1987).

Attachments are the framework within which people mature and thrive. From the moment of birth individuals develop in a social context. Beginning with the mother-infant bond, this matrix continually incorporates wider interpersonal and cultural influences. Children maintain constant touch with powerful protectors by being attached to their caregivers. They seek and need the assurance of a "safe base" to which they can return after exploring their surroundings. This security promotes self-reliance and autonomy and instills a sense of interrelatedness with others. Adults need a safe base too, but their options are wider and include ever-enlarging circles of affinity to people, skills, and cultural values (van der Kolk 1987).

However, after severe trauma, the ability to reestablish constructive communication is severely impaired. Frightened people (e.g., abused children, battered women, and hostages) will, in desperation, paradoxically seek increased attachment even when the only available attachment objects are the source of danger (Rajecki et al. 1978). Thus attachment bonds become stronger as much through fear as through safety.

Childhood Trauma

The earliest and perhaps most catastrophic psychological trauma occurs when caregivers who are supposed to be sources of safety and nurture sexually or physically assault their children. When this happens, the child becomes fearfully and angrily attached and unwillingly or anxiously obedient. The child is simultaneously terrified that the caregiver will attack and/or be unavailable for protection. Bowlby (1984) called this "a pattern of behavior in which avoidance competes with the desire for proximity and care and in which anger against the self or others is apt to become prominent" (pp. 10–11). Traumatized adults sometimes develop the psychological reactions of abused children, but are usually better protected against long-term effects. They know that they have been able to take effective action against stress in the past and that they have developed a range of coping resources.

In both children and adults, the threat of loss of attachment is followed first by "protest" (anger) and then by despair. The purpose of anger, especially intrafamilial anger, may be to maintain and control the quality of the attachment bonds. Family violence is potentially functional behavior distorted and exaggerated (Bowlby 1984). Individuals who have grown up in families where physical safety was not ensured rarely learn to use aggression appropriately to negotiate their emotional needs. They tend to respond to perceived deprivation as if it were a life-threatening situation and to react with excessive violence or, conversely, with all overt expressions of aggression inhibited and internalized (Cicchetti 1984; Green 1989).

In adulthood, these children from abusive homes often are exquisitely sensitive—anticipating the reactions of both potential protectors and victimizers and attempting constantly to please them and prevent abandonment or injury. The problems of these adults are compounded because they often have difficulty distinguishing between protectors and victimizers (Ferenczi 1955; Reiker and Carmen 1986). They simply do not know whom to trust. In therapy, for example, the dependency of these adults on the therapist may be a function of fear, not a result of a therapeutic alliance. In fact, it is exactly these individuals with a troubling past of prior trauma who are most vulnerable to sexual and emotional abuse from therapists and who most lack the ability to extricate themselves from such abusive relationships (Gutheil 1989; Russell 1984).

In addition, the absence of a safe base in childhood interferes with curiosity and the development of satisfactory friendships. Numerous studies have shown that anxious attachment to caregivers prevents the development of satisfactory peer relationships (Grunebaum and Solomon 1982; Sharp 1980). Victimized children approach their peers as potential sources of terror and bully or withdraw. Bereft of experiences in the pleasures and frustrations of peer relationships, they fail to establish the connections that largely determine human beings' later life satisfactions (Blos 1979). Regardless of parental assets or shortcomings, it is this area, peer relationships, that needs to be mastered and in which traumatized people often find the greatest gain from therapy.

Role of the Peer Group in Overcoming Trauma

In a study of group phenomena in concentration camp survivors, Shamai Davidson (1984) wrote: "It has become increasingly evident that cooperating for survival among members of the same species is a basic law of life. Throughout the history of man, sharing relationships have been the central mode of coping with and adjusting to the environment" (p. 555). When faced with external threat, people tend to band together in groups to protect themselves. The degree to which people seek this protection depends on both their internal sense of security and the intensity of the external threat. Becker (1973), discussing submergence in the group, said that "transference is the taming of terror" (p. 145). He quoted Freud's essay on group psychology (Freud 1921) to support his observation that the more terrifying the external threat, the stronger allegiance becomes.

Continuing this line of study, research has further shown that a cohesive support network strongly militates against the development of long-term symptoms of PTSD after potentially traumatizing experiences (Quarentelli 1985). In analogy to Freud's notion of trauma resulting in a rupture in the membrane of the mind (1919), Lindy and Titchener (1983) called this social support the "trauma membrane." For young children, the family can be a very effective source of protection against traumatization—that is, an effective trauma membrane—and most children are amazingly resilient as long as the family is emotionally and physically available. Even after individuals mature, they often continue to depend on the family to provide this trauma membrane. However, after traumatic events such as physical or sexual assaults by strangers, families often experience shame and guilt about having been powerless to prevent the traumatization of one of its members. Disillusioned and upset, the family members may then turn against each other (Solomon 1987).

Therefore, one of the most urgent tasks facing therapists of traumatized individuals and communities is the re-creation of a sense of safety and interdependence. Often, fellow victims provide the most effective short-term bond because the shared history of trauma forms the nucleus of retrieving a sense of community. Sharing a common experience in the past sets the stage for better understanding and bearing the continuing pain in the present.

Individual Versus Group Therapy

Although group interventions after large-scale traumatic experiences such as manmade or natural disasters are generally thought to be very effective (Lystad 1988; Raphael 1986; Solomon 1988), people with histories of chronic intrafamilial trauma initially benefit most from individual therapy. Disclosing the trauma, expressing related feelings, and establishing a trusting relationship with another person allow these individuals to explore emotions, to retrieve memories, and to understand current behaviors as reactivations of past experience. Provided that a degree of safety is established in the individual therapy relationship, a trauma victim can begin confronting the residual shame and vulnerability. Discussing the events and their impact on the patient's current life has an organizing effect. It allows patients to distinguish between past powerlessness and current options and to begin valuing current realities in a fresh light. This detailed examination of the patient's mental processes and memories cannot be replicated in the group therapy setting.

In individual therapy, however, there is an inherent inequality. It is a relationship between a therapist, the "helper," who implicitly has answers and is not helpless, and the patient, who needs help. In this setting the patient is continually confronted by his or her own passivity, dependency, and helplessness. Therefore, the individual therapy relationship has both strengths and limitations. Initially, it promotes a sense of safety, encouraging the fantasy of new strength as the relationship with the all-powerful therapist bestows a renewed sense of control to the patient (Pines 1981). But such emotional dependence conversely inhibits growth at later stages. Full-blown exploration of ambivalence and disappointment becomes difficult, especially for people for whom confrontation with powerful adults has been associated with fears of annihilation. Because trauma victims often have difficulty finding the right balance between initiative and dependency, support alone (as in an individual therapist relationship) may foster passivity and interfere with confronting the aggression.

Groups provide a setting for experimenting with different roles. In a group, positions of passivity alternate with those of activity and mutual support (Bard and Sangry 1987). Ventilating feelings and sharing experiences with people who have suffered through similar events promote the self-concept of being at once victim and survivor. Group therapists can encourage mutual support, explore resistances to taking an active role, and help patients to discuss hard-earned survival skills with others.

Principles of Group Therapy With Traumatized Patients

Group therapy has been used for victims of natural disasters (Raphael 1986; Lystad 1988), incest (Herman and Shatzow 1984), rape (Yassen and Glass 1984), spouse battering (Rounsaville et al. 1979), concentration camps (Danielli 1985), and war trauma (Lifton 1983; Parson 1984; Walker 1981). Regardless of the nature of the trauma or the structure of the group, the purpose of group therapy is to help individuals cope with the aftermath of trauma through the transformation, rather than reenactment, of their isolation, helplessness, hate, and pain. This is done by actively attending to the expression of the individual's, and others', histories and associated emotions.

As stated earlier, the task facing trauma-related groups is to explore and validate perceptions and emotions, to retrieve memories, and to understand current affects and behaviors as reactivations of past experience. Fear of reactivating the past is the central resistance in these groups, and many group problems are outgrowths of avoiding such recurrences. The most powerful protections against reactivating trauma are the very things undone by the trauma: predictability, structure, basic rules of safety, and continual awareness of the status of the therapeutic alliance.

There are two general categories of group therapy for people who have been exposed to catastrophic trauma. First are trauma-focused groups, which encompass a variety of short-term and long-term approaches. Groups that fall in this category include 1) acute crisis intervention for people affected by the same traumatic experience, such as a natural disaster, a kidnapping, or witnessing a homicide; and 2) extended homogeneous groups for people with a shared history of a past trauma, such as childhood incest, holocaust survival, war trauma, or having been held hostage. There are a large variety of self-help groups that define themselves according to the past traumas or the symptoms of their members.

In the second form of group therapy for this population, the long-term heterogeneous groups, the emphasis is less on the trauma itself and more on the exploration of interpersonal reenactments and the resolution of personality changes secondary to traumatization.

All these group modalities inherently focus on providing a safe place where physical or sexual assaults are unacceptable and where members can voice traumatic memories, expressing verbally what occurred and giving meaning to it. This is done by sharing grief about past helplessness and understanding the impact of the trauma on current feelings and relationships. Once the traumatic experiences have been located in time and place, individuals can begin differentiating between further life stresses and past trauma.

Acute Crisis Intervention Groups

In recent years, the mechanics of crisis intervention for victims of catastrophic trauma have been greatly improved, and this modality is now widely applied to communities hit by disasters (Raphael 1986; Lystad 1988; Solomon 1988). The essence of these groups is to provide a place where people can 1) feel safe from physical harm, 2) restore a sense of community and interpersonal belonging, 3) discern exactly what occurred, and 4) start giving voice to the meaning of the experience.

The mechanics of forming these groups need to be carefully considered, because every community has hierarchical structures and informal power relationships that need to be respected. Without the assistance of these structures, outside providers of group therapy are doomed to fail. Disaster intervention therapists must position themselves as consultants to existing hierarchical structures. They cannot vie for leadership with the natural spokespeople of the community. Furthermore, the natural leaders, in assuming their role, set an example in sharing the facts and feelings related to the disaster.

The identified community leaders need to be responsible for arranging the meeting time and place for all affected people. To set the frame for the crisis intervention, they also are responsible for explaining the details of the traumatic events and introducing the crisis intervention personnel. Once these personnel take the baton, they need to recapitulate what the community leaders have said and provide a simple introductory lecture about the expected psychological reactions to traumatic experiences. The lecture is best accompanied by easy-to-understand literature that will help affected individuals understand that they are not going crazy, but rather that their psychological reactions are normal responses to pathological events.

After these introductions, the affected group members are asked to go around the circle and detail the cognitive aspects of their experience: where they were, what they saw, and what they thought it meant. At this point, group members are actively discouraged from emotional reaction. This phase of the group process allows members to express their own experience in such a way that they make themselves understood and expand their connection with the group. The technique of going around the circle allows skilled mental health professionals to assess the vulnerability of each individual and the extent to which some individuals will need to be specifically invited for further therapy. Although people who cannot restrain their grief and anger are most easily identified (and most difficult to contain) at this point, it is the group members who pass the opportunity to speak, or who dismiss the seriousness of the disaster, who are perhaps most vulnerable to eventually developing PTSD.

After everyone has spoken, the members are asked to go around the circle a second time, this time emphasizing their emotional reactions to the events and to each other's stories. The group leader's task is to facilitate this process while promoting mutual support and containing the amount of emotion expressed. After 2 to 4 hours of allowing the group to express emotions and reactions to events (which inevitably unearths skeletons long since hidden in the communal closet), he or she gently brings the meeting to a close and arranges, with the community leaders, the site and time of the follow-up meeting(s). At the end of the second meeting, the details of further follow-up need to be negotiated, and a contract needs to be established about who will come and for how long. Generally, crisis intervention groups established in response to a community or workplace disaster meet with professionals not more than three or four times. After that, groups tend to disband, or the affected individuals take over the initiative for continuing the group, with professionals further utilized only as consultants.

Self-Help Groups

Self-help organizations for people with adult or childhood trauma, including parental addictions, have elaborate models of treatment that address many of the core issues of repetitive traumatization. These groups provide people with a cognitive frame for dealing with the residual sense of helplessness in predictable and ritualized human attachments. This process powerfully promotes a sense of meaning and belonging in the members. These groups focus on the development of "serenity"—a state of autonomic stability and of peace with one's surroundings. The groups teach that serenity is gained by developing spiritual values, that is, new meaning systems that transcend daily concerns and promote interdependence by helping people in (re)learning trust by surrendering and by making contact and developing interpersonal commitments. A support network, one that avoids the barriers that people create to bolster their individual differences and perpetuate social isolation, is formed.

In these circles it is said that "No pain is so devastating as the pain a person refuses to face and no suffering is so lasting as suffering left unacknowledged" (Cermak and Brown 1982). Everybody is encouraged to find words in which to frame the meaning of their personal experience. There is an emphasis on the here and now, with the knowledge that adults, in contrast to victimized children, can learn to protect themselves and can make a conscious choice about not engaging in relationships or behaviors that are known to be harmful. The underlying assumption is that conclusions drawn from a child's perspective retain their power into adulthood until verbalized and examined. In a group context, victims can finally learn that as children they were not responsible for the chaos, violence, and despair surrounding them, but that as adults there are choices and consequences (Cermak and Brown 1982; Sanford 1990).

The major drawback of self-help groups is that intragroup differences, competition, jealousies, and so forth cannot be addressed. All problems are viewed as being in the there and then, and the group is focused on survival in the here and now. Although this group approach is usually enormously helpful to a large variety of people with trauma histories, the lack of exploration of how the past affects present intragroup dynamics, dependency, and aggression is limiting. The group is handicapped in its attempts to effect the character change necessary to stop the likelihood that past trauma will continue to dominate the quality of contemporary interpersonal relations.

Time-Limited Homogeneous Groups

The essence of traumatization is the sense of having been deserted by all sources of protection. Traumatized individuals feel utterly alone and utterly ashamed of having been unable to prevent the trauma. This shame and self-blame tend to become the organizing forces in their lives, particularly in those who were assaulted by their own relatives. Making the past public is essential to overcome the shame and to abandon one's identity as a victim (Herman and Shatzow 1984; van der Kolk 1987); it requires active exposure and attention to other people's interests and difficulties.

The benefits of sharing one's experiences for the first time in the company of others who have undergone the same trauma cannot be overestimated. Individuals are allowed to express thoughts and feelings openly, to stop blaming themselves, and to give themselves permission to remember what happened. Group members lend each other words and facilitate the full experience of affects that often was unacceptable for so long. Sharing the trauma provides a sense of belonging and acceptance that was not possible before. The temporary illusion of fusion in groups of individuals who share a common trauma and the relative anonymity of the group effects temporary suspension of ambivalent and aggressive feelings. Thus the expression of emotions and memories becomes spontaneous and complete in a way that may not be achieved in individual therapy (Fox 1974; Pines 1983).

Furthermore, these groups encourage patients to use each other as mirrors to reflect traumatic memories and feelings. The groups are characterized by dependency rather than confrontation. Once group members overcome their initial distrust and shame, they rapidly establish a high degree of cohesion—a sense of us versus them (the dangerous world) (Pines 1985; van der Kolk 1985). The groups benefit greatly from a clear structure and boundaries. Because the groups are often quite stressful, members are required to have some social support and/or an individual psychotherapist and must be alcohol and drug free. Members contract to be present for the length of the group, usually 10 to 12 sessions and are asked to specify a realistic task that they will attempt to accomplish in this period. Frequently, they are given homework assignments.

Members are actively encouraged to fully share the memories of trauma and the progress of their self-imposed tasks within the group. The exploration of group process—including aggression, competition, and idealization—is interpreted as a resistance to the work of the group, which is the disclosure and sharing of trauma-related memories.

The intense feeling generated by disclosure promotes idealization of both the group itself and of the leader. The leader is often credited with much greater power than the leaders of other therapy groups. In the initial phases of homogeneous groups for trauma victims, group members tend to assume that they are all similar. This idealization seems gratifying for both therapist and members, but ultimately it operates as a resistance to overcoming helplessness and maintains the locus of control outside the individual. This intense pressure for sameness and fusion in groups of trauma victims and the difficulty in exploring intragroup aggression led Herman and Shatzow (1984) and others (Parson 1984; van der Kolk 1987) to recommend time-limited homogeneous groups followed by group therapy involving people with mixed diagnoses. The time limit prevents regressive fusion and avoids the formation of a block of victims united against a dangerous world, but conversely it promotes rapid bonding and sharing of emotionally sensitive material. As Parson (1985) remarked: "Since individuation is the goal of group treatment, persistent group we-ness is a resistance to growth and separateness." The fact that the group will terminate soon always is an important focus: uncontrolled farewells are the hallmarks of trauma. Allowing these groups to continue over time prevents members from learning to mourn and fosters the development of a victim identity.

Heterogeneous, Long-Term Groups

People whose trauma has become integrated into the totality of their personality usually continue to repeat the anger, dependency, and betrayal of their relationships with lovers, therapists, and bosses at the expense of gratifying peer relationships. In heterogeneous, transference-oriented trauma groups, the social expressions of these fears are invariably re-created and are readily observable by fellow members, the therapist, and the patients themselves. Those with adequate prior individual therapy are especially able to recognize and label their actions. The recapitulation of the affects and behaviors associated with the trauma of these patients in the group psychotherapy setting can lead to a capacity for interpersonal relatedness, boundary maintenance, conflict resolution, and intimacy. The work of the group includes, but is not confined to, sharing one's traumatic past fully as a part of one's life experience and tolerating other people's pain. Group members need to acknowledge both their trauma-related pain and their sadism. In order to facilitate attention to the details of the experience of others without automatically assuming sameness, it is advisable to recruit members from a variety of backgrounds.

Before unearthing the traumatic roots of current behavior, patients need to stabilize their current life situation. They must also gain reasonable control over the longstanding secondary defenses (e.g., alcohol and drug abuse and violence against self or others) that were originally elaborated to defend against being overwhelmed. The trauma can be dealt with only after some sense of safety and a capacity for self-care have been established. In contrast to traumatic events or relationships, which are unpredictable, uncontrollable, physical, and bewildering, therapy groups must have firm boundaries to be useful to traumatized individuals. Times of meetings, rules about absences and vacations, methods of payment, nature of outside contacts allowed, use or prohibition of physical contact in the group, and the amount of notice to be given before termination all need to be unambiguously clear and defined.

The members idealize the group and the leader at the expense of self-esteem. People with abusive backgrounds need to tackle the issue of safety before the group can truly be a therapeutic force for them. Disclosure of details of traumatic experiences promotes the development of a narcissistic alliance, which often becomes the germ that leads to an indispensable group cohesion. This sense of commitment to the whole transcends individual alliances and allegiance to the group leader. The gradual shift from a narcissistic alliance to an object-related working alliance is largely a function of the capacity of the group leader to tolerate and explore primitive and aggressive feelings, particularly those directed at disappointing parental transference figures.

When the group members discover that neither compliance nor idealization of the leader can ward off a repetition of trauma-related affects, a crisis of confidence occurs in which disappointment and aggression with the group and toward the leader need to be addressed. Traumatized individuals often elevate their therapists into cult heroes, which perpetuates a personal sense of helplessness. This helplessness is covered over by the illusion of the group's omnipotence through identification with a leader who is regarded without conscious ambivalence. The idealization must be vigorously addressed and interpreted. Only after the traumatized group member starts tackling the leader's real and imagined shortcomings can he or she really start to see himself or herself as useful and powerful. Only then do group members regain a sense of individual effectiveness (Alonso and Rutan 1984; Horowitz 1971). The group therapist must be prepared to absorb the full force of the negative transference that is unleashed when the group members become aware that the members, not the leader, are the agents of therapeutic change in the group—a step absolutely necessary for overcoming trauma-related learned helplessness (Pines 1985).

As individual members take increasing risks in revealing painful and traumatic experiences and become increasingly capable of tolerating and expressing aggressive and tender feelings without fear of annihilation, their self-efficacy and their ability to help others improve. Group focus on relationships among members allows new losses to be experienced as object losses with concomitant grief and sadness, rather than as narcissistic injuries with the accompanying feelings of helplessness, numbing, or vengeful rage. This transition must be made before the group can start receiving the full benefit of the strengths that many victims developed to survive catastrophic trauma. At this point, the therapeutic capacity of the group far surpasses the therapeutic benefits of the individual therapist.

Resistances

The central resistance in long-term trauma groups is the fear that the trauma will be reactivated by talking about it. Many group problems can be understood as outgrowths of avoiding such recurrences. It is important to realize that this concern is well founded: Traumatized people are prone to reexperience affects, behaviors, and memories of the trauma when exposed to stimuli that remind them of it. Avoiding acknowledgment of the trauma-related feelings, however, promotes acting out. The patients must learn that experiencing trauma-related feelings does not bring back the trauma and its accompanying violence and helplessness.

Group members deal with the current threat of reactivation with the same coping strategies employed for the original trauma. These include dissociation, passivity, and identification with the aggressor. Avoidance of revictimization comes in many guises. It can surface as avoidance of intragroup aggression by a commonly held illusion of sameness. In identifying with aggressors, members often actively demonstrate to the group how they were victimized, and they reenact their victimization as either subject or object with other members. Because traumatized families are characterized by sadism, passivity, revictimization, and attribution of blame to the weakest member of the family, these patterns invariably will make their appearance in the group.

People who have had to accommodate assaultive caregivers or lovers learn that dependency is hazardous (Pines 1983). Fearful of renewed betrayal and subjugation, many develop a "myth of self-sufficiency." They believe that they will become secure only if they can become fully self-reliant. They tend to hide underlying feelings of emptiness, loneliness, and fear by overfunctioning or with acts of bravado, including antisocial behavior. One common solution is to attach oneself to an even more troubled mate. In this relationship, the individual fulfills the dual purpose of hiding his or her own dependency needs and exerting a restitutive influence on someone who embodies his or her own sense of inadequacy.

Normal envy, competition, assertiveness, sharing, and intimacy are particularly delicate in trauma groups, because most patients have few or no recent experiences of successful negotiation around these issues. In one-to-one relationships, traumatized patients have great difficulty establishing the right to disagree and to express hateful feelings, believing they will annihilate themselves or the therapist. Thus for the sake of safeguarding the integrity of the individual relationship, large areas of a person's psychological life are sacrificed. In groups, it is easy to recognize the price paid for such avoidance. Confrontation, at best a thorny problem in individual therapy, can be modulated in groups by the simultaneous offer of support and empathic identification.

Throughout the life of the group, there is a tension between the insistence on acting out old and familiar patterns and the validation of current experience. The fundamental counterbalance to projections is empathy, which entitles people to their own distress (Alonso and Rutan 1984; Horowitz 1971). The group leader should avoid being seen as the fount of empathy, but he or she should quietly reinforce empathic stances by group members, so that the power of the group is located in the members, not in the leader.

Conclusions

Posttraumatic stress is not primarily concerned with unconscious intrapsychic conflicts, but rather with haunting memories that can affect victims' capacity for hope, intimacy, trust, competition, and aggression. Although the therapist is often drawn into serving the patients' dependent and narcissistic needs, posttraumatic symptoms themselves do not supply secondary gain. Interpretation alone cannot undo the damage caused by traumatic experiences, although it may clarify the past and help the patient deal with the consequences of the trauma (A. Freud 1974). Group psychotherapy reestablishes a peer group in which sharing and reliving common experiences may facilitate self-efficacy and the promises and limitations of trust. By experiencing the effect of others on themselves and vice versa, patients can learn to modulate their responses to others according to today's requirements, rather than the demands of past trauma. This facilitates the process of growing, which was arrested by the trauma.

References

Alonso A, Rutan S: The experience of shame and the restoration of self respect in group psychotherapy. Int J Group Psychother 38:3–14, 1984

Bard M, Sangry D: The Crime Victim's Book, 2nd Edition. New York, Brunner/Mazel, 1987

Becker E: The Denial of Death. New York, Free Press, 1973

Blos P: The Adolescent Passage. New York, International Universities Press, 1979

Bowlby J: Violence in the family as a disorder of the attachment and caregiving systems. Am J Psychoanal 44:9–27, 1984

Cermak TL, Brown S: Interactional group psychotherapy with adult children of alcoholics. Int J Group Psychother 32:375–389, 1982

Cicchetti D: The emergence of developmental psychopathology. Child Dev 55:1–7, 1984

Danielli Y: The treatment and prevention of long-term effects and intergenerational transmission of victimization: a lesson from Holocaust survivors and their children, in Trauma and Its Wake, Vol 1. Edited by Figley CR. New York, Brunner/Mazel, 1985, pp 295–313

Davidson S: Human reciprocity among the Jewish prisoners of the Nazi concentration camps, in Proceedings of the Yad Vashem International Historical Conference. Jerusalem, Yad Vashem, 1984, pp 555–572

Ferenczi S: Confusion of tongues between the adult and the child: the language of tenderness and the language of passion, in Final Contributions to the Problems and Methods of Psychoanalysis. London, Hogarth Press, 1955, pp 156–167

Fox RP: Narcissistic rage and the problem of combat aggression. Arch Gen Psychiatry 31:807–811, 1974

Freud A: A psychoanalytic view of developmental psycho-pathology. Journal of the Philadelphia Association of Psychoanalysis 1:7–17, 1974

Freud S: Introduction to psychoanalysis and the war neuroses (1919), in The Standard Edition of the Complete Psychological Works of Sigmund Freud, Vol 17. Translated and edited by Strachey J. London, Hogarth Press, 1954, pp 207–210

Freud S: Group psychology and analysis of the ego (1921), in The Standard Edition of the Complete Psychological Works of Sigmund Freud, Vol 18. Translated and edited by Strachey J. London, Hogarth Press, 1955, pp 69–143

Green AH: Child Maltreatment. New York, Jason Aronson, 1989

Grunebaum H, Solomon L: Toward a theory of peer relationships, II: on the stages of social development and their relationship to group psychotherapy. Int J Group Psychother 32:283–307, 1982

Gutheil T: Borderline personality disorder, boundary violations and patient-therapist sex: medico-legal implications. Am J Psychiatry 146:597–602, 1989

Herman JL, Shatzow E: Time limited group psychotherapy for women with a history of incest. Int J Group Psychother 34:605–610, 1984

Horowitz L: A group-centered approach to group psychotherapy. Int J Group Psychother 27:423–439, 1971

Lifton R: The Broken Connection. New York, Basic Books, 1983

Lindy JD, Titchener J: Acts of God and man: long term character change in survivors of disasters and the law. Behavioral Science and the Law 1:85–96, 1983

Lystad M: Mental Health Response to Mass Emergencies. New York, Brunner/Mazel, 1988

Parson ER: The role of psychodynamic group psychotherapy in the treatment of the combat veteran, in Psychotherapy of the Combat Veteran. Edited by Schwartz HJ. New York, Spectrum Publications, 1984, pp 153–220

Parson ER: Posttraumatic accelerated cohesion: its recognition and management in group treatment of Vietnam veterans. Group 9:10–23, 1985

Pines M: The frame of reference in group psychotherapy. Int J Group Psychother 31:275–285, 1981

Pines M: Psychoanalysis and group analysis. Int J Group Psychother 33:155–170, 1983

Pines M: Psychic development and the group analytic situation. Group 9:60–73, 1985

Quarentelli EL: An assessment of conflicting views on mental health: the consequences of traumatic events, in Trauma and Its Wake, Vol 1. Edited by Figley CR. New York, Brunner/Mazel, 1985, pp 173–215

Rajecki DW, Lamb ME, Obmascher P: Toward a general theory of infantile attachment: a comparative review of aspects of the social bond. The Behavioral and Brain Sciences 3:417–464, 1978

Raphael B: When Disaster Strikes: How Individuals and Communities Cope With Catastrophe. New York, Basic Books, 1986

Reiker PP, Carmen E: The victim-to-patient process: the disconfirmation and transformation of abuse. Orthopsychiatry 56:360–370, 1986

Rounsaville B, Lifton N, Bieber M: The natural history of a psychotherapy group for battered women. Psychiatry 42:63–78, 1979

Russell DEH: Sexual Exploitation: Rape, Child Sexual Abuse and Workplace Harassment. Beverly Hills, CA, Sage Publications, 1984

Sanford L: Strong at the Broken Places. New York, Random House, 1990

Sharp V: Adolescence, in Child Development in Normalcy and Psychopathology. Edited by Bemporad J. New York, Brunner/Mazel, 1980, pp 175–218

Solomon DS: Mobilizing social support networks in times of disaster, in Trauma and Its Wake, Vol 2. Edited by Figley CR. New York, Brunner/Mazel, 1988, pp 232–263

van der Kolk BA: Adolescent vulnerability to post traumatic stress disorder. Psychiatry 48:365–370, 1985

van der Kolk BA: Psychological Trauma. Washington, DC, American Psychiatric Press, 1987

van der Kolk BA: The compulsion to repeat the trauma: reenactment, re-victimization and masochism. Psychiatr Clin North Am 12:389–411, 1989

Walker JI: Group psychotherapy with Vietnam veterans. Int J Group Psychother 31:379–389, 1981

Yassen J, Glass L: Sexual assault survivor groups. Social Work 37:252–257, 1984

PART IV

Special Considerations

CHAPTER 17

Combined Individual and Group Psychotherapy

Kenneth Porter, M.D.

Introduction

Combined individual and group therapy is a unique treatment approach. More than just the sum of its parts, it stands on its own as a modality. Some therapists believe it to be the treatment of choice for many outpatient disorders. Combined therapy has its own history, mechanism of action, indications and contraindications, developmental stages, and approach to transference, countertransference, and resistance. In presenting the considerable literature on combined treatment, I try to balance my own point of view with that of other authors and to add clinical case material from my own and others' practices, so that theory may come alive for the reader.

History

Two pioneers in group therapy, Louis Wender and Aaron Stein, published an article in 1949 outlining the use of combined therapy in a psychiatric outpatient clinic in New York State (Wender and Stein 1949). Practitioners soon established combined therapy as a field in its own right. Over 25 articles outlined the theory of the new approach and its use for special patient populations and dealt with technical issues, including transference, countertransference, and resistance. In 1964 the *International Journal of Group Psychotherapy* recognized the growing stature of the field by publishing the first collection of articles on combined therapy, the proceedings of an American Group Psychotherapy Association symposium. This collection included articles and discussions by Aronson, Bieber, Cappon, Durkin, Rosenbaum, Sager, and Stein (Symposium on Combined and Individual Group Therapy 1964).

The 1970s were quieter. The decade was highlighted by the appearance of the first review articles on combined therapy, by Toby Bieber (1971) and Benjamin Sadock (1975), and the first book on the subject, a text by Ormont and Strean arguing in favor of "conjoint psychoanalysis" with two different therapists (Ormont and Strean 1978).

Since 1980 combined treatment has come of age. Three more major review articles by Scheidlinger and Porter (1980), Wong (1983), and Sadock (1985) were followed by another book, a comprehensive text by Caligor et al.(1984), by major articles including those of Alonso and Rutan (1982) and Swiller (1988), and by another major collection of articles and commentary, published in *Group,* including contributions by Alonso and Rutan, Bernstein, Caligor, Fieldsteel, Weinblatt, and Wright (Porter and Edwards 1990).

For readers particularly interested in the historical background of combined therapy, the literature has been reviewed several times by Wong (1983) and by myself (Porter 1980; Scheidlinger and Porter 1980).

Mechanisms of Action of Combined Therapy

There are two major processes through which combined therapy exerts its therapeutic influence. These may be called *complementarity* and *potentiation.* Complementarity refers to the fact that individual therapy and group therapy bring unique advantages to the therapeutic arena. Each provides something the other lacks. Potentiation means that each modality increases the effectiveness of the other, in addition to simply supplementing it.

Complementarity

Referring to complementarity, Sadock (1985) stated that

> Most workers in the field think that combined therapy has the advantage of both the dyadic setting and the group setting, without sacrificing the qualities of either. . . . The modality seems to bring problems to the surface

and to effect their resolution more quickly than might be possible with either method alone. (p. 1423)

Intrapsychic exploration.   Individual therapy allows for deep intrapsychic exploration. By the very fact of who is and is not present, individual treatment permits a deep level of intrapsychic work, including work on transference and genetic material, that is probably unmatched by any other psychotherapeutic modality. This seems especially important for the psychotic and severe pre-oedipal character disorders, including borderline and narcissistic syndromes. In all these conditions, according to our present understanding, the psychodynamic difficulties date from the years of childhood development primarily dominated by a dyadic relationship and hence may be effectively dealt with by returning to that situation therapeutically. There is considerable controversy about this position, which is discussed later in this chapter.

This principle is not confined to these more severe disorders, however, but applies to the broad range of character disorders seen in outpatient practice as well.

Interpersonal exploration.   Group therapy allows for broad interpersonal exploration. The mirror image of the capacity of individual treatment to deal with intrapsychic issues is the capacity of the group to deal with interpersonal issues. This has long been acknowledged as the major source of group therapy's effectiveness. Interpersonal exploration occurs in the following ways:

1. Multiple transferences can be explored. Group therapy allows a patient to work on multiple transferences simultaneously (for example, experiences of parents, siblings, or grandparents). This allows for both the resolution of multiple dyadic transference relationships and also the resolution of triadic transferences, with their attendant experiences of competitiveness and jealousy.
2. Group therapy allows for a corrective family experience. In group therapy there is the simultaneous nurturing presence of a range of family-like figures that may not have been present in earlier years.
3. Group therapy serves as a laboratory for risking new behaviors. The dyadic relationship in individual psychotherapy is deliberately structured to create a difference in roles between patient and therapist. This difference in roles, which includes (among others) differences in power and freedom of expression, is useful in promoting transfer-

ence, regression, and a concentration on intrapsychic issues in the patient and in promoting objectivity in the therapist. These advantages are bought at a price, however. Certain peer behaviors are not easily enacted by the patient toward the therapist. In group therapy, on the other hand, these role and power differences are not present among group members. This naturally allows for the group to become a testing ground for all those peer-oriented interpersonal skills that patients need to refine, such as effective self-assertion, constructive expression of anger, effective expression of dependency needs, and less guilt-ridden and anxiety-ridden expression of sexual feelings.

4. Group therapy resolves characterological difficulties unique to social situations. Group therapy allows for the emergence and resolution of obstacles to growth that are different from those that emerge in the dyadic situation. Therefore, it allows for the resolution of different resistances and elicits different aspects of our personalities and different difficulties. All group therapists regularly report surprise when a patient who is submissive in individual treatment turns out to be a "tiger" in the group, or when a relaxed individual therapy patient is overwhelmed by anxiety in group. Those aspects of an individual's personality that cause difficulty in social situations emerge spontaneously in the group, allowing their exploration and resolution. The psychotherapy group becomes a microcosm of society and hence can take on, where necessary, the social functions that may have been absent in the background of a patient. This may be especially important in the development of social values, a function for which society usually supplements the family in a child's maturation.

5. Group therapy provides special forms of ego support. The group situation allows for the provision of certain types of experiences that individual therapy, constrained by going for "bigger psychoanalytic game," usually does not provide (e.g., personal feelings by other group members, direct encouragement, and advice-giving).

Potentiation

So far I have discussed the ways in which group therapy and individual therapy with their own strengths naturally complement each other when joined together. Each modality adds capabilities that the other lacks. There are also ways in which the two modalities are not only additive but also magnify each other's strengths so that the resulting mixture is even more than simply the sum of its parts.

Effect of individual therapy on group therapy. Individual therapy can prevent group therapy dropouts. When an impulsive patient has a strong negative reaction to a group session that may not be apparent in the group, the therapist in an individual session can provide support and further exploration, at times avoiding a group dropout.

For this reason, many group therapists believe that concurrent individual treatment decreases the likelihood of dropouts from group therapy (see, for example, Caligor 1977). An important verification of this opinion was provided by Stone and Rutan (1984). These two senior group therapists provided their personal experience to the professional community in an article presenting data on the length of time their group therapy patients remained in treatment and on the reasons for differences in length of stay. For one therapist the dropout rate was 38% without concurrent individual treatment versus 11% when concurrent treatment was present. For the other, the corresponding figures were 56% and 19%. Concurrent individual therapy cut the rate of dropping out from group therapy to approximately one-third of the rate without individual treatment.

Individual therapy can explore deeper intrapsychic material after a group effectively confronts a patient's character defenses. The following case example illustrates both ways in which individual psychotherapy can potentiate group therapy:

Case 1

Ms. A started therapy at age 35 at the insistence of her fiance, who was already in treatment. Two of the issues that emerged were her feelings about two subsequent miscarriages, without apparent medical cause, and a fear of speaking in social situations that had bedeviled her for many years, prevented her from rising in her job, and caused her to drop out of numerous college classes. Understandably, Ms. A was frightened to start group therapy. She agreed with the recommendation when I made it, but was afraid she would not be able to prevent herself from shamefacedly leaving the session when she became anxious. After an initial period of several months of anxiety in the group, she became one of the group's most active and dedicated defenders.

What became clear in the group was the connection between Ms. A's anxiety and the emergence of a forbidden feeling, usually an angry or a competitive one. The group, and especially the women, repeatedly tried to work with Ms. A in a rather gentle way on her avoidance of these feelings. Each time this happened, she would come in to her individual session announcing quite forthrightly that she was being attacked, that she was not going to take it, and that she planned to leave the group. As she was quite impulsive, this was not to be taken as just empty words. Each time the possibility that she really did have angry and competitive feelings was explored in the individual session, and we clarified the genetic roots of this problem.

As a result of this work, Ms. A gradually made progress on her phobic behavior. In school she was able to stay in class and do well in a number of courses that previously were impossible for her to take, with a great lifting of shame and a feeling of pride and accomplishment. Perhaps coincidentally, she was also able to convince her husband to adopt a child, which was her lifelong dream, and which brought Ms. A great and sustained joy.

Effect of group therapy on individual therapy.   Group therapy facilitates the resolution of transferences that are difficult to resolve in individual treatment alone. Many patients, especially those suffering from pre-oedipal conditions, develop transferences in individual treatment that may be difficult to resolve. Examples are 1) the transference of the patient who "has no transference"—"I just don't have feelings like that for you" (this may be especially prominent in narcissistic or obsessional patients); 2) the extremely dependent, clinging transference; 3) the unremittingly demanding and angry borderline transference; and 4) the critical and guarded paranoid transference.

Group therapy facilitates the resolution of character defenses (resistances) that are difficult to resolve in individual therapy. In a therapy group, spontaneous emotional interaction is requested of every patient by the therapist. It is the equivalent of "the basic rule" of free association in traditional psychoanalysis. But because the patient has characterological defenses that, unbeknownst to him or her, interfere with his or her effective interpersonal functioning, the patient will be unable to fully comply with the request to relate freely and openly. In the group interaction character defenses will immediately emerge, such as withdrawal, intellectualization, projection, grandiosity, withholding, impulsivity, or seductiveness. These character defenses may be easier to work with in group than in individual sessions for the following reasons. First, the defenses may not show up in the individual situation if they are elicited more by peer interaction than by hierarchical interaction. Second, other group members may provide feedback and may also serve as objects for observation of what is denied in the self of the patient but may be more easily seen in another.

Group therapy creates a culture that supports the values of personal

growth. Contrary to those who see psychotherapy as a value-free enterprise, I believe that our therapy is constantly shot through with values and
that this is a necessary and useful aspect of our work. Certain values, such
as honesty, caring, and the importance of emotional life, seem inextrica-
bly connected to the psychological healing we perform. Because values
are transmitted by families and cultures, and because the therapy group
becomes a new "family" and "subculture" for the patient, the group also
becomes a carrier of positive values. I believe the support for these values
offered by the presence of the therapy group is itself an additional healing factor in combined therapy, as the following case example illustrates:

Case 2

Ms. B was able to stay in individual treatment at one point only because of
her strong tie to her therapy group. At first, therapy proceeded well. In
twice-weekly individual treatment, to which group was later added, Ms. B
developed a positive relationship with me and fell in love with and married
a man with whom she seemed happy. As her therapy deepened, however,
the situation changed. Over a period of years, she seemed unable to
change her job situation, and she developed a powerful negative transference with strong paranoid and masochistic elements that resisted all attempts at resolution. During this time she continued to work productively
in the group. Ultimately she terminated her individual treatment and continued only in the group, making it clear that she felt inches away from
terminating treatment altogether.

Case 2 has an apparently happy ending that I will relate later in the
chapter. For now what is important is that her strong ties to the group
enabled Ms. B to survive a difficult period in her therapy and to go on to
complete important psychological work that was almost left undone.

Objections to Combined Therapy

In spite of this impressive list of benefits associated with combined treatment, many therapists believe that combined therapy is an inferior approach. The objections have come from group therapists and individual
psychoanalysts alike. In each case the criticism has been the same: that
the combined modality interferes with the full effectiveness of the solo
approach, which is considered superior in efficacy.

Many of the earliest group psychotherapists were individual psychoanalysts who felt they had discovered a superior form of treatment in group therapy. Because of enthusiasm for their new discoveries, the natural tendency of new systems to reject the old, or hostility from individual psychoanalysts, many early group therapists rejected any admixture of individual treatment into the new group modality they had discovered. They felt that individual sessions would drain off the anxiety, transference, and other deep material that was necessary for the full functioning of the psychoanalytic group.

Wolf and Schwartz (1962), although not uniformly rejecting combined therapy, stated their belief that exclusive group therapy was preferable. Foulkes (1964) did the same, although at least in certain stages of his work he practiced a dilute form of combined treatment (seeing group patients individually every 2 months). Ezriel's position (1957) was similar. More recently, Whitaker and Lieberman (1964) and Yalom (1975) also agreed. It is of interest that many of these group therapists preferred a pattern of intensive group therapy for their patients with groups meeting twice weekly or more frequently, rather than the once-a-week format most common now in the United States.

On the other side of the argument, many traditional individual psychoanalysts have maintained for years that the use of group therapy concurrently with psychoanalysis would significantly vitiate the individual treatment. This point of view was based on the idea that the therapy group would become an arena for the acting out of conflicts that properly belonged within the analytic sphere; therefore, a proper transference neurosis, considered essential for the curative action of psychoanalysis, would either not develop or would not be analyzable.

This position has gradually diminished in importance for a number of reasons. In the case of individual psychoanalysis, the emphasis on the development of a transference neurosis as the sine qua non of a successful analysis—as opposed to the interpretation of transference more broadly understood—has gradually diminished. At the same time, the accumulated experience of psychoanalytically oriented group therapists that it is indeed possible to work in depth with transference in the group setting also has tended to make this argument obsolete. Some psychoanalytic group therapists, such as Durkin and Glatzer (1973), even argued that it is possible within the group to develop and resolve a full transference neurosis.

In summary, I believe the original discovery of group psychotherapy led to a rigidification of positions among both individual and group therapists regarding the efficacy of each other's methods. As time has softened earlier positions, and as each field has grown more mature, less defensive, and more flexible, there is less enmity and more appreciation by analysts and group therapists alike of each other's contributions and less antagonism to combined treatment as well.

Indications and Contraindications for Combined Therapy

Who Should Be in Combined Therapy?

Clinicians fall into two camps when discussing the indications for combined treatment. There are those, including myself, who believe that combined therapy is basically the treatment of choice for most disorders seen by psychotherapists on an outpatient basis. These would include most personality disorders (including borderline and narcissistic conditions), most impulsive or addictive disorders (relating to substances, food, sex, and behavior), most depressive and anxiety disorders, and many outpatient psychotic conditions (Scheidlinger and Porter 1980). A somewhat different position, but one that also recommends combined therapy for a broad range of conditions, was taken by Caligor et al. (1984), who advocated the use of combined treatment to facilitate the working-through process of psychoanalytic treatment in general.

The other and, judging from the literature at least, more prevalent position is that combined therapy is a valuable form of treatment, with specific indications that differ both from the indications for group therapy alone and from the indications for individual psychoanalytic treatment. Good examples of this position can be found in the articles by Alonso and Rutan (1982) and Wong (1983).

Alonso and Rutan (1982) listed several types of patients for who combined treatment is indicated, including patients who cannot produce sufficient material in either individual or group treatment alone, patients who wish to work more deeply (intrapsychically) or broadly (interpersonally) than either solo modality will allow, patients who are frightened or in crisis and who need the support possible in the combined modality, and patients who elicit major countertransference difficulties.

Who Should Not Be in Combined Therapy?

Interestingly enough, there is greater agreement in the field on the contraindications for combined treatment. There are basically four types of patients for whom combined therapy is contraindicated (Alonso and Rutan 1982).

Patients referred for combined therapy as a resistance to a difficulty in either their individual psychotherapy or their group psychotherapy. Alonso and Rutan (1982) stated this position very clearly:

> First and foremost, it is an error to add another modality when such an addition is a resistance to something in the original therapy. That is a fundamental error all too often made. The first consideration one should make when a patient is being considered for the addition of group therapy to individual therapy for example, is, "does this request represent the wish to avoid confronting something important in the individual therapy?" That avoidance, by the way, can often be on the part of the referring therapist, as well as on the part of the patient. (pp. 273–274)

However, even these wise words must be tempered with a word of caution. Occasionally one gets a referral for group therapy from an individual therapist, for example, and it becomes apparent that some difficulty exists in the individual treatment with which both patient and therapist are struggling. At times it does not seem possible to be of help to the individual therapist directly, and indeed the referral may be a conscious or unconscious request on the part of one or both parties for help. As we live in an imperfect world, sometimes it may be the better part of clinical wisdom to proceed with combined treatment, knowing that one is offering both patient and therapist a potential exit from an otherwise untenable situation.

Certain severely borderline or narcissistic patients who cannot tolerate the anxiety induced by group treatment.   For a new patient in group therapy, the group is a less protected environment than the individual session. Two common sources of anxiety are the emotional honesty that prevails in the group, which can stimulate intolerable unconscious feelings in the new patient, and the experience of sharing the therapist with other group members, which can deprive the new patient of a selfobject tie with the therapist that was previously used to maintain emotional stability. Many severely borderline and narcissistic patients may experience so much anxiety in the group setting that only individual treatment is productive. For some of these patients, combined treatment may be useful after a prolonged period of individual treatment has strengthened the ego. For others, combined treatment may never be appropriate.

Patients not appropriate for group therapy in accordance with the usual contraindications for group. These include patients who are extremely paranoid, shy, monopolistic, psychopathic, psychotic, suicidal, or in crisis. Naturally these criteria are not absolute and should be applied with flexibility by the clinician to meet the needs of specific individual situations.

Patients with focal neurotic symptoms who either have no significant underlying personality disorder or no interest in changing an underlying personality disorder. In our present state of knowledge such individuals may be treated with behavior therapy (which, of course, can be carried out in a time-limited behavior therapy group), pharmacotherapy, or classical analysis, depending on the resources and inclination of both patient and therapist.

Initiation of Treatment

The most common way to start combined therapy is for a patient already in dyadic treatment to enter a group led by his or her individual therapist or by another therapist. This probably reflects the fact that in the private practice of psychotherapy, individual treatment is still considered the norm, and even most group therapists spend a large part of their professional time in the practice of individual psychotherapy. (In clinics and agencies exigencies of time and money often necessitate a choice between individual or group treatment for a given patient, and combined therapy is less common.)

Ways to Initiate Combined Therapy

Starting group and individual therapy simultaneously. In most cases, starting group and individual therapy simultaneously may overload both patient and therapist with more issues than can be productively handled. It seems simpler, and less stressful for all parties, to take on one new challenge at a time. However, as Alonso and Rutan (1990) pointed out, starting both modalities at once does have the advantage of giving a clear message that group therapy is equal in value to individual therapy. It also avoids the patient's feeling of losing an exclusive relationship with the therapist if he or she were to enter a group after having been in individual therapy only.

Starting with group therapy and adding individual therapy.   Combined therapy can certainly be initiated with group treatment, with individual therapy added later. Indeed, this is probably the most useful way to proceed for two groups of patients. First, patients who have had prolonged experiences with individual treatment, either successful or unsuccessful, may be disinclined to initiate yet another period of individual therapy. Where individual treatment has been successful but incomplete, group therapy may be correctly perceived as offering fresh opportunities to approach previously unsolved problems. Where individual treatment has been less successful, group treatment may be either correctly or incorrectly seen as a completely different approach that may prove effective where individual treatment did not. Under these circumstances, it is often clinically wise to support the patient's choice to start group therapy alone. In the therapist's mind the possibility of combined therapy may remain as a potential for the future. The second group of patients for whom initiating combined therapy with group therapy alone may be appropriate are those with a strong fear of intimacy, for whom the prolonged contact of one-to-one treatment may at first prove intolerable.

Starting combined therapy with individual treatment and then adding group therapy.   This is the more usual way to initiate combined therapy. It has several advantages. First, the initial issues of starting treatment can be handled in the individual therapy framework. The urgent practical problems with which people usually enter treatment, the task of forming a working alliance, and the beginning emergence of transference and resistance do not have to burden the therapy group, which is freer to concentrate on its own here-and-now activities. Second, the anxieties stirred up by entry into the therapy group can be dealt with in the context of a more secure therapeutic alliance with the therapist and a more experienced and reflective ego in the patient. Third, by the time the patient enters group therapy, it is likely that the therapist will possess a fairly good understanding of the patient's major characterological and transferential issues.

A pattern of combined therapy commonly practiced today in the United States is for the individual therapist and the group therapist to be the same person. The theory and practice of this pattern of combined therapy were clearly outlined in an early article by Aronson (1964) and more recently in the book by Caligor et al. (1984).

Issues in Initiating Combined Therapy

The individual therapist needs to consider several issues when adding group therapy to a patient's treatment plan. These include 1) the timing of the recommendation; 2) when a session added to the patient's schedule should be group rather than individual; 3) the manner of the recommendation, and what is actually said to the patient; and 4) the technical question of whether the frequency of the patient's individual sessions should be decreased and the related question of whether the patient's fees should be decreased if the patient requests it.

The timing of adding group to individual treatment.   The traditional recommendation for when to add group to individual therapy was succinctly stated by Caligor et al. (1984):

> The therapist considers adding group when he or she feels that aspects of the therapy best dealt with in individual therapy have been accomplished; when there is a collaborative understanding of history as related to current functioning; when there is an awareness of the quality of the transference; and when there is a solid working alliance. (p. 40)

Whether an additional session should be individual or group.   Another issue that frequently arises, especially for the psychoanalytically oriented therapist, is whether to add an additional individual session to a patient's weekly treatment schedule rather than a group session, if an intensification of treatment is being considered. Here clinicians probably need to be guided by a combination of factors, including their own ideological preference for group or individual treatment, the preference and resistance of the patient, the nature of the patient's difficulties, exigencies of time and money, and how often the patient is already coming to individual treatment, to name just a few possible considerations.

In my own experience, I tend to be guided by what seem to be the patient's needs and by how well the patient is working in individual treatment. When the primary focus of the therapeutic work is intrapsychic rather than interpersonal, insofar as such a distinction can be made, and when the patient is working well in dyadic treatment, my inclination would be to recommend the addition of an individual rather than a group session. On the other hand, when the patient is struggling with interpersonal conflicts, and/or when the individual treatment seems not very productive, I may be inclined to recommend an additional session of group therapy, hoping that it will add a dimension to the treatment as well as facilitate the individual sessions.

How the recommendation should be made.   What can and should be said to the individual psychotherapy patient when the subject of group therapy is broached? Of course it is easiest for the clinician if the patient initiates the discussion, but this occurs in the minority of cases. Otherwise, if the therapist raises the subject, it is often useful to connect the recommendation to material that is current in the patient's treatment. If the choice of group therapy is a sound one, it should reflect ongoing dilemmas in the patient's life, and it will be most comprehensible to the patient if this connection is made manifest. Examples of this connection would be the recommendation of group therapy when the patient has been working on issues of isolation, difficulty being in touch with feelings, or interpersonal conflicts.

Some patients are immediately quite responsive to the idea of group therapy. When the patient is not responsive, it is usually best to explore whatever resistances may be present. If after this, the patient is still negative, it is best to drop the subject, respecting the patient's wishes and leaving open the possibility (in the therapist's mind, at least) of returning to the issue at a later date.

When the therapist is puzzled by apparently excessive resistance on the part of the patient to entering group therapy, it may be that a part of the patient's dynamics is not being understood by the therapist, as the following case example illustrates:

Case 3

Ms. C entered individual treatment in her late twenties. She desperately wanted to attend law school but had tried repeatedly to gain admission and failed. The child of concentration camp survivors, she had grown up with a sickly younger sister who had recently managed to enter law school herself. Growing up, the girls had contended with a narcissistic mother and a loving but depressed father. Both parents lived under the influence of their

World War II experiences, and the girls clung to each other in a highly competitive yet symbiotic existence, providing for each other what was unavailable from their parents.

During Ms C's treatment I repeatedly, and at times quite forcefully, recommended that she add group therapy to her treatment. The combination of her intense sibling rivalry with her sister plus her ongoing difficulty in relating to men seemed to make group therapy a natural for her. However, somewhat to my puzzlement, she steadfastly refused.

After 8 years her treatment changed dramatically when during one session I lost my temper with her, related to a longstanding pattern in her transference of objectifying me while maintaining an arrogant attitude. This unfortunate and useful event opened up profound issues in Ms. C's treatment. It became apparent that the lack of involvement with me that she had maintained throughout the 8 years had not prevented her from achieving certain goals, but it had limited her capacity to work out deeper interpersonal issues. As I understood better her transference resistance, and her therapy deepened, I understood why Ms. C had resisted group therapy for so long. Without being able to articulate it, she sensed that crucial issues needed to be raised and resolved in her transference relationship with me before she would feel secure enough to risk further anxiety in the group setting. The original recommendation on my part had been a technical error.

At times the clinician's judgment about adding group to individual therapy may be correct but premature. Caligor (1990) gave an excellent example:

George, a man in his early thirties, had come into treatment because of his use of cocaine and a series of brief intense affairs with women. . . . In three-times-a-week treatment, George made remarkable progress. He quickly formed an attachment, stopped the coke and slowed up on the race to get away from women. . . . However . . . in relationships with women he continued to first idealize and then be completely disillusioned. . . . It seemed like good timing for the introduction of group. Although George understood the history of his problems, he was experiencing minimal anxiety in the therapy session, where he felt safe. . . . Adding group seemed to be a good way of getting a more conflicted experience into therapy. The patient was anxious about the suggestion but he was willing to try it on the therapist's recommendation with the condition that if he didn't like it he would discontinue after a few sessions. At George's entry into the group he was obviously disorganized and confused to an extent that surprised his therapist. In his individual session George reported that he was re-experiencing some of the kind of anxiety that had initially brought him to treatment. . . . The group continued to generate unbearable anxiety for George. He did discontinue, going back to individual sessions only, where he gradually resumed productive treatment. A year and a half later he entered group at his own request. Functioning on a more integrated level, he was able to use the group productively. (pp. 20–21)

Whether the frequency of sessions and fees should be changed when the individual patient adds group to his treatment. A frequent issue that arises when a patient adds group therapy to individual therapy is a request from the patient to reduce the intensity of individual therapy. It has been my experience that in theory it is best to maintain the previous level of individual sessions. In fact, however, for reasons of both time and money, a patient may not always be able to adhere to this guideline.

The question of fees is dealt with differently according to the philosophy and needs of each clinician. In principle there seems nothing wrong with reducing fees somewhat to enable a patient to attend a more intensive therapy schedule, but the clinician needs to be alert to countertransference issues that involve a sense of coercing or "bribing" the patient.

Conjoint Therapy

Conjoint individual and group treatment (i.e., when the individual therapist and the group therapist are different people) is a common approach under two conditions: 1) when group therapy is desirable for a patient receiving individual treatment, and the patient's therapist does not lead therapy groups, and 2) when individual therapy is desirable for a patient receiving group therapy, and the group therapist either does not do individual therapy or has no available time.

Conjoint therapy has a number of distinct advantages. An especially clear article summarizing this approach (Ormont 1981) and a major book (Ormont and Strean 1978) exclusively devoted to conjoint therapy presented a detailed and sophisticated model for this form of treatment. As Alonso and Rutan (1982) concisely summarized it:

Ormont and Strean argued strongly for the use of two different therapists when group therapy and individual therapy are combined. They stressed the advantages to the patient of having multiple transference objects, multiple observers, multiple interpreters, multiple emotional resolvers, multiple therapeutic settings, multiple counter-transference reactions, and multiple ego states. (p. 275)

Among all of these advantages, the most important ones seem to be the opportunity for the patient to be exposed to different, potentially mutually enriching therapeutic approaches and the opportunity to work with multiple transferences, especially toward a male and female therapist, as the following case example illustrates:

Case 4

Mr. D, a single man in his early thirties, entered conjoint therapy when his analyst referred him to me for concurrent group therapy. A moderately successful attorney, Mr. D had had 4 years of analysis but remained unable to have a sexual or emotional relationship with a woman, although he was clearly heterosexual. A childhood with a narcissistic mother and a violent, abandoning, alcoholic father had left him with a combination of narcissistic and oedipal difficulties that so far had precluded successful heterosexual function.

Although this case had multiple factors that were difficult to tease apart, one factor that seemed to play a role was the difference in approaches of Mr. D's analyst and myself. Mr. D's analyst was experienced as warm and caring although he focused his interpretations at the oedipal level. I, on the other hand, was experienced as tough and fatherly, especially in the group context, where I encouraged the group to focus on Mr. D's narcissistic defenses against interpersonal involvement. The combination of a maternal approach that focused interpretively on oedipal factors and a confronting approach that dealt with narcissistic issues seemed of benefit to this patient.

However, the difficulties of the conjoint approach should not be underestimated. On the therapists' side, these include the possibility of major substantive disagreements between the two clinicians. On the patient's side, there is the danger of severe transference splitting, that is, the patient's dealing with the normal complexity of both loving and hating each therapist by directing positive feelings exclusively towards one therapist and negative feelings exclusively towards the other.

When conjoint therapy is being practiced, an open channel of communication must exist between both clinicians, and this must be understood and accepted by the patient. In my experience, this channel may be used for frequent phone consultations between the two therapists or may lie virtually unused for months or even years, except for very brief occasional chats. What is crucial is not how frequently the channel is used but that all parties are aware of and respect its existence. Virtually every instance of failed conjoint therapy in my own experience was character-ized (in retrospect, unfortunately) by insufficient communication be-tween myself and the individual therapist of the patient.

Which is preferable, combined or conjoint individual group therapy? Each clinician will probably reach his or her own conclusion; my own opinion is that it is probably not a crucial question. In fact, it is usually decided by the practical needs of the therapeutic situation (who is avail-able for what), and in my experience there is nothing wrong with that. Most experienced clinicians have probably seen enough excellent in-stances of each form of treatment, and enough questionable instances, to have overcome whatever initial biases they may have had on the issue.

The Middle Phase of Treatment: Working Through

Crucial to combined therapy is working through, that is, the session-to-session, repeated exploration of unconscious conflicts that can grad-ually lead to healing of the personality. I would like to concentrate on one particular aspect of working through, the different ways in which individual and group sessions may articulate with each other in forming a unified approach to treatment. In exploring this area I would like to make use of a traditional distinction between insight and supportive ap-proaches to psychotherapy. (Dewald's classic text [1964] presents a thoughtful exposition of this position by a traditional psychoanalyst.) Insight-oriented (also referred to as uncovering or reconstructive) ap-proaches modify ego defenses to allow unconscious experience to be integrated into conscious awareness. Supportive approaches (which in-clude what have sometimes been termed guidance and counseling) aim at strengthening conscious functioning through relieving the forces of shame and guilt that inhibit the ego and through providing education to enhance capacities for skillful living (Slavson 1964).

The key to successful working through in combined therapy is for the clinician to understand that individual and group sessions may be com-bined in four different ways: 1) both modalities may be used for insight, 2) both modalities may be used for support, 3) individual sessions may be used for insight and group sessions for support, and 4) group sessions may be used for insight and individual sessions for support. Through the flexible use of these four patterns, the clinician may obtain the optimal therapeutic benefit from combined psychotherapy.

Termination

The ending of combined individual and group therapy poses interesting challenges for patient and therapist alike. In addition to provoking the usual experiences, both joyful and painful, that accompany the end of therapy, combined treatment allows for the creative use of two simultaneous modalities of treatment. In a thoughtful review of termination of combined therapy, Fieldsteel (1990) described the possible forms the process may take.

Ending Both Treatments Simultaneously

Ending both treatment modalities at once highlights the issue of termination for the patient. This might be appropriate when both patient and therapist feel that the treatment is reasonably complete or when a patient has unresolved issues relating to loss that the therapist or patient might wish to highlight, as the following case example illustrates:

Case 5

Mr. E, a 21-year-old student, entered treatment for difficulties with relationships and public speaking. During the course of treatment he selected a career in dentistry, completed his studies, established himself successfully as a professional, met and married a woman whom he felt delighted to be with, had a child whom he deeply loved, and generally expanded his capacity to enjoy life. Termination of individual and group therapy simultaneously was planned 12 months in advance. As might be predicted, the ending of treatment evoked deep and painful feelings of loss and anger. An important feature of the treatment was that it had started quite early in my career, and so it included a number of interventions that in retrospect seemed less than optimal. As Mr. E patient grew in maturity and confidence, he was able to confront me on these issues, expressing considerable anger and hurt. This material emerged particularly during the termination period, which therefore was quite useful as a time to review and, as far as possible, correct the previous distortions. At the agreed-on time Mr. E finished his treatment with what seemed to be an appropriate mixture of sadness and joy. Several indirect follow-ups at 2- and 4-year intervals indicated that he was continuing to do very well.

In Case 5, it was actually the patient who made the suggestion to terminate group and individual therapy at once. The ensuing year was useful in highlighting the issue of loss—the central issue in his childhood and in his treatment. I believe that the patient intuitively sensed that ending both therapeutic modalities simultaneously was the ideal procedure for eliciting deeper aspects of his remaining difficulties. As is so often the case, the patient chose wisely.

Ending Individual Therapy Before Group Therapy

This form of termination intuitively appeals to both patient and therapist. It seems to match the rhythm of childhood maturation, as the individual emerges from closeness with parents to the adolescent stage of intense peer relationships. This type of termination may be appropriate for two types of patients:

1. The patient whose transference does not develop toward clear resolution, and for whom a kind of "weaning" seems appropriate for a modified resolution.
2. The patient whose transference in individual therapy deepens into a transference neurosis that does not seem capable of resolution within the individual therapy framework. In these instances, the partial termination (the shift to solely group therapy) decreases the intensity of the transference and may allow for movement, as the following case example illustrates:

Case 6

Mr. F, a plumber, entered couples therapy at age 30 with his wife. They were locked into a sadomasochistic marriage of several years' duration. He was a hard-drinking, hard-drugging, hard-motorcycle-driving, overweight macho man who on several occasions had physically assaulted his wife. He was also among the most intelligent and motivated patients I have ever worked with. After a number of years of treatment, the couple divorced and Mr. F continued in combined therapy. Gradually his life improved. He stopped drinking and using drugs, he gave up the motorcycle, and he remarried very happily. The new relationship seemed remarkably free of the conflicts that had destroyed his first marriage.

Mr. F's therapy seemed to include a full exploration of his transference. However, he remained grossly overweight, unable to advance in his work, unable to relate constructively to his teenage daughter, and plagued with periods of feeling extremely empty and depressed. Both Mr. F and I felt that there was further work to be done, and we agreed that he should terminate individual treatment and continue in group alone. This led to an elaboration of negative and dependent aspects of his transference that seemed unavailable in the individual context. Concurrent with this, Mr. F was able to advance significantly at work for the first time in his career.

Ending Group Therapy Before Individual Therapy

This type of termination is more unusual in the course of combined treatment, and it is probably most prevalent when positive work has been accomplished in treatment, unresolved transferential issues remain, and the dyadic relationship seems capable of sustaining deeper exploration.

Transference in Combined Therapy

Transference is the unique core of psychoanalytic treatment. Of all the central procedures of analysis (including, among others, the resolution of resistance, the interpretation of the unconscious, and the maintenance of technical neutrality by the analyst), only making the resolution of transference the heart of treatment clearly distinguishes psychoanalytic treatment from all other forms of treatment.

Advantages of Combined Therapy

Combined individual and group treatment provides the clinician with potent weapons in the struggle to help the patient liberate himself or herself from the compulsive grasp of transference. Reviewing some of what is discussed in an earlier section (Mechanism of Action of Combined Therapy), combined therapy allows for the following:

Multiple transferences can be explored simultaneously. The following example illustrates this point:

> One woman, raised by a single mother, experienced unbearable competition from her older sister for the mother. In group, she re-experienced the helplessness she had felt when at home with the mother and sister. Alone with the therapist she felt quite safe and comfortable. She was at ease with the group members as soon as they walked out of the therapy room and away from the therapist. But when the group and the therapist were present, she felt anxious, tense, unsafe, and nearly unable to communicate. (Caligor 1990, p. 22)

"Family" transferences can be resolved.   Patients often refer to their therapy group as being like a family, either in the negative sense ("you're just like my family!") or in the positive sense ("this group is like the family I never had!"). A patient can have a transference to an entire family that differs from the transferences to each of its members. This aspect of emotional experience is usually not accessible in dyadic treatment alone.

A particular transference may be diluted and so be more amenable to resolution.   This position is not universally accepted, however. After an excellent historical review of this issue, Wong (1983) explained:

> Various opinions exist regarding the transferences in combined treatment. Some clinicians believe that the transference becomes diluted and split, contaminated and inhibited in its development, and less intense and made more difficult to manage in combined treatment. Others feel that the transference manifestations are not greatly affected, or become more intense and that there may be a reinforcement of positive as well as negative components. The manifestations of transference are also influenced by the actual relationship between the patient and therapist in each of the two treatment settings, the timing of the combined treatment, the patient's personality, the composition of the group, and the style of leadership of the therapist. (pp. 78–79)

Group therapy may elicit transference patterns that differ from those seen in individual treatment alone.   A case of Caligor (1990) nicely illustrates this common phenomenon:

> Peggy, a 32-year-old compliant woman patient, always a "good girl" and avoidant of competition with her mother, insisted on presenting herself in the therapy dyad as inadequate and unable to cope, despite repeated interpretations regarding the defensive nature of this behavior. Upon entry to group there was a decided shift, a composure, a clear use of social skills, and a kind of assertiveness that the therapist had heard about but never experienced. Although she remained deferential to the analyst in the group, the change to a group context evoked different and more developed aspects of this woman's behavior. (p. 19)

Indeed, it is also important to bear in mind that a patient may actually develop two different transferences to the same therapist in the two settings that comprise combined treatment. Caligor (1990) explained this phenomenon:

Some patients continue to experience the therapist very differently in the two modalities. Frequently the pattern is that the patient perceives the therapist as understanding and responsive in the individual session but not to be counted on in the group. For some . . . the gratification of the individual session with the complete and undivided attention of the analyst masks the negative transference. However, with the change to a group setting, competitive feelings and envious fantasies emerge, and a good deal of anxiety and tension surface. (pp. 19–20)

Transference can be elucidated and resolved in many more ways in combined treatment. First, the patient may feel more comfortable with transference feelings after having seen other group members express similar feelings to the leader. Second, other members may encourage the patient to express crucial transference feelings more completely. Third, if the patient is dealing with negative feelings about the therapist, the patient's fear of retaliation may be diminished by being in the public arena of the group and by sensing the unspoken support of other group members. Fourth, the fact that other patients may have transference reactions to the therapist that differ from those of the patient may help the patient gain perspective on his or her distortions. Finally, the patient has the use not only of the therapist's understanding of the transference but also of the insights of fellow patients.

An instructive example of the use of combined individual and group therapy to resolve a difficult transference was presented early in the literature on combined treatment by Jackson and Grotjahn (1958). They reported in their summary of the case:

The case of an oral dependent and demanding character neurosis in a woman is described. A combination of group and individual analytic psychotherapy was used. In individual therapy, a typical transference neurosis developed and was properly interpreted, but the interpretations remained therapeutically ineffective. It became obvious that the essential trends of the individual situation offered too much oral gratification to the patient, so that she accepted interpretations by incorporating them like mother's milk and not by integrating them at a mature level of functioning. Because of her nonparticipation, the patient obtained little benefit from the group psychotherapy until the transference neurosis was established in individual analytic therapy. Only then, when she transferred her neurosis from the individual to the group situation, could the therapist, who no longer was standing exclusively in the focus of her neurosis, calmly observe and simultaneously interpret her behavior and productions with the help of the other members of the group as assistant therapists. The gratification could be diminished, the transference entrenchment loosened, and integration achieved. The individual sessions could then be used to supplement the process of working through after it was started in group psychotherapy. It appears doubtful that any other therapy would have achieved as dynamic and therapeutic a result as the combined treatment method. (p. 383)

What is unique about the combined therapy situation is that the traditional advantages of group therapy are combined with the traditional advantages of individual psychotherapy in exploring a transference situation in depth. In this way, combined treatment may truly be said to revivify, and allow to be modified, the earliest pathogenic situation of the patient's life, which usually occurred in both a dyadic and a group (familial) context.

Levels of Transference in Combined Treatment: Multiple Targets

A patient in combined treatment has three main targets for his or her transference:

1. The therapist
2. The members of the therapy group
3. The group as a whole

Types of Transference in Combined Therapy: Narcissistic Transferences and Object Transferences

Since the development of self psychology, we have been able to conceptualize with clarity the rich array of transference reactions present in our patients. We may think of transference patterns as falling into two broad categories: object transferences and narcissistic (or selfobject) transferences.

Object transferences.   This term refers to the traditional psychoanalytic notion of transference. In an object transference we experience the other person (object) as a whole person, separate from us, but we confuse them with our experience of someone from the past. For example, in my practice a common pattern is for a patient to experience a paternal object transference to me, a maternal object transference to the group as a whole, and specific sibling object transferences to group members.

Selfobject transferences (narcissistic transferences). In this type of transference, the other person is experienced not as a separate person but as a part or function of our own self—hence the term "selfobject."

Transference to the group as a whole. Transferences to the group as a whole can easily be overlooked in the multiplicity of factors that a therapist and group are attempting to integrate at any given moment. In an important article published over 25 years ago, Scheidlinger (1964) suggested that, in the state of regression that the therapy group may induce, patients may relate to the group as a whole on an unconscious level as a pre-oedipal mother.

Working with Transference in Combined Treatment

The basic principles of resolving transference in combined treatment do not differ substantially from those appropriate for the individual analytic setting, although their application may differ in the combined treatment situation. Some of these principles are as follows:

Nature of the intervention. In accordance with current thinking regarding psychoanalytic technique, narcissistic (selfobject) transferences are best dealt with by allowing them to flower, with the therapist or group trying to provide, to whatever extent is realistically possible, the heretofore missing selfobject function. When this is not possible, the therapist or group tries to empathically clarify the realistic limits of the situation. Object transferences are best dealt with by interpreting their unconscious meaning.

Timing. As in the dyadic treatment setting, timing is all. Interventions regarding transference that come when the intensity of the patient's transference is too low will produce only an intellectual effect; interventions that come when the transference intensity is too high will get lost in the emotional storm.

Working through. Transference is clarified and ultimately resolved through a process of repetitive exploration. The group becomes a laboratory for the patient to experiment with healthier ways of relating. The availability of group therapy to aid in the working through of transference conflicts is a major advantage of the combined treatment model over the traditional dyadic analytic model, which at times can remain an overly intellectual process that is not fully translated into behavior by some patients (Caligor et al. 1984).

Importance of an attitude on the part of the therapist that is both neutral and caring.   Freud's original recommendation (1915) of analytic neutrality was intended to safeguard the analyst from excessively siding with any intrapsychic agency of the mind. But as many writers have pointed out, the tradition of neutrality in the work has often been misinterpreted to mean that the analyst should remain emotionally uninvolved (Greenson 1967). In combined therapy, even if it were desirable for the therapist to be emotionally uninvolved, it is virtually impossible. The requirements of face-to-face interaction with eight patients dilute the analytic incognito, which would in any case appear forced and stilted even if it could be maintained. This poses interesting issues for the psychoanalytic clinician doing combined individual and group therapy, as the dyadic situation requires a certain distance on the part of the analyst in order for the transference to flower, and the group situation elicits more of the analyst's realistic emotional behavior.

In actual clinical experience, the dilution of the analytic incognito does not pose great difficulty. Along with many other psychoanalytic authors, I believe that the involved stance required of the therapist in combined treatment is a plus in itself. Technical neutrality can be combined with a caring attitude on the part of the therapist without any impairment of therapeutic efficacy and, indeed, with an actual benefit to the healing aspects of the relationship between patient and therapist. The group portion of combined therapy does not interfere with the full development of a transference, nor with its effective resolution in the dyadic situation.

Resistance in Combined Therapy

All the resistances present in both dyadic treatment and group treatment are present in combined therapy. These have been well documented in the analytic literature. (See, for example, Greenson's traditional exposition [1967] and the insightful book on resistance in group therapy by Leslie Rosenthal [1987].) But of great interest to the practitioner of combined therapy are those resistances particular to the combined treatment situation. Alonso and Rutan (1990) highlighted many of these in their recent and excellent discussion, "Common Dilemmas in Combined Individual and Group Treatment."

Transference Splitting

This relatively common occurrence in combined treatment can take two obvious forms: an overemphasis on positive feelings in the individual situation, to the exclusion of negative feelings, which then emerge in the group; and the maintenance of a distant relationship in the dyadic situation, with more affectionate feelings emerging in the group.

Transference splitting, often considered an undesirable occurrence, actually constitutes a major reason to recommend combined treatment for patients with significant pre-oedipal pathology. When individual or group treatment alone is employed with such patients, transference splitting will occur anyway, with one component of the transference being acted out beyond the framework of treatment, often with destructive erotic or aggressive consequences for the patient. Combined treatment may be said to facilitate the possibilities for splitting, but from another point of view it only contains the already existing tendency within a more carefully managed therapeutic framework than is available to the practitioner of solo group or analytic treatment. By expanding the boundaries of the therapeutic situation to include both individual and group therapy, combined treatment may actually facilitate the intelligent clinical management of transference splitting.

What is the best approach to dealing with this particular resistance? In my experience, the first priority is to support the patient in fully expressing his or her feelings in whatever modality they may appear. This task takes precedence over other considerations. Then, once the patient can fully express the relevant feelings in the modality that feels most comfortable, the therapist can gradually address the absence of certain feelings in each modality, thereby gradually resolving the splitting defense.

Keeping Secrets From the Group

Frequently patients will choose to discuss a certain issue only in their individual sessions and will expressly avoid bringing it up in the group. Alonso and Rutan (1990) commented:

> It is never easy to solve the delicate question of how to protect the patient's dignity and to avoid unnecessary shame on the one hand, and how to avoid participating in and encouraging unhealthy secrets from the group on the other hand. It is a truism that it is never worth humiliating the patient for the sake of some technical or theoretical purity. (p. 7)

In dealing with this situation, the two most extreme positions should be avoided. First, one might simply let the situation be, as if there were no problem. In the long run this will produce a patient who is less than a full participant in group and will tend to vitiate the power of the combined modality. At the other extreme, a therapist might take the position that no confidentiality exists between individual and group sessions and that either the patient or the therapist should be free at any time to bring up material from either modality in the context of the other. This position, although it resolves the resistance, runs headlong into normal considerations of decency, tact, and therapeutic empathy, and it thereby may win a battle but lose a war (or a patient).

What seems to work best in this area, as in so many others, is a judicious middle position, recognizing the right of patients in individual treatment to withhold material from the group, but viewing this as a resistance to be tactfully and gradually resolved over a period of time.

The clinician must always give attention to the viability of the group context. When a patient cannot bring certain material up in the group, this may indicate a group resistance. The group itself may be unable to hear certain material from a number of different patients. If the therapist realizes that this may be the case, the proper arena for exploration will, of course, not be the individual session but the group, where the resistance can be explored and resolved on a wider basis.

Wanting to Leave One Modality of Treatment

Often a patient in crisis will announce a desire to leave either group or individual treatment and continue in the other form of therapy. Is this always, sometimes, or never resistance, and how may it be handled?

Basically, the problem here is to distinguish between a resistance on the part of the patient and a normal aspect of the patient's evolving therapeutic career, which may involve terminating one of the modalities of combined treatment as a step toward eventual full termination. Even if the clinician, after careful consideration, believes the patient's request to be a resistance, the words of Alonso and Rutan (1990) are well worth noting:

> When all is said and done patients need to know that they can act out and not be excommunicated for it; it is incumbent on the therapist to manage his/her own countertransference in order to remain in empathy with the patient's solution, and avoid retaliation or abandonment in the crisis. (p. 9)

Countertransference

My impression is that, for the therapist who has been seeing patients for a number of years, countertransference difficulty, rather than inadequate theoretical or technical knowledge, is at the heart of most problems in treatment. Yet in most articles or books on combined treatment, countertransference is barely discussed. This seems to result from the difficulty experienced by most of us, with a few exceptions, such as Racker's well-known work (1968), in saying anything theoretically interesting about countertransference. Combined therapy is rife with opportunities for both the constructive and destructive use of countertransference. The chief difficulty, from the therapist's point of view, is that he or she is both more exposed and more confused than if he or she were practicing either modality alone. The therapist is more exposed because individual psychotherapy patients relate to the therapist in the more transparent and less controlled environment of the group, and because group therapy patients can present the therapist privately with their intense feelings. The therapist is more confused because his or her patients' transferences and resistances can often shift abruptly and without warning or explanation from group to individual to group session.

Combined therapy allows the therapy group to assist the therapist in resolving unconscious countertransference difficulties.

Case 2 (*continued*)

The case of Ms. B illustrates the use of combined therapy in helping the therapist avoid treatment-destructive countertransference difficulties. Ms. B was a social worker in her late thirties who entered treatment because of difficulties with men, subsequently married, developed an apparently unworkable transference, and terminated individual treatment while continuing productive work in the group. Around the time she terminated individual treatment Ms. B almost terminated treatment totally, and her group explored with her the causes for this situation. The group quickly hit on the fact that Ms. B had felt there were certain issues she could not raise with me.

What then ensued was a long and painful period in the group during which, with much encouragement from the group and me, Ms. B gradually made it clear that she had felt mistreated by me. She felt I had been critical of her, that I had not allowed her to express anger, that when she had tried to express anger I had interpreted this as her problem, and that in the group and individually I had been authoritarian and defensive. As this incident occurred during a period in my career when I was reviewing and revising my way of working as a therapist, I was able to recognize the validity of many of her criticisms, although of course there was transference distortion present. The group confirmed that there was truth as well as distortion in Ms. B's point of view.

There is no doubt in my mind that without combined individual and group treatment, Ms. B as a patient and I as a therapist would have been unable to break out of the unresolved difficulty we found ourselves in. The group helped give Ms. B the courage of her convictions to confront me and enabled me to see the validity of her point of view.

A well-run analytic group can be counted on, in most instances, to be a fair witness to the difficulties encountered by the therapist with one of the group members. The group will pick up patients' resistances, encourage them to express their deeper feelings, acknowledge the validity of their observations, correct their transference distortions, pick up the therapist's defensiveness, and also support the therapist when he or she honestly acknowledges difficulties. Although the group also can be swayed by distortions and needs the leadership of the group therapist, for the most part it can be an honest broker in helping its therapist resolve the countertransference difficulties that may be operating outside of his or her awareness.

Conclusions: Combined Therapy and the Therapist's Professional Fulfillment

We have reviewed, with case examples, the history, mechanism of action, indications and contraindications, treatment stages, and transference, countertransference, and resistance aspects of combined individual and group psychotherapy.

One further aspect of combined therapy bears mentioning, and that is the effect of practicing combined treatment on the therapist's enjoyment of his or her own professional life.

The entire subject of what inhibits and facilitates our enjoyment of our work as therapists is rarely touched on in the professional literature, although it is hardly a minor matter. This lack of discussion in the literature is balanced by its being incessantly discussed during informal social and professional contacts. A certain puritanical tone tends to pervade discussions of this subject, as if "therapeutic work" is not meant to be enjoyed by the therapist, as if therapy should consist of pain and suffering on both sides of the couch or circle, and as if enjoyment on either side suggests self-indulgence, acting out, or transference gratification.

To my mind, this is a prescription for unfulfilled psychotherapists and unhealed patients. Truly effective psychoanalytic work is enriching to both patient and therapist. In this enterprise the practice of combined individual and group psychotherapy has much to recommend it. This is not to say that a lifelong practice of either psychoanalysis or group therapy alone cannot be equally rewarding, What combined therapy does uniquely offer, however, is the opportunity for the therapist to express, in a balanced way, quite different aspects of his or her professional identity. Individual treatment allows the clinician to be thoughtful and profound; group therapy allows him or her to be more active and more socially engaged. For these reasons, combined therapy keeps professional practice interesting, varied, and rewarding for patient and psychotherapist alike.

References

Alonso A, Rutan JS: Group therapy, individual therapy, or both. Int J Group Psychother 32:267–282, 1982

Alonso A, Rutan JS: Common dilemmas in combined individual and group treatment. Group 14:5–12, 1990

Aronson ML: Technical problems in combined therapy. Int J Group Psychother 14:425–432, 1964

Bieber TB: Combined individual and group psychotherapy, in Comprehensive Group Psychotherapy. Edited by Kaplan HI, Sadock BJ. Baltimore, MD, Williams & Wilkins, 1971, pp 153–169

Caligor J: Perceptions of the group therapist and the drop-out from group, in Group Therapy 1977: An Overview. Edited by Wolberg LR, Aronson ML, Wolberg AR. New York, Stratton Intercontinental Medical Book Corp, 1977, pp 112–128

Caligor J: A current look at transference in combined analytic therapy. Group 14:16–24, 1990

Caligor J, Fieldsteel ND, Brok AJ: Individual and Group Therapy: Combining Psychoanalytic Treatments. New York, Basic Books, 1984

Dewald P: Psychotherapy: A Dynamic Approach. New York, Basic Books, 1964, pp 99–112 and passim

Durkin HE, Glatzer HT: Transference neurosis in group psychotherapy: the concept and the reality, in Group Therapy 1973. Edited by Wolberg L, Schwartz E. New York, Intercontinental Medical Book Corp., 1973, pp 129–144

Ezriel H: The role of transference in psychoanalytical and other approaches to group treatment. Acta Psychother 7:101–116, 1957

Fieldsteel ND: The termination phase of combined therapy. Group 14:27–32, 1990

Freud S: Further recommendations in the technique of psychoanalysis: observations on transference-love (1915), in Collected Papers, Vol II. Translated by Riviere J. New York, Basic Books, 1959, pp 377–392

Foulkes SH: Therapeutic Group Analysis. New York, International Universities Press, 1964, pp 37, 78, 232

Greenson R: The Technique and Practice in Psychoanalysis. New York, International Universities Press, 1967, pp 216–224

Jackson J, Grotjahn M: The treatment of oral defenses by combined individual and group psychotherapy. Int J Group Psychother 8:373–383, 1958

Ormont LR: Principles and practice of conjoint psychoanalytic treatment. Am J Psychiatry 138:69–73, 1981

Ormont LR, Strean H: The Practice of Conjoint Therapy: Combining Individual and Group Treatment. New York, Human Sciences, 1978

Porter K: Combined individual and group psychotherapy: a review of the literature, 1965–1978. Int J Group Psychother 30:107–114, 1980

Porter K, Edwards N (eds): Special section: combined individual and group psychotherapy. Group 14:3–34, 1990

Racker H: Transference and Counter-Transference. New York, International Universities Press, 1968

Rosenthal L: Resolving Resistance in Group Therapy. Northvale, NJ, Jason Aronson, 1987

Sadock B: Combined individual and group psychotherapy, in Comprehensive Textbook of Psychiatry/II, 2nd Edition, Vol 2. Edited by Freedman AM, Kaplan HI. Baltimore, MD, Williams & Wilkins, 1975, pp 1877–1881

Sadock B: Group psychotherapy, combined individual and group psychotherapy, and psychodrama, in Comprehensive Textbook of Psychiatry/IV, 4th Edition. Edited by Kaplan HI, Sadock BJ. Baltimore, MD, Williams & Wilkins, 1985, pp 1403–1427

Scheidlinger S: Identification, the sense of belonging and of identity in small groups. Int J Group Psychother 14:291–306, 1964

Scheidlinger S, Porter K: Group therapy combined with individual psychotherapy, in Specialized Techniques in Individual Psychotherapy. Edited by Karasu T, Bellak L. New York, Brunner/Mazel, 1980, pp 426–440

Slavson SR: A Textbook in Analytic Group Psychotherapy. New York, International Universities Press, 1964, pp 98–109

Stone WN, Rutan JS: Duration of treatment in group psychotherapy. Int J Group Psychother 34:93–109, 1984

Swiller H: Alexithymia: treatment utilizing combined individual and group psychotherapy. Int J Group Psychother 38:47–61, 1988

Symposium on combined individual and group psychotherapy. Int J Group Psychother 14:403–454, 1964

Wender L, Stein A: Group psychotherapy as an aid to outpatient treatment in a psychiatric clinic. Psychiatr Q 23:415–424, 1949

Whitaker DS, Lieberman MA: Psychotherapy Through the Group Process. Chicago, IL, Aldine, 1964, pp 211–214

Wolf A, Schwartz E: Psychoanalysis in Groups. New York, Grune & Stratton, 1962, pp 179–206

Wong N: Combined individual and group psychotherapy, in Comprehensive Group Psychotherapy, 2nd Edition. Edited by Kaplan HI, Sadock BJ. Baltimore, MD, Williams & Wilkins, 1983, pp 73–83

Yalom I: The Theory and Practice of Group Psychotherapy, 2nd Edition. New York, Basic Books, 1975, pp 415–419

CHAPTER 18

Ethical and Legal Issues in Group Psychotherapy

Maria T. Lymberis, M.D.

Introduction

Group therapy encompasses a wide spectrum of psychiatric practices that involve a variety of settings, goals, and time frames. This chapter addresses ethical and legal aspects of psychiatric group therapy practice as opposed to self-help groups, corporate groups, or self-improvement groups. Group therapy with nonpsychiatric medical patients and group psychotherapy by mental health professionals who are not psychiatrists are essentially governed by the same ethical and legal principles that apply to psychiatric group practice.

From the ethical and legal perspective, group therapy is a form of medical practice. As such, it is governed by the following factors that apply to all types of medical practice:

- The ethical principles that form the foundation of competent care
- The patient's constitutional rights
- The federal and state laws and the decisions and directives of the courts and other, nongovernmental agencies that regulate the practice of medicine

Professional Ethics

In the past 15 years ethical issues have been at the forefront of professional and public concern. For over 2,000 years, the Hippocratic tradition has been the foundation of medicine (Dryer 1988). In the United

States the American Medical Association (AMA) first revised and adopted its own version of the Hippocratic Oath in 1847. Since then there have been several revisions (1903, 1912, and 1957). In all these revisions the fundamental tenets of the tradition were maintained.

The Hippocratic tradition was based on a religious calling. The Hippocratic sect first defined who the physician was, not by what the physician knew, but by how the physician applied knowledge in human moral terms. The focus was service to the individual patient. The physician was to function exclusively as the patient's agent. The needs and interests of the patient took precedence over those of the physician. Physicians were specifically required to keep absolute confidentiality and to abstain from sexual relations with patients. The focus was on the sanctity of the doctor-patient relationship, which was based on honesty, trust, and dedication and which was for the sole benefit of the patient.

In the 1980 AMA revision of medical ethics, several aspects of the Hippocratic tradition were significantly modified in keeping with contemporary realities (American Psychiatric Association 1989), including

1. Our view of knowledge is no longer absolute and certain, and medical decisions are now based on a risk-benefit analysis.
2. The physician is no longer an absolute authority, and the paternalistic attitude of the Hippocratic tradition has given way to the current view of the patient as a full partner in medical treatment. The basis of the doctor-patient relationship is now informed consent. Informed consent is a process that runs throughout the entire treatment.
3. Although the exclusivity of the doctor-patient relationship, the hallmark of the Hippocratic tradition, is still affirmed, confidentiality is no longer absolute but "within the constraints of the law."
4. The physician is no longer exclusively dedicated to the individual patient nor functions exclusively as that patient's agent. Now, physicians recognize a responsibility to participate in activities contributing to an improved community.

Clinical practice is based on ethical principles. Although legal requirements and local regulations affecting clinical practice may vary in different cities and states, practitioners have to address these requirements from the perspective of the ethical principles that govern clinical practice. Whenever the external requirements conflict with the ethical standards, practitioners are to obtain consultation from their professional association's ethics committee and from their malpractice attorneys.

Constitutional Rights of Patients and Treatment

Since the beginning of the twentieth century, a major change has taken place in the way North American medicine is practiced. This shift led to dramatic advances in scientific knowledge and technological innovation, but it also led to the need to safeguard individuals' rights. Civil libertarians have turned to the Constitution in their attempts to support the rights of patients.

Medical treatment in today's reality is best viewed as a legally regulated societal function. All forms and varieties of medical treatment can be rendered only with the informed consent of the patient. (For a detailed discussion of informed consent, see Chapter 6 of Dryer's book [1988].) The patient is a full partner in the treatment process. Legal requirements should be viewed as posing technical challenges that represent clinical problems. Legal interventions are the last resort and, if necessary, should be framed as part of the therapeutic endeavor to safeguard the therapeutic alliance. Both the patient and the therapist function within the same social context. Legal interventions are for the protection of both the patient and the therapist and should not conflict with the goals of treatment.

Legal Aspects of Practice

General Remarks

Medical practice has always been governed by law. Currently, professionals face a very high standard of accountability, not only because of the threat of malpractice but also because of the monitoring of professional practice through the National Data Bank. The National Data Bank began operation in the fall of 1990 with physicians and dentists, but eventually it will include *all* licensed health care practitioners throughout the United States. The mandatory reporting of disciplinary actions against practitioners and of malpractice awards or settlements has already had an impact on the entire health care field. The emphasis is on prevention and risk management. Suits now primarily involve allegations of negligence for improper management of psychopharmacological treatment, suicide, inappropriate hospitalization, patient abandonment, and sexual involvement. Malpractice suits for negligent psychotherapy, per se, are uncommon because the standard of care is so diverse, given the multitude of psychotherapeutic schools and the fact that causation is very hard to establish. Negligent psychotherapy is usually associated with other allegations.

Sexual Misconduct

Although the Hippocratic tradition clearly held that sexual involvement with any patient was unethical, the reality is that, like child sexual abuse, sexual relations between health care practitioners and patients have been one of those dark secrets that one made every effort to forget, to not see, and to not hear.

There are powerful societal and professional resistances against the confrontation of this problem. Most surveys done today among psychologists, psychiatrists, and other mental health professionals have reported an incidence of sexual involvement with patients of around 5%–10%. The California Senate Task Force on this issue (California Legislature 1987) stated that "with 38,000 licensed mental health practitioners" in the state the incidence of sexual involvement with patients constituted "a public health problem" (p. 1).

Sexual involvement with patients involves abuse and exploitation of the vulnerable and less powerful by the more powerful and less vulnerable. As in childhood incest, it is not necessarily the sexual act itself that causes the damage, but the violation of trust.

As of 1990, all professional associations of health care providers specifically had addressed the issue of sexual involvement with patients and uniformly viewed such behavior as unethical. The American Psychiatric Association was the first medical specialty organization to focus attention on ethical issues in clinical practice and specifically on sexual misconduct. In 1973, the first edition of *The Principles of Medical Ethics with Annotations Specifically Applicable to Psychiatry* was issued. The 1989 revision (American Psychiatric Association 1989) includes sections relevant to this problem:

> *Section I, Annotation 1:* The patient may place his/her trust in his/her psychiatrist knowing that the psychiatrist's ethics and professional responsibilities preclude him/her gratifying his/her own needs by exploiting the patient. This becomes particularly important because of the essentially private, highly personal, and sometimes intensely emotional nature of the relationship established with the psychiatrist.
> *Section 2, Annotation 1:* The requirement that the physician conduct him-

self/herself with propriety in his/her profession and in all the actions of his/her life is especially important in the case of the psychiatrist because the patient tends to model his/her behavior after that of his/her therapist by identification. Further, the necessary intensity of the therapeutic relationship may tend to activate sexual and other needs and fantasies on the part of both patient and therapist, while weakening the objectivity necessary for control. Sexual activity with a patient is unethical. Sexual involvement with one's former patients generally exploits emotions deriving from treatment and therefore almost always is unethical.

Section 2, Annotation 2: The psychiatrist should diligently guard against exploiting information furnished by the patient and should not use the unique position of power afforded him/her by the psychotherapeutic situation to influence the patient in any way not directly relevant to the treatment goals.

In 1990, the AMA House of Delegates adopted Policy 32.0045:

On Sexual Misconduct in the Practice of Medicine: It is the policy of the AMA that (1) Sexual contact or a romantic relationship with a patient concurrent with the physician-patient relationship is unethical. (2) Sexual or romantic relationships with former patients are unethical if the physician uses or exploits trust, knowledge, emotions or influence derived from the previous professional relationship. (3) Education on the issue of sexual attraction to patients and sexual misconduct should be included throughout all levels of medical training. (4) Disciplinary bodies must be structured to maximize effectiveness in dealing with the problem of sexual misconduct. (5) Physicians who learn of sexual misconduct by a colleague must report the misconduct to either the local medical society, the state licensing board or other appropriate authorities. Exceptions to reporting may be made in order to protect patient welfare. (6) It should be noted that many states have legal prohibitions against relationships between physicians and current or former patients. (CEJA Rep. A, 5-90; see also Current Opinions Section 8.14.)

The American Psychological Association's *Ethical Principles of Psychologists* (1981 [revised 1989]) included the following:

Principle 6a: Sexual intimacies with clients are unethical.
Principle 6d: Psychologists do not exploit their professional relationships with clients, supervisees, students, employees, or research participants, sexually or otherwise. Psychologists do not condone or engage in sexual harassment.

In *NASW Policy Statements: Code of Ethics* the National Association of Social Workers (1980) specifically noted

Section II, item 5: The social worker should under no circumstances engage in sexual activities with clients.

Section II, item 4: The social worker should avoid relationships or commitments that conflict with the interests of clients.

The American Association for Marriage and Family Therapy *Code of Professional Ethics* (1988) included

Section 1.2: Marriage and family therapists are cognizant of their potentially influential position with respect to clients, and they avoid exploiting the trust and dependency of such persons. Marriage and family therapists therefore make every effort to avoid dual relationships with clients that could impair their professional judgement or increase the risk of exploitation. Examples of such dual relationships include, but are not limited to, business or close personal relationships with clients. Sexual intimacy with clients is prohibited. Sexual intimacy with former clients for two years following the termination of therapy is prohibited.

The *Code for Nurses With Interpretive Statements* (American Nurses Association 1985) included

Section 3: The nurse acts to safeguard the client and the public when health care and safety are affected by incompetent, unethical or illegal practice of any person. Sexual involvement between nurse and client is both unethical and unprofessional.

Regardless of theoretical orientation, a finding of negligent psychotherapy can result from failure to maintain clear treatment boundaries. Boundary violations include inappropriate extratherapeutic actions such as seeing patients outside of the regularly scheduled sessions or making sexually suggestive comments. Sexual involvement between a therapist and a patient is unequivocally unethical, illegal, and in some states a criminal act that can result in years of litigation, censure from one's own professional association, loss of license, a jail term, and severe financial, emotional, and personal hardship to the professional and damage to the patient.

Focus on Ethics and Group Therapy

There are no data on the incidence of sexual involvement among group therapy patients either during or subsequent to group therapy. Such involvements may expose the therapists of the involved patients to malpractice suits on the basis of negligent group psychotherapy. It is the therapist's responsibility to set and maintain clear group therapy boundaries. Patients who attempt to or actually violate these pose a major technical therapeutic challenge for any therapist. Specific techniques are needed for managing such patients, including obtaining consultation and referring the patient for individual therapy. Malpractice suits for negligent group psychotherapy may be difficult to win. However, the stress of a malpractice suit is extremely taxing on the involved professional, causing major disruptions in one's personal, family, economic, and professional life.

Finally, patients may disclose in the course of group therapy a sexual involvement with a prior or current therapist. The management of such disclosures presents specific technical problems. The therapist has to be knowledgeable about the applicable state laws and reporting requirements. Consultation with the professional ethics committee and/or an experienced professional in this area is strongly recommended. Such patients often go through very severe regressions with manifestations of complex symptoms as they are coming to terms with their past or present abusive experience. In the absence of legally mandated reporting requirements, it is the patient's decision regarding what, if anything, to do about such experiences.

Confidentiality Issues

Confidentiality in clinical practice is one of the ethical duties of every practitioner or health care provider. Legally, confidentiality (i.e., the right to privacy) is a constitutional right of every citizen. In addition, there are specific statutes involving physician-patient privilege and, in most states, specific statutes dealing with psychotherapist-patient privilege.

Patient Records and Confidentiality

In most states, there are specific statutes that govern access to medical or health care records or summaries of those records. These statutes include procedures for disclosure directly to patients, as well as reasons for denial of such disclosure requests. Usually patients who are denied access may designate a health care professional who can review the records. Therapists are urged to obtain legal consultation from their malpractice carrier in all cases involving requests for medical records, even if it seems that there is proper patient authorization and/or court order for such release.

In the past, there was considerable debate about keeping psychiatric records. Therapists felt that the best way to protect their patients confidences was by not keeping any records. Today, however, medical records are viewed as part of the standard of practice and are required. The record must document the need for care, the type of care, and the patient's response.

Problems of Boundary Violations and Multiple Agentry

The psychotherapist-patient relationship is a fiduciary one. As a fiduciary the therapist knows that the patient's needs and interests take precedence over those of the therapist. However, there are situations where the therapist's allegiance to the patient is in conflict with demands from the institution or other professionals. This is a double-agentry situation.

Until recently therapists were not aware of how the organizational structure in which they work affects their professional function as clinicians. In the past, patients were seldom informed in cases of multiple agentry. However, the situation is rapidly changing. Double agentry conflicts are now recognized to exist in some practice settings (such as managed care) where economics and corporate policies, rather than clinical assessment and specific patient needs, dictate the type and level of care that patients receive. In addition, double-agentry conflicts are found in cases involving the duty to preserve confidentiality and the need of the practitioner to publish, as well as between service and research obligations. These are now handled with specific notification and authorization by the patient or patients involved.

Currently, special attention is focused on dual relationships with patients that represent a whole spectrum of treatment boundary violations other than sexual transgressions. Whenever the doctor-patient relationship is altered by the initiation of any other type of relationship with the patient or by the assumption of any other role vis-à-vis the patient, a boundary violation can result.

There is a spectrum of boundary violations. Some are therapeutically required and justified for optimal patient care. Some are part of a pattern of multiple repeated violations, the slippery slope phenomenon, which often culminates in sexual misconduct. Examples of boundary violations include assuming the role of "real friend" in the patient's life by participating in the life of the patient outside of the therapy by attending dinners and social functions; lending a patient money; investing in a patient's business or having the patient invest in the therapist's business; entering in joint business ventures with the patient; revealing to the patient personal problems and traumas and disclosing feelings, particularly sexual feelings and arousal about the specific patient; and employing a patient in one's practice, to name just a few. When such transgression fulfills narcissistic needs of the patient or is part of collusive acting out, it may take years for the patient to recognize the reality of the violation. The dynamics are similar to those seen in patients who have been sexually involved with their therapists. Damage to patients can be extensive.

Denial, idealization of the therapist, and identification with the therapist, as well as other types of transference-countertransference configurations, tend to make recognition of the transgression very difficult for both patients and therapists. Such recognition may take years.

Studies on nonsexual transgressions are currently being reported by various professional organizations. The *Ethics Newsletter* of the American Psychiatric Association's Ethics Committee (1990a) included specific recommendations regarding boundary violations stemming from religious or ideological commitment of the therapist. Namely, religious convictions and beliefs of therapists should not be presented as treatment recommendations but should be explicitly acknowledged as such. The American Psychiatric Association's Ethics Committee (1990b) also addressed some of the nonsexual boundary violations that result in exploitation of patients. Five different patterns were described: exploitation for financial reasons, exploitation for family reasons, exploitation for fame or notoriety, exploitation by "living through a patient," and exploitation by interpretation.

Priorities need to be set when dealing with ethical dilemmas. The treatment needs of the individual patient may, at times, conflict with those of the group. The therapist has to be guided by the fiduciary and ethical duty to each and every patient, while at the same time ensuring the preservation of the safety and integrity of the group. Clinical skill and experience are the fruits of repeated trials in the clinical field.

Special Considerations in the Practice of Group Psychotherapy

Members of therapy groups are vulnerable to abuse not only by therapists but also by other group members. Member-to-member exploitation is possible in the areas of sex, money, self-aggrandizement, and so forth. Members are protected from abuse by group therapists by the standards and laws discussed above. How are they protected from abuse by one another?

There is no specific legal requirement for protection of the individual group member from member-to-member abuse in group therapy. The usual legal requirements that apply to all forms of psychiatric treatment also apply to group therapy. Situations could arise when a group member could become violent and present a clear threat toward another specific group member or members. The clinical challenges of the *Tarasoff* requirements—the duty to warn and the duty to protect potential victims—present major treatment problems, particularly in outpatient settings. Group therapy is no exception. (For a full discussion of these issues, see Beck 1988.)

The competence of the group leader is the best defense against member-to-member exploitation. The leader must have clear guidelines about permitted and prohibited member-to-member interactions. These must be explicitly communicated to group members and documented in appropriate records. When exploitative behavior arises, it must be pursued in the context of the therapy. If this behavior proves intractable, consideration must be given to terminating group membership for one or both parties engaging in such behavior.

Appropriate consultation with colleagues, ethics committees, and legal advisers is strongly recommended.

Careful and thorough records of all therapeutic interventions and consultations are essential.

The basic governing principle is that of competent care. Group members cannot be protected from every risk of member-to-member exploitation, but it is essential that the group leader exercise and document due diligence and clinical judgment.

Patient Care Principles in Group Therapy

Adequate records for each group therapy patient must be maintained. These records must contain

- The initial evaluation.
- The diagnosis.
- The indications for group therapy.

- Documentation of informed consent of the patient for group therapy. Patients have to be informed that this is only one type of treatment among others and that other options may specifically be recommended on further evaluation during group therapy.
- A copy of each group therapy session summary.
- A quarterly clinical summary of the patient's progress.

Reevaluation should be done and documented on every patient who fails to use the group therapy successfully after a reasonable period or whose conditions worsen significantly while in group treatment. Such reevaluation may include consultative discussions with colleagues and, when appropriate, direct evaluation of the patient by a consultant.

In view of the fact that specific psychopharmacological treatment is now available for a variety of psychiatric symptoms and conditions, patients should be informed that a consultation with a psychiatrist is indicated if patients either have a specific psychiatric diagnosis on entering the group or manifest symptoms suggestive of such diagnoses in the course of group therapy.

Billing practices should ensure that the name and qualifications of the therapist who actually runs the group treatment are stated, as well as the name and qualifications of the supervisor or director.

Conclusions

The practice of group therapy requires that the therapist uphold all of the relevant ethics set by professional organizations and by law for medical and mental health professionals and reviewed in this chapter. In addition, the group therapist has the unique responsibility of exercising due diligence in protecting group members from injury and exploitation by one another. Both these areas, particularly the latter, are evolving rapidly, and the responsible group therapist must remain informed about current developments.

References

American Association for Marriage and Family Therapy: Code of Professional Ethics. Washington, DC, American Association for Marriage and Family Therapy, 1988

American Medical Association: Current Opinions: The Council on Ethical and Judicial Affairs of the American Medical Association. Chicago, IL, American Medical Association, 1990

American Nurses Association, Committee on Ethics: Code for Nurses With Interpretive Statements. Kansas City, MO, American Nurses Association, 1985

American Psychiatric Association: The Principles of Medical Ethics with Annotations Especially Applicable to Psychiatry. Washington, DC, American Psychiatric Association, 1989, p 2

American Psychological Association: Ethical Principles of Psychologists. Washington, DC, American Psychological Association, 1981

American Psychiatric Association's Ethics Committee: Ethics Newsletter, Vol 6, No 1. Washington, DC, American Psychiatric Association, 1990a

American Psychiatric Association's Ethics Committee: Ethics Newsletter, Vol 6, No 2. Washington, DC, American Psychiatric Association, 1990b

Beck JC (ed): Confidentiality Versus the Duty to Protect: Foreseeable Harm in the Practice of Psychiatry. Washington, DC, American Psychiatric Press, 1988

California Legislature: Report of the Senate Task Force on Psychotherapist and Patients' Sexual Relations, prepared for the Senate Rules Committee, March 1987. Sacramento, CA, Joint Publications, 1987

Dyer AR: Ethics and Psychiatry: Towards Professional Definition. Washington, DC, American Psychiatric Press, 1988

National Association of Social Workers: NASW Policy Statements: Code of Ethics. Washington, DC, National Association of Social Workers, 1980

Additional Readings

Apfel R, Simon B: Sexualized therapy: causes and consequences, in Sexual Exploitation of Patients by Health Professionals. Edited by Burgess AW, Hartman CR. New York, Praeger, 1986, pp 143–151

Bergmann MS: Platonic love, transference love, and love in real life. J Am Psychoanal Assoc 30:87–111, 1982

Gabbard G: Sexual Exploitation in Professional Relationships. Washington, DC, American Psychiatric Press, 1989

Gartrell N, Herman J, Olarte S, et al: Psychiatrist-patient sexual contact: results of a national survey, I: prevalence. Am J Psychiatry 143:1126–1131, 1986

Marmor J: Some psychodynamic aspects of the seduction of patients in psychotherapy. Am J Psychoanal 36:319–323, 1976

Person ES: The erotic transference in women and in men: differences and consequences. J Am Acad Psychoanal 13(3):159–180, 1985

Sanderson B (ed): It's Never OK: A Handbook for Professionals on Sexual Exploitation by Counselors and Therapists. St Paul, MN, Minnesota Department of Corrections, 1989

Schoener G, Milgrom JH, Gonsiorek JC, et al (eds): Psychotherapists' Sexual Exploitation of Clients: Intervention and Prevention. Minneapolis, MN, Walk-In Counseling Center, 1989

Stone AA: Sexual misconduct by psychiatrists: the ethical and clinical dilemma of confidentiality. Am J Psychiatry 140:195–197, 1983

CHAPTER 19

Establishing Groups in an Individual Office Practice

Arnold Cohen, Ph.D.

Introduction

Most clinicians start their practices by working with individuals. This chapter discusses many of the pertinent issues that arise when starting a group in an office practice. It attends to the theoretical, technical, and pragmatic issues a clinician encounters when beginning a psychotherapy group.

Historically, group therapy has been seen as a second-class therapy and, therefore, has not had primary importance in training programs. Redl (1963) confirmed the notion of group therapy being seen as second class:

> . . . It has been gradually conceded that clinical work in groups, if done well and by appropriately trained therapists, could at least take over what the analyst wouldn't be too eager to deal with anyway, and group therapy has come a little closer to the position psycho-therapy is allowed to hold in relation to "analysis proper." (p. 135)

Things have changed in recent years. Group therapy has become a much more accepted and valued form of treatment. However, it continues to be the stepchild of individual psychotherapy. As Anthony (1971) suggested, it is difficult to gain admission into the "therapeutic club." Rivalry is intense and the competitive feelings one can have about which modality is "the best" may remain unspoken but nonetheless powerful.

Besides the theoretical and training constraints, there are practical impediments to beginning groups in an office practice. It takes a considerable amount of time, energy, and coordination to bring together six to eight individuals. This is a daunting challenge, and it contributes to the reasons why group therapy is often not a part of a beginning clinician's outpatient practice.

So the beginning clinician embarks on a practice mostly treating individuals. How does it happen that this person becomes interested in diversifying the practice to include group therapy? A therapist may respond to several factors:

- There is a need for group therapy in the community, and he or she may want to respond to that need.
- For certain patients in the practice (those whose primary concern is with their interpersonal relationships), group therapy is the treatment of choice, rather than individual therapy.
- Attendance at a seminar or workshop on group therapy may stimulate curiosity about running a group.
- Experience in the clinician's training group may become more integrated, and the therapist may wish to offer that experience to certain patients.
- The financial constraints on many patients may press for a more economical treatment.

Once a person has developed an interest in starting a group, he or she must then determine what needs to be done to get it started in an office practice. Below are some of the theoretical, technical, and training issues to consider when adding a psychotherapy group. Theoretical considerations regarding combined individual and group therapy are taken up in Chapter 17 of this volume. Pragmatic issues, as well as these dynamic issues, confront the therapist who is about to start a group.

What a Therapist Needs to Know Before Starting a Group

Before the first group session there are several steps a therapist can take to prepare himself or herself for leading the group. Some of the more important ones are

- Learning basic theory
- Attending workshops, seminars, and training programs

- Figuring out the community needs and one's referral sources
- Figuring out the type of group he or she is interested in running

Learning Basic Theory

Group theory has evolved considerably over the last two decades. Scholars have developed a much better understanding of how groups function and how they affect individuals. Although there is no one correct theory of group psychotherapy, most therapists have come to use a combination of group dynamic, interpersonal, and intrapsychic psychodynamic theories as the foundation of group psychotherapy practice (Rutan and Stone 1984). Yalom's book (1975) on group therapy is considered a "must read" book for any beginning practitioner wanting to learn about group theory. Yalom took an interpersonal theoretical position. Rutan and Stone (1984) offered a general overview of psychodynamic group theory and practical guidelines for starting a psychodynamic psychotherapy group.

In addition to these two excellent books, the *International Journal of Group Psychotherapy* is a rich source of current information about group psychotherapy. It is the official journal of the American Group Psychotherapy Association (AGPA) and publishes research of current interest to practitioners.

It is important to learn the conceptual differences between running a therapy group and conducting individual psychotherapy. Although knowledge of individual therapy helps in the work with groups, it is not enough to run a group effectively. In a therapy group one can enter the patients' world on three different levels: the intrapsychic, the interpersonal, or the group as a whole. It is these multiple levels of intervention that make group therapy unique and different from working with people individually.

Workshops, Seminars, and Training Programs

Throughout the country there are organizations that promote the learning of group psychotherapy. The major national professional organization is AGPA. This multidisciplinary organization sponsors a variety of training opportunities for learning about group psychotherapy. The most comprehensive of its programs is designed as a mentor program. A mentor is an AGPA fellow (an experienced group therapist). A trainee is assigned to a mentor who helps him or her find supervisors and courses to take to satisfy the requirements for a certificate of completion. Mentoring can be done at the national or local level.

Besides its training program, AGPA has an annual conference each February that brings together many of the most prominent group therapists nationally and internationally. At this week-long meeting, one can attend workshops, forums, or lectures or participate in intensive group experiences. These meetings are held at different locations around the country. The national training program and annual conference of AGPA are excellent places to meet colleagues and learn about group psychotherapy.

In addition to the national organization, many local organizations are affiliated with AGPA. These local organizations, like AGPA, sponsor a variety of events for people interested in learning more about group therapy. Becoming a member of a local organization is a way to have contact with other professionals, maintain a network, conduct research, and in general remain involved in current issues in group psychotherapy.

Community Need and Referral Sources

In addition to the criteria listed above, it is useful to take into consideration the community need when starting a group. What groups are already being run in the local professional community? What kinds of groups would provide an additional needed service? It is especially useful to speak to colleagues and locate the gaps in the community. Calling colleagues and agencies and learning about the landscape of one's community is time consuming, but in the long run it probably ensures success in building a group. One does not want to start a group that has no referral base and is set up to fail. This leads to the next critical element in planning to start a group: identifying the more likely referral sources and what types of patients they are likely to refer. These last two criteria, community need and one's referral network, are critical to the potential success of starting a group.

What Type of Group to Lead

Several factors should be taken into account when deciding what type of group to lead: Should the group be time limited or ongoing? Should the group be issue specific or not? What level of functioning should the patients have?

A time-limited group carries with it a very different commitment than an ongoing therapy group. The goals for short-term therapy groups typically include the following (Klein 1985):

- Amelioration of distress
- Prompt reestablishment of the patient's previous emotional equilibrium
- Promoting efficient use of the patient's resources
- Developing the patient's understanding of his or her current disturbance and increasing coping skills for the future

The therapist's role in time-limited groups is to be active, directive, managerial, and flexible.

In an ongoing long-term group the commitment of the therapist is to help the patients resolve characterological concerns and work on interpersonal skills. Therefore, the expectation is that patients will stay for a considerable length of time, because character changes slowly. The role of the therapist is to promote group cohesion and to allow the patients safe regression and the open expression of affective responses. Most time-limited groups are issue specific, whereas most ongoing groups are not. This has consequences for the type of group that evolves. Although some clinicians believe that putting people together around similar symptomatic issues helps to generate group cohesion, this is not necessarily true. Early on there may be a feeling of togetherness because of the similarity of life experience; however, as a group progresses and character traits and pathology emerge, the bond around symptomatology fades. People develop genuine trust because of who they are, not because of what they have done or experienced.

When putting a group together, it is very important to consider and plan the level of functioning of the patients. The themes of a group (what patients talk about) are related to the patients' level of functioning. Some groups struggle with fundamental issues of trust for years, whereas others struggle with power and anger, and others struggle with intimacy. It is helpful to have patients cluster around a similar level of functioning so they can learn and relate to one another's experience. However, it is also effective to have enough differences in life experience and personality style that people can see other ways of dealing with similar situations. It is this balance of similarity and difference that needs to be taken into account when putting a group of people together in treatment. For example, it would probably not be a good idea to put schizophrenic patients together with well-functioning neurotic patients. The discrepancy between their internal experiences would be too great to build a bridge. However, it may be an excellent idea to place a patient with an obsessive-compulsive personality style in the same group with another who has a hysterical personality style. They have a lot to learn from each other in terms of interpersonal styles and defensive functioning, and their capacity to relate to one another would probably be enhanced.

What a Therapist Needs to Do to Start a Group

In addition to the steps one needs to take to learn about group theory, community needs, referral sources, and so forth, one must think about certain practical considerations when beginning a group. These include

- Office arrangements
- Leadership considerations
- Pregroup interviews
- Supervision

These practical considerations should be addressed in a logical and thoughtful way if the group is to succeed.

Office Arrangements

When a therapist considers beginning a group, office size, location, and community laws become critical factors. The ideal group size is between 6 and 10 people; therefore, the office must be big enough to accommodate this many people.

Related to the size of the office is the issue of furniture. If most of a therapist's practice is with individuals, couples, and families, it is likely that he or she will have to find additional furniture. Because most of a therapist's time may be spent seeing people individually, he or she will want the office to feel comfortable when there are only two people in the room. Finding a way to change the office around or have additional space must be considered.

Another piece of the puzzle that must be attended to is the location of the office. If the office is in a business area, parking is not a problem. However, in a home office, parking can often be a difficult problem. Having 6 to 10 cars coming to one's office weekly can create neighborhood concerns and lead to problems. Check zoning regulations; in some communities therapists need a variance to see more than a given number of people per session. Nonetheless, most of these practical obstacles can be overcome with a little creativity and a strong measure of resolve.

Leadership Considerations

There are many leadership considerations when one sets out to start a group. These include leading alone or with another therapist, fees, the group contract, and setting a date and time.

Individual leadership or coleadership?   Although it is a common phenomenon to have two therapists leading a group in clinic settings, it is not as common to have two therapists leading a group in private practice. Many therapists prefer leading groups with another person. There are advantages and disadvantages to both models of leadership, which I briefly outline below.

Rutan and Stone (1984) noted several potential advantages to coleadership:

- A fuller and more complementary view of the group
- Watching and learning from a colleague
- Availability of ongoing coverage during illness and vacation
- Peer support and consultation
- Replicating the two-parent family
- An opportunity for imitating, modeling, and identifying with the behavior of therapists working out conflict
- Training value because coleadership can lessen anxiety, provide a sense of support, and allow for shared responsibility. (See Chapter 26 of this volume.)

Many of the arguments listed above are actually arguments that can be used against cotherapy. In fact, some people suggest that the disadvantages of cotherapy generally outweigh the advantages of this model. The disadvantages of cotherapy are as follows:

- Reducing anxiety is a problem because cotherapy does not allow a therapist the opportunity to confront the same anxiety as the patient, which allows for a stronger empathic connection.

- Children (patients) can encourage parents (therapists) to fight or love each other as a way of deflecting feelings from themselves (transferences and projections).
- Energy is drained away from patients because of the need to attend to the cotherapy relationship.
- Fees must be shared.
- Divergent development of therapists may impede the group process.

The need to attend to the cotherapy relationship is an important aspect of cotherapy. Attending to this need can be very rewarding or extremely cumbersome. As in any relationship, over time leaders develop differently and ultimately may not be compatible. These issues should be factored into a therapist's decision about the style of leadership to determine what suits him or her the best.

Fees.   Whether one leads individually or with another person, there are several aspects of leadership that must be worked out before the start of a group. Fees and a group contract are two elements that should be clarified before interviewing patients.

Two issues that arise concerning fee payment are the need for a policy concerning missed sessions and whether to offer a fee reduction.

In a group a person's seat cannot be filled in case of an absence. Therefore, the policy of paying for one's seat is often used. This option, although appearing to be rigid and self-serving, can in fact be useful to both the patient and the therapist. It reduces absenteeism and allows patients to explore the myriad feelings surrounding missed sessions.

In a group, fee reduction is a complicated and difficult clinical issue. A patient with a fee reduction occupies a special position in the group. This unique position will reverberate among the patients and should be discussed by the group as a whole so that everyone has the opportunity to express and learn about their feelings. Often this situation provides an excellent opportunity for working through the conflict between altruism and envy among the members.

The group contract.   The contract is an essential element of a group. It binds individuals into a therapeutic entity. Early theorists suggested that without an explicit agreement a group may become a destructive force. With an agreement a group may become a positive therapeutic force.

A contract is between the leader and the individuals as well as between the individuals and the entire group. A breach of contract affects everyone in the group. Below is a model contract that works well with psychodynamic therapy groups.

Each patient is asked to agree to the following:

1. Be present each week, be on time, and remain throughout the entire meeting.
2. Work actively on the problems that brought you to the group.
3. Put feelings into words, not actions.
4. Use the relationships developed in the group therapeutically and not socially.
5. Remain in the group until the problems have been resolved.
6. Be responsible for the fee for each session.
7. Protect the names and identities of fellow group members.

The contract is the foundation on which the therapeutic alliance is based. It needs to be carefully fashioned to meet the appropriate needs of the particular patients and the structure of a given group.

Pregroup Interviews

It is easy to put off starting a group. One of the most common excuses is that "I don't have enough members to begin." Setting a date often rectifies this problem. A deadline often acts as a catalyst to getting the group off the ground. A deadline gives patients who are waiting and potential referral sources a sense that the group does exist. Colleagues are not apt to refer to a planned but nonexistent group.

Meeting with patients before they start in the group is crucial. Making a beginning alliance with each member is often a critical factor in helping patients get through the difficult times during their early group experience.

In the pregroup interview one needs to learn about the patient. This includes finding out about the person's history, learning about the presenting problem, and discovering what his or her interpersonal history has been like. During the interview it is also important to educate the person about group therapy, respond to his or her fears and anxiety, and present him or her with the group contract. A careful discussion of each aspect of the contract will allow the patient to voice concerns and the therapist to make a fuller evaluation of that patient's capacity to work in this particular group.

Supervision

Leading a group can be a very exciting and rewarding experience. However, it can also be a very difficult and unpleasant experience. Transference and countertransference issues abound in groups. The more people there are in the room, the more opportunity there is for displacement and projection.

It is extremely helpful to be supervised by an experienced group therapist when leading one's first therapy group. The opportunities for mistakes abound in therapy groups, and it is a clinician's professional and ethical responsibility to acquire supervision when learning a new modality of treatment. In addition, it is a relief to know that there is someone with whom the clinician can discuss the myriad ways of getting into trouble when leading a therapy group and who can help resolve the difficulty.

Summary

The experience of beginning a group in an office practice is exciting, anxiety producing, and difficult. Little attention has been paid to this specific issue in the group therapy literature.

There are theoretical, technical, training, and pragmatic issues that must be attended to before starting a group. These range from the more pedestrian or practical concerns of office size and location, to creating and sustaining a collegial network, to acquiring good supervision and training. Attention to these parameters can enable the clinician to add a powerful new modality with which to serve his or her patients and to add a positive and exciting dimension to one's clinical options.

References

Anthony EJ: Comparison between individual and group psychotherapy, in Comprehensive Group Psychotherapy. Edited by Kaplan HI, Sadock BJ. Baltimore, MD, Williams & Wilkins, 1971, pp 104–112

Klein R: Some principles of short-term group therapy. Int J Group Psychother 35:309–330, 1985

Redl F: Psychoanalysis and group therapy: a developmental point of view. Am J Orthopsychiatry 33:135, 1963

Rutan JS, Stone W: Psychodynamic Group Psychotherapy. Lexington, MA, The Collamore Press, 1984

Yalom I: The Theory and Practice of Group Psychotherapy, 2nd Edition. New York, Basic Books, 1975

PART V

Gender Issues in Groups

CHAPTER 20

Women in Group Psychotherapy

Patricia Doherty, Ed.D.
Pamela L. Enders, Ph.D.

> It is questionable how much any individual woman
> before the women's movement was helped by indi-
> vidual therapy or advice. What became essential
> was for women to see themselves collectively, not
> individually, not caught in some individual erotic
> and familial plot and, inevitably found want-
> ing. . . . I suspect that female narratives will be
> found where women exchange stories, where they
> read and talk collectively of ambitions, possibili-
> ties, and accomplishments.
>
> Carolyn Heilbrun
> *Writing a Woman's Life*

Introduction

It wasn't so long ago that two psychoanalysts, Karen Horney (1935) and
Clara Thompson (1941), attempted to convince their colleagues to consider the influence of cultural attitudes and pressures on the psychological formation of women. This "culturist" orientation was rejected by
traditional psychoanalysis but experienced a renaissance in the 1970s.
At that time the social structure was sufficiently fortified by the women's
movement to allow other analysts to pick up where Horney and Thompson left off.

The power of the women's movement in the context of the turmoil of the 1970s turned our attention once again to the impact of society and culture on women's psychological development. Today it is the rare psychotherapist who will not consider, to some degree, sociocultural factors in the assessment and psychotherapy of a patient, male or female. It is important to note that consideration of sociocultural factors alone is as detrimental to the patient as is the exploration of intrapsychic factors exclusively. The patient is best served when the therapist attends to

- Sociocultural factors (the world in which a person lives)
- Interpersonal experiences (the way the person interacts in that world)
- Intrapsychic dynamics (the motivations and conflicts that affect the patient's interactions and color his or her perceptions)

Of course, it is erroneous to think that these are discrete entities. A more useful approach might be to imagine a tricolored piece of fabric where the different colored threads contribute to the beauty and integrity of the whole. At one moment, the viewer might appreciate the blue tone more than the red or yellow; later, the yellow will seem more compelling. Still, one can never completely cease to apprehend the harmonious, blending impact of all three colors. Similarly, in conducting psychotherapy or in developing theory, we believe that failure to regard all three factors (sociocultural, intrapsychic, and interpersonal) will result in an incomplete understanding of the patient.

Group psychotherapy provides an ideal setting in which to see, to explore, to understand, and to work through all of the three factors mentioned above. Insofar as the group represents a microcosm of society, one will see sociocultural biases emerge, allowing the patient to experience those constraints in the group, to recognize whether and how she might be participating in perpetuating such biases, and to discover new ways of understanding and dealing with those pressures. The following case example illustrates how one patient had to confront his own preconceived notions about homosexuality:

Case 1

Ms. A and Mr. B both entered a group at the same time and quickly formed a strong bond. Later, when Ms. A "came out" in the group, Mr. B said, "I don't know how to relate to you now that I know you're a lesbian." Ms. A insisted that she was still the same person. After a silent moment, Mr. B said,

"I guess it makes me feel rejected as a man. . . . I feel if I were a better man you would like us (men) better."

The interpersonal dimension comes alive in groups as the patient interacts with other members and the group leader. Such interactions can be understood and addressed from a number of theoretical orientations, including the interpersonal learning approach espoused by Yalom (1970) and object relations theory. A group can provide a broader context in which the patient's intrapsychic problems can be examined.

In this chapter we 1) present a brief historical overview of the psychological development of women, 2) consider the application of current theory to working with women in group therapy, 3) explore the advantages and disadvantages of homogeneous versus heterogeneous groups, and 4) address the role of the female leader.

The Psychological Development of Women

Housewife[1]

Some women marry houses.
It's another kind of skin; it has a heart,
a mouth, a liver and bowel movements.
The walls are permanent and pink.
See how she sits on her knees all day,
faithfully washing herself down.
Men enter by force, drawn back like Jonah
into their fleshy mothers.
A woman *is* her mother.
That's the main thing.

The poem by Anne Sexton (1981) conveys the isolation and alienation of some housewives but it also captures, in a few lines, what theorists have been struggling with in volumes; that is, the complex relationships between a man and a woman and between men, women, and their mothers. Given our current sociocultural environment, a woman is still seen, by herself and others, as an object and not a subject with her own sense of

---

[1] "Housewife" from *All My Pretty Ones* by Anne Sexton. Copyright © 1962 by Anne Sexton. Reprinted by permission of Houghton Mifflin Company. All rights reserved.

authority and agency. It is easy to see how difficult it can be for a woman to be judged mentally healthy.

Diagnosis and assessment are dependent, in part, on the conscious or unconscious inclusion of gender-role analysis. Traditionally a "normal" woman (at least a white, middle-class woman in the United States) is one who exhibits behaviors and traits such as nurturance, compliance, dependency, passivity, ambivalence about her sexuality with the wish to be desired but a fear of actively desiring, a strong wish to please others, and a tendency to focus on interpersonal relationships (Brown 1986).

Although these qualities and behaviors are what our society has traditionally associated with women, the picture becomes complicated when we consider the dichotomous theorizing within the psychoanalytic community, which generally perceives development as a linear progression from dependence to independence and which considers separateness as the pinnacle of mental health. An individual's wish and ability to form attachments are relegated to a lower slot on the hierarchy of health (Spieler 1986). Where does this leave women?

According to Susan Spieler (1986) and others (Chehrazi 1987; Zilbach 1987), Freud's theory of personality is androcentric and therefore, "the feminine sense of self is seen as essentially crippled because it is not masculine" (Spieler 1986, p. 34). Briefly, Freud believed that the little girl, like the boy, has a primary masculine (phallic) sexuality but that the girl, who lacks a penis and has only a clitoris, experiences penis envy and feels inferior. She becomes passive, masochistic, and narcissistic (Deutsch 1945) and blames her mother for her genital inferiority. Mother is rejected and the girl turns to father, who has the magical penis. The girl does not develop a strong superego because she does not suffer from castration anxiety (she has already been castrated). The wish for father's baby is, according to Freud, a substitute for the real prize, his penis. The wish for pregnancy is understood as a derivative of penis envy and not as an identification with mother as primary nurturer (Bernstein and Warner 1984).

Freud's theory on female sexuality has been strongly criticized by his peers and by our contemporaries. Charlotte Perkins Gilman referred to his work as a revival of "phallic worship" (Donovan 1985), whereas Karen Horney (1926) rejected the importance that penis envy played in female development. Horney (1926) also stated that men experience envy of women's reproductive capacities. Clara Thompson (1942) specifically addressed the importance of cultural influences in personality problems and said that penis envy is the result of the greater prestige and power of men in our society:

> I have pointed out that characteristics and inferiority feelings which Freud considered to be specifically female and biologically determined can be explained as developments arising in and growing out of Western woman's historic situation of underprivilege, restriction of development, insincere attitude toward the sexual nature, and social economic dependency. The basic nature of woman is still unknown. (p. 339)

Most of the early theoretical contributions were based on hypotheses about infant development generated by the clinical material of adult analyses, usually conducted by men. Infant observation was rare, and empirical studies were lacking. The belief that the path of development for boys and girls was the same (i.e., that it was essentially masculine for both) persisted in spite of the few dissenting voices.

The 1960s heralded new ideas based on infant observation. Stoller (1968) introduced the term "core gender identity," the felt sense that one is a girl or a boy, which occurs long before the onset of the phallic phase of psychosexual development. Core gender identity is shaped by biological, sociological, and psychological forces. This research brings into question Freud's notion that both girls and boys start out as "little men."

Some clinicians and theorists proposed a separate line of development for females (Miller 1976; Gilligan 1982; Jordan and Surrey 1986; Stiver 1986; Zilbach 1987), which emphasized the importance of relationships, affiliation, caretaking, and interconnectedness. Although agreeing that these qualities are indeed critical for women, Zilbach (1987) sought to find an equivalent female concept with the power of the masculine concept of the phallus. She called this "active engulfment." In her view, there is a center of core or primary femininity that is transformed over time, in social and familial interactions, into characteristics of nurturance, embracing love, affiliation, and interrelatedness.

Jordan and Surrey (1986) used the term "self-in-relation" to describe their idea, which has as its central thesis the notion that "women organize their sense of identity, find existential meaning, achieve a sense of coherence and continuity, and are motivated in the context of a relationship" (p. 102). Carol Gilligan summarized this idea and compared women with men by indicating that masculinity is defined through separation, whereas femininity is defined through attachment.

Certainly, an obvious problem with any dichotomous structuring of affiliation and nurturance versus autonomy and achievement is the implication that men do not find meaning in the context of relationships (Lerner 1988). Generalizations and misinterpretations are just as much a problem for feminists as they are or have been for traditional theorists. These women have, however, helped us challenge a tendency to pathologize female development and have offered a more positive perspective on the mother-daughter dyad. But it is just this focus on the mother-daughter dyad that troubled Lerner, who believed that we need to conceptualize development as taking place within a system that includes several individuals, not just two. Enlarging the scope of development from a dyadic to a systemic model fits in well with group therapy, where one can witness a recreation of life's myriad relationships. Without an appreciation of the family system, Lerner worried that just as mothers might be praised for their nurturing capabilities, so too they could be castigated for their failure to nurture correctly.

Chodorow (1978) wrote extensively on this subject in her book *Reproduction of Mothering,* in which she discussed the problems inherent in a society where women do most of the mothering. Mother can be perceived by her child as a narcissistic extension whose sole reason for existence is to gratify the child's needs and wants. Mother (woman), then, will be viewed as the other or object. She will rarely be seen as a subject, a self with her own set of needs, wants, motivations, and ideas. Males and females are likely to harbor the perspective that women are objects, not subjects. Later, we will see how group therapy can provide an opportunity for men and women to see women as subjects with their own sense of agency and authority. In other words, group therapy can facilitate the demythologizing of women.

Jessica Benjamin (1988) incorporated some of Chodorow's thinking along with the research of Daniel Stern (1985) in her work on intersubjectivity. Like Chodorow, Benjamin was concerned with the extent of female mothering and with the failure to see women as subjects. She stressed how important it is for the child to recognize mother as an independent subject instead of the object of attachment or the object of desire. To Benjamin (1988), recognition was central to human existence: " . . . to recognize is to affirm, validate, acknowledge, know, accept, understand. . . . " (p. 15). Mutual recognition is crucial to the intersubjective view because it implies that we have a need to recognize the other as a separate person who is like us yet is distinct. "The recognition a child seeks is something the mother is able to give only by virtue of her independent identity" (Benjamin 1988, p. 24). The mother should not be just a mirror but must embody an independent other who responds in her own different way.

According to Benjamin (1988), the intersubjective view refers to what happens in the field of self and other, but she warned that "without the intrapsychic concept of the unconscious, intersubjective theory becomes one dimensional, for it is only against the background of the mind's private space that the real other stands out in relief" (p. 21). She also stated: "To claim anything more for intersubjectivity would invite a triumph of the external . . . a relational psychoanalysis should leave room for the messy, intrapsychic side of creativity and aggression. . . . " (Benjamin 1990a, p. 45).

The theory of subjectivity as outlined by Benjamin seems to incorporate, in many ways, the three factors originally deemed important by us: sociocultural, interpersonal, and intrapsychic. We now show how this theory of subjectivity can be applied to understanding the way women interact in and can benefit by group psychotherapy.

Advantages of Group Therapy for Women

If we believe that the isolation of women has, in part, contributed to the overwhelming feelings of depression, defectiveness, and loneliness they often experience, then it is readily clear that a group can be a haven of comfort and support—a reprieve from isolation.

It was this sense of isolation experienced in the context of sweeping social and cultural changes that led to the development of consciousness-raising (CR) groups in the late 1960s. CR groups offered hope and promise of increased power to women in the 1960s and 1970s (Bernardez 1983; Kirsh 1974, 1987). These groups (ranging from 5 to 12 members) were designed to promote a feeling of sisterhood, commonality, support, and relief from the belief that one was defective simply because one was a woman. The main ideology of CR groups was that problems experienced by women were the result of living in a sexist society where roles were rigidly defined and where one encountered prejudice because of one's gender. The focus of discussion was on the impact of sociocultural factors on a woman's life. Change, it was believed, could occur only if society itself changed. It was thought that by making women aware of the external causes of their distress, they would feel empowered to produce change in the outside world. The structure of CR groups reflected feminist ideals: nonhierarchical, democratic, accepting, supportive, and emotional rather than intellectual in character. Hence, the typical CR group was leaderless, with each woman viewed as being her own authority. Hierarchy was eschewed.

Over the years, these CR groups have evolved into what are now variously called, support groups, rap groups, and discussion groups. They may have a particular theme, such as "a young mothers' support group," but the roots are in the early CR groups. The important legacy of CR groups is the fact that they alerted us to the powerful impact of sociocultural pressures on people's lives. The minimal research on the effectiveness of these groups leaves us wondering how they specifically changed women's lives, but the anecdotal "evidence" supports the belief that many women found CR groups helpful.

One of the things that made CR groups distinctive is also what makes them problematic: that is, the intense focus on external factors, often at the exclusion of exploring internal dynamics. For some groups, clinging to ideology at all costs may have unwittingly perpetuated sexual dichotomies and polarities. Still, because of CR groups, it is hard to imagine ignoring the sociocultural factor today.

As useful as CR groups may be, they are not psychotherapy. The ideology, structure, goals, and process differ between the two modalities (Kravetz 1987). Psychotherapy focuses more on a person's internal world and/or interpersonal dynamics with an appreciation for the impact of the sociocultural context rather than the stronger emphasis on external factors that occurs in CR groups. Psychotherapy also seeks to define and heal the psychopathological aspects of the individual's personality organization. Group psychotherapy operates in a defined context with a leader and a clear contract that allows for the freedom and safety necessary to effect in-depth change. Through the interpersonal exchange and the leader's interpretations, unconscious material emerges in the "workplace" of the group. This milieu allows for multiple transferences, a plethora of responses, and a variety of models. The therapy group provides a laboratory in which to experiment with new behavior and to examine and reorganize character traits and defenses as these are played out in the group context.

Women's Groups Versus Mixed Groups

Some writers have claimed that women's groups are superior to mixed groups (male and female members) in numerous ways (Burden and Gottlieb 1987; Walker 1987), including the "lack of unconscious sexism," an increased sense of warmth and closeness, and more freedom to talk openly. Women in single-sex groups are said to bring up "taboo" subjects (e.g., sex) earlier than they do in mixed groups. However, these claims are largely unsubstantiated by empirical data. Unfortunately, like much of the literature on psychotherapy in general, the claims are based on observations that were not made in a systematic way and were not derived from objective measures.

In a review article assessing women's groups, Kathleen Huston (1986) concluded that, although the structure and goals of women's groups may be unique, not much else can be determined about how they differ from mixed-sex groups in terms of process and outcome. She cautioned, however, that the lack of research does not mean that women's groups are not uniquely effective. Huston urged that feminists move from presenting theory alone to validating their theoretical positions by conducting empirical studies.

Although it is probable that some women may fare better in a women's group, the question remains: under what circumstances and for what set of problems should a woman patient be treated in a women's group rather than a mixed group?

Theoretically, it seems that a single-sex group with same-sex therapist(s) makes sense for early adolescents "to promote progressive ego development, gender identification with ego ideal figures, and a protective period of vicarious preparation for heterosexual relations" (Kennedy 1989, p. 39). Women who have experienced incest or sexual abuse usually feel more comfortable and are freer in expressing their feelings and telling their stories in women's groups (Herman and Schatzow 1984). The same can be said for women who have been battered or otherwise abused by men.

Women's groups may be especially helpful for women who are at points of transition in their lives and who require the extra boost of female support in order to move ahead. Obviously, a request by a woman to be placed in a women's group shouldn't be ignored, but neither should the therapist act on such a request without first carefully exploring the meaning and usefulness of such a request. Problems with single-sex groups include perpetuation of gender polarities with unwitting (at best) support for the continuation of gender-role mythology; a tendency to encourage blaming the absent gender for one's problems; increased susceptibility to fusion either between members or with the same-sex leader; and the fact that single-sex groups do not resemble the real, heterogeneous world in which we live. Outside of the group therapy literature, however, there is evidence that a single-sex environment can be beneficial to young women's development. This is especially true in the classroom, where it has been shown that girls and young women flourish in an all-female environment and are more likely to speak out with confidence than they are in a coeducational school (Krupnick 1985).

Single-sex groups can promote particular countertransference difficulties for a leader who is of the same sex and who may not acknowledge and not welcome a homoerotic transference (Alonso 1987). In mixed groups, "the erotic fantasies emerge in the heterosexual displacement, and can later be brought into focus as homoerotic for the member who is of the same sex as the leader" (Alonso 1987, p. 161).

A Women's Group Becomes a Mixed Group

The following case example illustrates how the addition of men to an all-female group can change the tenor and tone of a group. Initially, the absence of men facilitated closeness and openness, but also inhibited expression of aggression—especially toward the female leader.

Case 2

A group that began with four women members and one woman leader developed a positive cohesiveness early on with considerable openness, an ability to be confrontative, and a capacity to express a wide range of feelings. Occasionally, one or another of the women wondered when "the men" would enter the group. There were jokes about how the group mirrored society in that "a good man is hard to find."

Finally, after several months, the leader announced that a new member, a man, would be joining the group. The women greeted the news with a pause, some laughter, and then numerous associations to brothers who were the favored siblings, fathers who were sexually abusive, men who were violent, and boyfriends who were male chauvinists. The women also told tales of disrupted friendships with women because of men. Would it be necessary for them to disconnect with each other in order for them to connect to a man?

Ms. C, who had few women friends and who generally preferred men, said, "It feels too close in here with all these women. We're too much alike. It feels yucky with all this closeness. Sticky. I get all these associations to menstrual blood and milky breasts." "Gee," Ms. D said, "you make it sound like a steamy jungle scene with bouncing boobs like National Geographic!"

When the new member arrived, two of the four women were absent. They were ill with the "flu" (or, perhaps, flew). On their return they were told by Ms. E that "we were flirty" with the new man. The talk in that session centered on issues of power and equality. Eventually two other men joined the group. For the first time, the women were able to address their anger and dissatisfaction with the female leader.

The Power of Groups to Demythologize

Sex-role stereotypes or myths limit all of us in subtle and blatant ways. These limitations affect the perceiver and the perceived. Both sexes have an investment in these myths, and hence little allowance is made for movement outside of these stereotypes. Group psychotherapy provides a safe place for members to try out new out-of-role behaviors and to assess the impact of these behaviors on other members and themselves. Furthermore, in listening to group members of another sex, myths about the opposite sex that were held dear by the listener can be challenged and eventually altered, as is illustrated in Case 3:

Case 3

Ms. F, an intelligent and competent businesswoman, had experienced a recent painful breakup of a relationship with a man. What made this especially difficult for her was the fact that she was 40 years old and desperately wanted children. She had seen this relationship as her last hope for marriage and a family. In her fury at her ex-lover, she berated all men for treating women terribly. She complained that there were no decent men left and that men ignored women's feelings and needs. Ms. F directed all this to the women in the group, shunning the men entirely. The men shifted in their seats, uncomfortable at being iced out by Ms. F and the other women. The leader eventually noted how the women were ignoring the men.

This simple intervention initially caused some anxious giggles among the women and sighs of relief among the men, but it encouraged the two sexes to face each other and opened the possibility for dialogue. The men expressed their genuine sadness about Ms. F's breakup and responded with heartfelt sensitivity to her predicament. Mr. G acknowledged that it was true that, even though he was 41, he didn't feel the same urgency women did to have children by a certain age. Mr. G had experienced pressure to make a commitment to a woman who, like Ms. F, wanted children before it was too late. He was not in love with this woman and did not want to marry her but also was unprepared to end the relationship. He had decided all women just wanted to hook a man so they could control him (as his mother had dominated his father). Until he had listened to Ms. F, he hadn't realized how exquisitely painful it was for women to deal with the prospect of a childless life. But what could he do, he wondered. He really didn't want to marry the woman, yet how could he go on hurting her?

Ms. F was moved and surprised to see how responsive the men were to her sadness. She was especially touched by Mr. G's dilemma and saw that her former lover was in a similar predicament (i.e., that he didn't love her enough to marry her and that the breakup may have been hard for him as well). "Maybe all men aren't shitheads after all," Ms. F said.

We can see that this mixed-sex group was actively dealing with myths about the other sex. The myths that all men were indifferent to the feelings and needs of women and that all women wanted to control men were questioned and analyzed because of the group context. The power these myths had over the attitudes and actions of the group members was diminished, and (at least for Ms. F and Mr. G) new understanding and appreciation of the complexity of heterosexual relationships were achieved.

Although it is true that such myths are the product of our sociocultural arrangement, to say that this vignette describes the success of groups in dealing with sociocultural biases in vivo is only part of the story. The fact that the women were initially shunning the men illustrates how interpersonal behavior, as it is recreated in the group, can be an accomplice to heartache. In other words, by actively ignoring them, the women weren't giving the men the chance to prove that they could be sensitive and responsive. Later in the group, the women wondered how often they unconsciously shunned men to prove to themselves how unfeeling men were and how wonderfully sensitive women were. They saw how their interpersonal actions served to block intimacy.

On an intrapsychic level, Mr. G was able to begin to see how his identification with his weak and ineffectual father led him to perceive all women as similar to his abusive mother. On the other hand, Ms. F had, like her mother, viewed all men as "selfish clods" resembling her father. Mr. G's response to Ms. F freed her up to recall several instances where her father had displayed kindness to her.

Women as Objects to Women as Subjects

Subjectivity, the felt sense that one has an independent identity that is actively recognized by another, is an important developmental achievement. This can be powerfully promoted in group therapy. The need for mutual recognition is critical to healthy development and is crucial to the intersubjective view as espoused by Jessica Benjamin (1988, 1990a, 1990b). The child has a need to see mother as an independent subject and not as an extension of himself or herself. Because of powerful culturally supported fantasies about mothering, women are seen as objects—objects of attachment or objects of desire (Benjamin 1988; Chodorow 1978, 1989). Females are likely to grow up believing that they have no right to express their own desire but must take pleasure only in being desired. They may fail to realize that they can actively desire something for themselves. Because women may not see themselves as subjects, they will not see other women as subjects. Men's behavior may confirm or dispel these notions. The following case example illustrates how group therapy can alter a person's sense of self from that of an object to that of a subject:

Case 4

Ms. H, a 35-year-old executive, had a number of unsatisfying relationships with men in which she ingratiated herself to please them. Ms. H's mother had told her (and had shown her in her marital relationship) that a woman must do everything possible to entice a man and to keep him happy. In the group, Ms. H tended to ask the male members for the "male perspective" on questions such as the following: Are men "disgusted" if a woman cries? What does a man think of a woman who "gives in" too easily? What do men feel about a woman who is assertive? Initially the men were pleased to offer their advice. Eventually, they encouraged Ms. H to explore more how she felt about such things rather than try to figure out what men wanted. Ms. H was surprised to learn that other people might have an interest in what she thought and felt. One day, she reported to the group that she had decided not to have a second date with a man she had met recently. She said, "I always thought that if a man wanted me, I had to acquiesce. It never occurred to me that I could decide whether or not I wanted him!" Ms. H began to see herself as something other than an object of desire; she began to believe in her own subjectivity and her own ability to have some control over her destiny.

Woman as Container and Expresser of Affect

It is not unusual for much of the affective work of a group to be done by the women, with the men serving as observers, learning vicariously about their feelings (MacNab 1990). Women are generally more adept at acknowledging and expressing a whole range of feelings. In a group, one can see one gender's wish to split off unacceptable feelings and provoke the other gender to contain and express the emotion. In some instances, women who cannot tolerate their hostility manage to evoke these feelings in the men, whereas men, who eschew dependency, form intense relationships with helpless women who hold these feelings for them. The following case example illustrates how one man was able to reclaim his own feelings only after a woman in the group first expressed them for him:

Case 5

> Mr. I described his childhood experiences of physical abuse and recalled how he avoided more extensive beatings by functioning as the "good little boy" while he observed his older sister "get it." While he was recounting several incidents of humiliating treatment, Ms. J began to cry and said, "I feel so sad . . . what a terribly sad childhood!" Mr. I paused and looked at Ms. J and then became teary himself. As he finally claimed and expressed his own sadness, Ms. J remarked that she no longer felt the distress. In noting how he "got" Ms. J to contain and express his feelings for him, Mr. I said, with some surprise, "Now I know why I felt so anxious and guilty when my sister got pregnant and left home; she took it (the abuse) for me all those years!" Mr. I also related incidents of relationships with women where he maintained an intellectual distance and the women expressed the emotion. One of the women in the group noted how that happened all the time in the group setting.

Woman as Group Leader

Gender raises certain expectations about power and intimacy. We look at, expect from, project onto, and interact with men and women differently depending on our own gender. Specifically, persons in positions of authority evoke different responses because of their gender. Group work is affected by the gender of the leader (Reed 1983) in various ways. But what is this effect when the group leader is a woman?

According to Broverman et al. (1970), feminine characteristics (e.g., warmth, dependency, and emotionality) are less valued than masculine characteristics (e.g., strength, independence, autonomy, and rationality) by students and clinicians alike. Because the qualities of women are deemed inferior, women are assigned (by women and men) lower status than men. Furthermore, many of these feminine qualities are in conflict with the leadership role (Reed 1983), which demands autonomy, strength, and objectivity.

Maleness is the more valued state, and leadership is the more valued role. Thus the woman as leader is somewhat of an anomaly; although she is "inferior," she presumes to be competent to exercise a function socially ascribed to the opposite sex—to be number one in the group. This position is incongruent with both the status and the role of a woman. The female authority poses a conflict for female group leaders and group members of both sexes because the position reverses their world view (Gornick 1986). To the extent that the group experience duplicates the family and social experience, these roles are played out in the group. If the roles in the group are altered, intrapsychic and interpersonal changes in the group members will occur. The following case example illustrates how a group responds to a female leader asserting her authority:

Case 6

In a mixed-sex group led by a woman, Mr. K came late to his first group meeting. He often canceled at the last minute. He met another member for coffee during the leader's vacation, and when the news broke in the group the other members felt betrayed and jealous of the special connection. The leader reminded Mr. K and the other member that their behavior was in violation of the therapeutic contract. The men were initially angry with the leader's strong stance but then expressed amazement. The women were relieved.

As Alonso and Rutan (1979) pointed out, a woman therapist occupies a position of power and authority, a role that is dystonic from a cultural point of view. The confusion in stereotypes may generate anxiety for women patients who may wish to identify with the woman leader but who see her as a tough act to follow. Men may fear to identify with a woman leader because their sense of masculinity is threatened. The female leader must be aware of and work through her own inferiority feelings as well as her ambivalence about the role and status conflict in order to face the challenges that will necessarily be presented by the group. Otherwise, she will simply reinforce rather than work through the stereotypes.

The female leader may stir up wishes and expectations of the all-perfect mother: selfless, totally uncritical, accepting, and soothing. Indeed, the leader may derive considerable gratification from the admiration she receives in being the perfect mother, and she may hesitate to step out of that role to be appropriately confrontative or to maintain firm limits and boundaries. Certainly, cultural roles demand that all women be caretakers, and the woman leader must be certain not to rely on or expect her female group members to help her with the nurturing in the group, especially vis-à-vis the men (Westkott 1986). The men may feel entitled to be the recipients of female nurturing. The group and the leader may be reluctant to set aside the fantasies of the perfect mother. The leader who has not resolved this issue for herself will not be prepared to deal with the inevitable anger and disappointment of the group as it discovers the leader's shortcomings. The following case example illustrates the positive outcome of a group in which the leader who invited her group's anger:

Case 7

> A few weeks after two new members joined a group, making a total of seven members, Ms. L complained that she preferred the smaller group. She believed the leader wanted the extra money and didn't take into consideration the feelings or needs of the group. The leader had a "cushy job" and didn't have to drive 30 miles to get home in bad weather. One member asked Ms. L how many people were in her family. "Seven," she replied, "and one dog," she added, glancing at the leader. The group laughed, recognizing the parallel association. The leader said, "Hmm, and one dog . . . a bitch?" This invitation to be angry with the leader unleashed a flood of associations from group members concerning mothers who were greedy, narcissistic, abusive, or negligent. Various group members began comparing their mothers with the mothering ability of the group leader. Ms. L said that she had always been fearful of her mother's wrath and that her mother would never tolerate any expression of anger from her children. Her mother had to be right. Finally Ms. L said, "Maybe my mother wasn't that strong after all if she couldn't handle a little lip from her kids. Maybe real strength is in being able to accept what your kids have to say."

Research on the impact of the therapist's gender on the outcome of psychotherapy has been mostly conducted with the dyadic model. One study found that regardless of the patient's gender, women therapists were found to have established more effective therapeutic alliances than male therapists (Jones and Zoppel 1982). The therapeutic-alliance factor gauged the therapist's interest in, acceptance of, and respect for the patient, as well as the extent to which the therapist's manner was seen as warm and attentive. Patients who saw same-sex therapists were more likely to view the therapist as neutral or nondirective than those in cross-gender pairings. Interestingly, female patients, regardless of the therapist's gender, were more likely to experience feeling deprecated by the therapist. Overall, there was some evidence that women therapists were more successful in attaining the therapeutic goals, especially with women patients.

The advantage of the above study is that it was based on actual and not analogue psychotherapy experiences. It did not address how women are perceived in groups. In another study that assessed affect responses to male and female leaders, it was found that female leaders elicited more negative nonverbal affect from group members than did male leaders offering the same initiatives (Butler and Geis 1990). In fact, it appeared that if a woman merely offered a substantive contribution it was sufficient to elicit displeasure in others. The authors suggested that "leadership and gender expectations are prescriptive as well as descriptive" (p. 54).

One recent study on groups found that women patients in particular perceived female-led groups as less effective for them than male-led groups (Boston Institute for Psychotherapy, unpublished research report, March 1991).

Previously, Bernardez and Stein (1979) stated that female group members may feel anger at the second-classness of the female authority and that the male members may rebel rather than "submit" or be placed in a subordinate position to the female leader. Because the leader has a different role from the other female members, she may by subjected to the typical responses accorded a token figure (i.e., one who is set apart and whose behavior is studied closely) (Reed 1983).

The female leader is given a variety of signals as to how the group wants her to respond. She should be warm and accepting, never angry or critical. If she steps out of the stereotypical response, confusion and conflict ensue. If she does not, the stereotypes live on. Groups with female leaders provide more opportunities for working through alternatives for both genders, whereas groups with male leaders may tend to reinforce stereotypes (Mayes 1979; Reed 1979). This last case example illustrates how difficult it can be for group members to accept a woman leader who acts in a nonstereotyped fashion:

Case 8

Ms. M arrived 5 minutes late for her first group meeting. She brought presents to the therapist: chocolate-covered strawberries and lilacs. She surreptitiously met with another group member during the therapist's vacation. She ran up a bill. For each incident, the female therapist explored the behavior and reinforced the contract, resulting in the rest of the group becoming angry that so much time was being spent on this. When Ms. M nonchalantly said that she was going to file for bankruptcy and that her bill would never be paid, the therapist said that Ms. M could continue only if she paid in cash each week. When she arrived with a check one week, the therapist said, "this was not the contract." Ms. M responded, "So, you want me to leave?" "No, but we have an agreement," the therapist said. Ms. M stormed out of the room. The group members' reactions were mixed; the women were relieved by the leader's firm stand but felt concerned that Ms. M would not return. The men were angry at the leader and felt protective toward Ms. M.

Summary

In this chapter we have looked at the development of women through a sociocultural, psychological, and interpersonal lens. Traditionally, the psychoanalytic literature presented a deficit model of development in which women were viewed as defective. However, even in the earliest days of psychoanalysis, powerful theorists such as Karen Horney were challenging this view of women as inherently inferior and envious. In more recent years, due to the evolution of theory, the entry of women as contributors to the literature, and the change in the sociocultural climate, a great deal of attention has been given (mostly by women) to women's psychological development. These theories have emphasized a separate line of development for women. A woman's need to be a whole person in her own right—to claim her own "agency" and not be considered and treated as an extension of men or mother—has been brought to the fore. Concurrently, women have attempted to move from the more conventional roles, and in so doing, they have experienced new levels of conflict and anxiety, for which they have sought help from clinicians and each other. Because women have more often looked to a group for advice, succor, and support, group psychotherapy is an obvious setting for the treatment of women in distress.

We have explored the ways in which group psychotherapy is particularly beneficial to women. Clinical options have been addressed, such as the kinds of groups that have evolved over time. Research, though spotty, does point out the benefits and drawbacks of single-sex and mixed-sex groups. The role of the female leader has been similarly examined. The woman group leader brings powerful tools to group therapy but must also struggle to overcome cultural inhibitions related to power and authority in herself and to deal with the anxieties a powerful woman may raise in her patients. We now have a direction and a mandate that call for more formalized research on how women can be helped through the process of group therapy and how the role of the female leader can affect that process.

References

Alonso A: Discussion of "women's groups led by women." Int J Group Psychother 37:159–162, 1987

Alonso A, Rutan JS: Women in group therapy. Int J Group Psychother 29:481–491, 1979

Benjamin J: Bonds of Love. New York, Pantheon Books, 1988

Benjamin J: An outline of intersubjectivity: the development of recognition. Psychoanalytic Psychology 7:33–46, 1990a

Benjamin J: The alienation of desire: women's masochism and ideal love, in Essential Papers on the Psychology of Women. Edited by Zanardi C. New York, New York University Press, 1990b, pp 455–479

Bernardez T: Women's groups, in Handbook of Short-Term Therapy Groups. Edited by Rosenbaum M. New York, McGraw-Hill, 1983, pp 119–138

Bernardez T, Stein TS: Separating the sexes in group therapy: an experiment with men's and women's groups. Int J Group Psychother 29:493–502, 1979

Bernstein AE, Warner GM: Women Treating Women: Case Material From Women Treated by Female Psychoanalysts. Madison, CT, International Universities Press, 1984

Broverman IK, Broverman DM, Clarkson FE: Sex role stereotypes and clinical judgments of mental health. J Consult Clin Psychol 34:1–7, 1970

Brown LS: Gender-role analysis: a neglected component of psychological assessment. Psychotherapy 23:243–248, 1986

Burden DS, Gottlieb N: Women's socialization and feminist groups, in Women's Therapy Groups: Paradigms of Feminist Treatment. Edited by Brody CM. New York, Springer, 1987, pp 24–39

Butler D, Geis FL: Nonverbal affect responses to male and female leaders: implications for leadership evaluations. J Pers Soc Psychol 58:48–59, 1990

Chehrazi S: Female psychology: a review, in The Psychology of Women: Ongoing Debates. Edited by Walsh MR. New Haven, CT, Yale University Press, 1987, pp 22–38

Chodorow N: The Reproduction of Mothering: Psychoanalysis and the Sociology of Gender. Berkeley, CA, University of California Press, 1978

Chodorow N: Feminism and Psychoanalytic Theory. New Haven, CT, Yale University Press, 1989

Deutsch H: The Psychology of Women. New York, Grune & Stratton, 1945

Donovan J: Feminist Theory. New York, Ungar, 1985

Gilligan C: In a Different Voice. Cambridge, MA, Harvard University Press, 1982

Gornick LK: Developing a new narrative: the woman therapist and the male patient. Psychoanalytic Psychology 3:299–325, 1986

Heilbrun CG: Writing a Woman's Life. New York, Ballantine, 1988

Herman J, Schatzow E: Time-limited group therapy for women with a history of incest. Int J Group Psychother 34:605–616, 1984

Horney K: Feminine Psychology (1926). New York, Norton, 1967

Horney K: The problem of feminine masochism. Psychoanal Rev 22:241–257, 1935

Huston K: A critical assessment of the efficacy of women's groups. Psychotherapy 23:283–290, 1986

Jones EE, Zoppel CL: Impact of client and therapist gender on psychotherapy process and outcome. J Consult Clin Psychol 50:259–272, 1982

Jordan JV, Surrey JL: The self-in-relation: empathy and the mother-daughter relationship, in The Psychology of Today's Woman: New Psychoanalytic Visions. Edited by Bernay T, Cantor DW. Hillsdale, NJ, Analytic Press, 1986, pp 81–104

Kennedy JF: Therapist gender and the same-sex puberty age psychotherapy group. Int J Group Psychother 39:255–265, 1989

Kirsh B: Consciousness-raising groups as therapy for women, in Women in Therapy: New Psychotherapies for a Changing Society. Edited by Franks V, Burtle V. New York, Brunner/Mazel, 1974, pp 326–354

Kirsh B: Evolution of consciousness-raising groups, in Women's Therapy Groups: Paradigms of Feminist Treatment. Edited by Brody CM. New York, Springer, 1987, pp 43–53

Kravetz D: Benefits of consciousness-raising groups for women, in Women's Therapy Groups: Paradigms of Feminist Treatment. Edited by Brody CM. New York, Springer, 1987, pp 55–66

Krupnick CG: Women and men in the classroom: inequality and its remedies. Teaching and Learning May:18–25, 1985

Lerner HG: Women in Therapy. Northvale, NJ, Jason Aronson, 1988

MacNab RT: What do men want?: male rituals of initiation in group psychotherapy. Int J Group Psychother 40:139–155, 1990

Mayes SS: Women in positions of authority: a case study of changing sex roles. Signs 4:556–568, 1979

Miller JB: Toward a New Psychology of Women. Boston, MA, Beacon Press, 1976

Reed BG: Differential reactions by male and female group members in the presence of female authority figures (Ph.D. dissertation). Cincinnati, OH, University of Cincinnati, 1979

Reed BG: Women leaders in small groups: social psychological perspectives and strategies. Social Work in Groups 6:35–42, 1983

Sexton A: The Complete Poems. Boston, MA, Houghton Mifflin, 1981

Spieler S: The gendered self: a lost maternal legacy, In Psychoanalysis and Women: Contemporary Reappraisals. Edited by Alpert JL. Hillsdale, NJ, Analytic Press, 1986

Stern DN: The Interpersonal World of the Infant: A View from Psychoanalysis and Developmental Psychology. New York, Basic Books, 1985

Stiver IP: Beyond the oedipus complex: mothers and daughters (Work in Progress #26). Wellesley, MA, Stone Center Working Paper Series, 1986

Stoller RJ: The sense of femaleness. Psychoanal Q 37:42–55, 1968

Thompson C: The role of women in this culture. Psychiatry 4:1–8, 1941

Thompson C: Cultural pressures in the psychology of women. Psychiatry 5:331–339, 1942

Walker LJS: Women's groups are different, in Women's Therapy Groups: Paradigms of Feminist Treatment. Edited by Brody CM. New York, Springer, 1987, pp 3–12

Westkott M: Historical and developmental roots of female dependency. Psychotherapy 23:213–220, 1986

Yalom ID: The Theory and Practice of Group Psychotherapy. New York, Basic Books, 1970

Zilbach J: In the I of the beholder: towards a separate line of development in women. Paper presented at the annual meeting of the American Group Psychotherapy Association, New York, February 1987

CHAPTER 21

Men in Group Therapy

Steven Krugman, Ph.D.
Samuel Osherson, Ph.D.

Introduction

The following case example illustrates the therapeutic potential of group for men:

Case 1

Six group members entered the room for the beginning of a psychotherapy session. Each of the members found a seat, as usual, except for Mr. A, a 33-year-old architect. Mr. A did something unusual: for the first time in his 2 years in the group he sat next to the therapist. Another group member, Mr. B, spotted the difference immediately and offered a friendly verbal poke: "Think you can tolerate being so close to Daddy, [Mr. A]?"

Mr. A spent much of his time in the group talking of his conflict about his father, who died during Mr. A's adolescence after a lengthy illness. Much of Mr. A's alienation from father figures, including bosses, was based in his fear that to be close to a father he had to act crippled and impotent.

Emboldened and playful, Mr. A exclaimed, "I don't want to be next to Daddy, I want to be in his seat." Gesturing towards the male therapist he said, "I want his power." Mr. A. looked sheepish at what he said, suddenly anxious at the direct expression of his wish for manly power.

Ms. C, a fellow group member, applauded, "Go for it, [Mr. A]!" He seemed visibly relaxed at the confirmation and turned to the therapist, "Did I upset you saying I wanted your seat?"

"It's hard for you to imagine that I could cherish your potency," suggested the therapist.

Later, Mr. A returned to this theme: "I've never felt that it was okay to be strong and demanding as a man, but I've always felt ashamed of myself.

This group is the first time that I've felt like I don't have to hide my inadequacy."

In this brief group interaction Mr. A. began to experiment more directly with leadership skills in the group, to examine his legitimate wishes for power and self-confidence, and to restore self-esteem damaged by the internalization of a painful relationship with his parents.

Special Challenges and Opportunities for Men in Group Therapy

Group psychotherapy offers the male patient a flexible modality within which to address a broad range of issues, ranging from problems of a social and interpersonal nature to those involving deeper levels of psychopathology. Group therapy is a powerful milieu in which to deal with the defenses and vulnerabilities men bring to treatment.

Men present special challenges for the psychotherapist (Meth and Pasick 1990). A man's sense of self frequently resides in his ability to feel competent and in control. The emphasis in psychotherapy on self-disclosure and affective expression may lead male patients to feel vulnerable and in danger of losing their sense of masculinity (Osherson and Krugman 1991).

Entering psychotherapy puts men in a bind: to do so is an admission that their life is not working and that they are not living up to widely held ideals of male self-sufficiency and stoicism. Traditional male sex role norms generate expectations for self-reliance, high tolerance for distress, and the disavowal of dependent needs (Balswick and Peek 1971; Lewis 1984). Many men need formidable evidence that life is not working (Osherson and Krugman 1991). Even then, there are men who will enter treatment only under duress, coerced by a partner who threatens to leave them if they won't or by the court, which orders them to do so as a part of their probation.

Central to the presenting problems many men bring to therapy are difficulties in forming and maintaining intimate interpersonal connections. These difficulties are rooted in male developmental experiences that leave men ambivalent about intimacy.

Group therapy offers male patients a particular kind of opportunity to address many of these dilemmas in a compelling and challenging environment. It is an environment that mitigates against some resistances men experience in individual psychotherapy while creating a host of new ones. Potentially, group therapy provides an opportunity for men to acknowledge and work with their weaknesses in a context that recognizes and affirms their masculine strivings and attendant conflicts.

In this chapter, we write about psychodynamic psychotherapy groups. At the same time, much of what we discuss pertains to men participating in a broad range of group situations—from board rooms to baseball teams, from Alcoholics Anonymous to men's groups. Female therapists will also recognize many of the behaviors and self-presentations we describe. Female therapists also experience other aspects of male self-presentation and group behavior (see Chapter 20).

In contrast to individual psychotherapy, group therapy may be experienced as less intense, more social, less individually exposing, and more readily rationalized. Whereas individual therapy (especially with a male therapist) invokes a kind of face-to-face intimacy of which many men feel distrustful, group therapy disperses and diffuses the encounter. The group experience is reminiscent of being part of other social, athletic, and work-related groups. Here men can learn new interpersonal skills in a safe and supportive setting. Vicarious learning (Yalom 1975) and social modeling facilitate new behavior. The group space allows the member to emerge at his own rate and control the sense of exposure (MacKenzie 1990). This is particularly important for shame-sensitive men. The curative factors that make group therapy effective have special impact on men. "Universality," "comembership," and "altruism" are particularly salient (Wright 1987). These experiences also help diminish the sense of personal isolation that is so characteristic of many male patients.

Men's "resistance" to psychotherapy is rooted, in large measure, in their propensity to feel shame over experiences of inadequacy. For men it is particularly humiliating not to be able to take care of oneself—to have to acknowledge one's dependency on others. Anxiety over feeling dependent, and being seen as dependent, shapes men's battles over attachment that characterize early phases of psychotherapy. The group milieu multiplies the experience of exposure and sense of personal risk. Over time, the frank acknowledgment that the patient needs therapy—that the man needs the group—represents a important hallmark of growth and change. It suggests that the deeply held male belief that to be in need is to risk all has been successfully challenged and that counterdependent defenses have begun to give way.

The therapy group is often experienced as a narcissistic injury at multiple levels: from the very need to be in a group to the forced identification with other group members; from the amplification of one's own inadequacies to the revelation of them to others; from the growth of a dependent relationship on the group to the penetration of interpretations in front of others. Male patients' growing capacity to tolerate the presence of the group reflects the relaxation of defenses and the willingness to risk revealing the self.

Male Characterological Defenses in the Group Setting

Across the life cycle, boys unto men struggle with conflicts around attachment, aggression, and self-esteem (Levinson 1978; Osherson 1986). These three dilemmas are profoundly interconnected, and it is their very interconnectedness that proves so problematic. It is important to recognize that women, too, struggle with these same dilemmas. Yet each gender wrestles with the particulars in parallel but distinct ways. For example, issues of self-esteem are obviously central to the emotional well-being of both men and women. For women, however, it is more likely to be the self-in-relationship that is the central source of their sense of self-worth, whereas for men it is the self-in-accomplishment that is the most likely source of concern.

Attachment

Case 2 illustrates the role of group in the separation-individuation struggle of men:

Case 2

Mr. D, a 38-year-old postman, had remained deeply devoted to his aging mother. His social life was otherwise quite limited. When she died, he found himself quite depressed and extremely isolated. Mr. D's father had been an unreliable figure in the family. Even as a boy, Mr. D's longstanding attachment to his mother had always precluded the development of peer relations. In group therapy he began to confront the shyness and embarrassment over his lack of social experience.

For boys and for girls to establish a solid sense of selfhood, they must begin to separate from their mothers. For many boys this transition from the intense primary identification with mother, which is so characteristic of small children, to a more independent sense of masculine identification is a troubled one (Chodorow 1989). Wright (1987) observed that from this perspective ". . . most men have had a major separation-induced emotional trauma inflicted on them in early life, and carry a serious shame and humiliation based handicap with them forever after" (p. 242).

This "emotional" leave-taking is never easy, but it becomes all the more problematic without the facilitating support of an engaged and emotionally available father. For most boys the psychological and physical movement away from mother as a source of primary identification toward father is fraught with difficulty (Osherson 1986). Fathers are surrounded by mystery and uncertainty. Boys misidentify with them, constructing a sense of manhood on partial images of power, strength, and inhibition of feeling. Basic attachment and security are traded for the sense of growth as the boy masters the skills and challenges of boyhood.

Aggression

Along with the basic problems inherent in the process of separation and differentiation is the overlapping concern regarding aggression—one's own and that of others. The oedipal struggle provides the boy with the opportunity to disidentify with mother and make the transition to a same-sex identification with father. Boys must learn to evade paternal and peer aggression while learning how and when to use their own in defense and attack. During this time boys are intently focused on the models provided by other boys and adult men. Recent developmental research (Jacklin 1989) has indicated that elementary school boys find the reinforcements offered by peers far more powerful than those provided by either girls or teachers. Sex role stereotypes and schemata (Bem 1981) offer important developmental support from latency into young adulthood. The codes of male behavior teach shame avoidance (Krugman S, Osherson S: Shame and its role in male development, unpublished paper, September 1990) and the substitution of verbal jousting for physical confrontation. Male patients often turn toward verbal aggression (e.g., sarcasm) at moments of vulnerability, as Case 3 illustrates:

Case 3

Mr. E was referred to therapy because his caustic style interfered with his customer relations. He would become defensive almost as soon as he revealed how frustrated he was with himself for "getting in his own way." If a group member moved toward him, he would lash out critically, charging that the other had problems too.

At the heart of the male developmental struggle is the difficulty of integrating aggression with attachment. Men develop a set of psychological defenses against feeling vulnerable and "clingy." To successfully socialize as a male means to suppress, if not repress, dependent yearnings for parental nurturance and protection. The stereotypically well-socialized male adopts a stance that communicates relative self-sufficiency and invulnerability (Komarovsky 1974). Competitive feelings may override and suppress attachment needs. Over time, the therapy group challenges this aspect of the male persona, giving permission for attachment to coexist with competitive and self-protective concerns.

Self-Esteem

As boys strive to consolidate their masculine identification, vulnerability and weakness associated with femininity become a threat to self-esteem. In their effort to separate from mother and become like father, feelings, behaviors, and experiences that cast doubt on this effort generate shame and embarrassment. To reassert their threatened masculinity, boys and men resort to aggressive displays and postures to reassure themselves and intimidate others. As the following case example illustrates, feeling powerful enhances self-esteem; feeling diminished is humiliating:

Case 4

Mr. F was easily affronted. Group members told him he put them off because he had to be approached with such care to avoid offending him. Soon after he missed several sessions without an apparent reason. When he returned, he had great difficulty talking and making eye contact. He had been fired and was too proud and humiliated to let the group know.

Narcissistic defenses that support the denial of dependent needs and obsessional defenses that avoid dysphoric feelings are coping defenses that are widely used by men. These maneuvers disguise emotional neediness and cover over vulnerable feelings by preventing self-disclosure, constraining social contact, and inhibiting intimacy. Male posturing ("machismo" in all its variations), substance abuse, overwork, and violence become common compensatory responses to despair, shame, and loss.

An alternative path of development for men lies in the direction of what Erikson (1950) termed "generativity." This requires a freeing up of the psychological and interpersonal resources that enable men—and women as well—to lead richer, more satisfying lives. For this to occur, defensive rigidity needs be reduced, and men's capacity to accept themselves, "warts and all," must be enhanced. A sense of secure identity precedes the capacity for intimacy.

Group Stages and Individual Differences

Let us follow four men through their progress in a mixed psychotherapy group, while attending to the evolving stages of group therapy on the one hand and the unfolding of individual defenses on the other. Mr. G used aggression to isolate and protect himself from shame:

Case 5

Mr. G was 42 years old and had been in group therapy for nearly 3 years. When he joined the group, he described himself as being cut off from his family of origin, socially withdrawn, and quite frightened of becoming close to anyone. On occasion he became intensely suspicious of women with whom he worked, wondering whether they could read his mind. He used alcohol to soothe himself and make even minimal social contact bearable. Mr. G had grown up with a mother who was prone to psychotic episodes during which she could be extremely intrusive. His father, a friendly salesman and an optimist, helped Mr. G develop some degree of distance from his mother. However, he was often overwhelmed by his wife and denied. He avoided dealing directly with the reality of his marriage and its impact on Mr. G. As a result, Mr. G learned to use hostility as a means to keep his mother at bay and express his great disappointment in those around him. His gender identity was fragile, forcing him to isolate himself to the point of paranoia. (See Rice 1987.)

Mr. H, on the other hand, coped with his dependent needs by denying them. He adopted a rather aggressive passive-dependent stance to further express his deep ambivalence over wishing to be connected to others:

Case 6

Mr. H, 36 years old, was the middle child in a large Catholic family that taught him the values of self-sacrifice, "service," and "turning the other cheek." He came to the group after several unsuccessful courses of individual treatment. Despite a growing weight problem and career stagnation, his passive-dependent stance had stymied all previous efforts at change. In and out of the group, Mr. H was endlessly helpful and attentive to the needs of others. When he began, he could hardly identify a need of his own; he would talk with great feeling about the plight of others and how ministering to them drained him. He had been in the group for 18 months.

Mr. I, by contrast, used his aggressive stance to support his self-esteem and ward off his deep and fearful dependent yearnings:

Case 7

Mr. I was an explosive man who talked with great feeling about how hard his growing up had been. His father, a domineering, frightening man, had cowed the family into submission. Mr. I was his mother's secret ally and confidant while striving to live up to his father's harsh demands and expectations. Four years into the group his own harsh superego had begun to relax. His deep sadness and underlying wish to be liked and cared for emerged in the group with considerable power. Where he had raged against insults, real and perceived, he now cried, full of hurt and a lifetime of injustice. Where his intimidating father had occupied center stage, he now began to experience his anger at his mother for requiring that he protect her rather than the other way around.

Mr. J's smooth presentation provided few opportunities to get to know him very well. Occasionally the veneer would separate, revealing a lonely and alienated man with deep insecurities:

Case 8

Mr. J was a "well-adjusted" homosexual involved in a steady, long-term relationship. He had grown up the only child of a Southern belle who had married "beneath" her family's expectations. Mr. J's father was an accountant whose lack of success forced the family to move again and again throughout Mr. J's childhood. Although Mr. J found acceptance in the homosexual community and success at work in a graphic design firm, he remained a deeply unhappy man with a pit of sadness and self-doubt that he could neither plumb the depths of nor drain. He felt that he held himself apart from others in order to protect some secret self. After about 6 months in the group, he had established himself as savvy and occasionally a wise fellow with a Teflon coating. People liked him, except for one man who found his homosexuality very threatening and a woman who mistrusted him from the moment he walked in the door.

These men brought to group treatment a deep sense of personal inadequacy that was rooted in a profound fear of and estrangement from affects: the men's own feelings and those of others. Men come into treatment when their isolating defenses have left them feeling internally barren, loveless, and at times desperate. They come when they have begun to experience intolerable levels of feeling—be it depression, anxiety, rage, or unbearable yearning. For many, relationships with women hold out both the promise and the threat of self-disclosure and vulnerability. However, the threat that organizes their defenses lies not with women, per se, but with closeness to others, male or female (Meth and Pasick 1990).

Group therapy challenges the self-representations of many obsessive-compulsive and passive-dependent avoidant men. The threat comes in several forms: the group itself, the presence of women, the competition with other men, and the transference to the leader. Ultimately, the male patient's capacity to maintain his psychic equilibrium is challenged by the powerful, often primitive, affects stimulated by membership in the group.

Entering the Therapy Group

On entering a mixed psychotherapy group, the male patient is confronted consciously by his competitive and aggressive wishes and fears and unconsciously by his dependent yearning and counterdependent defenses (Agazarian 1981; Rutan and Stone 1984). A man among other men in the presence of women is caught between his wish to be noticed and chosen by the women (or woman of his choice) and his need to connect with the other men. He also may be in touch with deep feelings of anger toward women for the power they have exercised in his life. Typically the men orient toward the women and triangulate with the other men. They jockey for position. Consciously, and more importantly unconsciously, they play to the women. As Sternbach (1987) and others have observed, " . . . in mixed groups men are likely to begin by utilizing women as objects of nurturance, mediators of emotional vulnerability, and as support people" (p.2). The competition is over getting taken care of. The following case example illustrates the interpersonal process at work as a male group member's use of distance activates a female member to pursue him:

Case 5 (*continued*)

Mr. G maintained his distance while gradually letting the group know more and more about his circumstances. He would have remained more aloof had it not been for Ms. K. She found his distance, his situation, and his drinking problem utterly compelling. Mr. G would come forward after not having spoken in weeks—as much out of the wish to be a "good group member" as out of an inner sense that he needed to share himself and break out of the killing isolation of his life. He'd let on a bit about some details at work, just to give the flavor of it. Ms. K would seize hold, pursuing for details, wanting know "more about you because I care about you." Mr. G would grow sullen and silent. "Leave me alone," he'd finally say. "This makes me uncomfortable. I don't know why you're interested in me this way." The group supported him as he learned to say, "No, I don't want to talk about it now, with you."

Like Mr. G, Mr. H responded to the anxiety-arousing demands of being a new member by doing what he knew best:

Case 6 (*continued*)

Mr. H talked for months about the sick and dying people he needed to care for in his family. He would also offer to help the women get their folding chairs set up and put away. The group kidded him about his selflessness to no avail. He didn't get the irony. After about 6 months, several of the men grew overtly impatient with him. One woman who had had a stranglehold on the role of "most helpful group member" became increasingly provocative. The group was divided between those members who were antagonized by Mr. H's posture and those who saw him as a helpless soul needing all the help he could get. After a brief flirtation with the faction "sympathetic" to his plight, Mr. H increasingly engaged the more sadistic members, fighting to explain himself while being disregarded and disdained by them.

Mr. I, who so often felt out of control in his family, used the first meeting as an opportunity to take control by claiming a familiar, if intimidating and unpopular, role:

Case 7 (*continued*)

When another member's remarks hinted at class and ethnic prejudice, Mr. I "blew her out of the water." When some members confronted him on his intimidating style, he all but threatened them physically. The group reassured itself and Mr. I as well with a reaffirmation that this was a talking group; no acting out was allowed. After a time, Mr. I could acknowledge how awful it was to see his father in himself. Contained by the group contract and by the readiness of some members to respond to him in a genuine fashion, Mr. I began to feel his longing to make contact. He began to recognize how this blustery style he'd learned from his father was an immigrant's response to not knowing what to do and not being able to say, "I don't know."

Mr. J had spoken in front of dozens of Alcoholics Anonymous meetings. He could talk about his "feelings" on national television:

Case 8 (*continued*)

From the first Mr. J was an active, attentive group member. He spoke movingly about his own successful struggle to accept his homosexuality and break his dependence on drugs. Some found him self-righteous and preachy. Mr. J's "Teflon-like" response had begun to irritate one subgroup of members. They charged him with being aloof. He felt misunderstood. After about 6 months in the group he became the object of a series of confrontations regarding his slipperiness. Throughout this time the group in general was dealing with some very charged material. Toward the end of one particularly intense meeting Mr. J announced, "This is my last session." The group reacted with shock and fury. He came one more time to "honor" his commitment to the contract.

The Early Group

In the dependent, preaffiliative phase of group development (Agazarian 1981), men deal with their anxiety and sense of being out of control in a variety of ways. They ask questions about the rationale and the group contract. They engage the leader by "challenging" his or her "assumptions." They pick fights; they withdraw. The real message is "notice me." Some men take the beginning of group to be the occasion for a kind of ritual mating dance in full sex-role display. Gender roles are quite prominent. Before too long, however, counterdependent defenses mount. After all, what is taking place is not a "worthy" competition among adult male adversaries, but rather a struggle for a special place in mother's gaze, or better yet, on her lap. Nor is the competition simply or even primarily for the admiration of the group. The more disturbed the group population is, the more intense is each member's yearning for the leader's sole and undistracted attention. Few men are able to openly acknowledge their wish to be seen and treated as "special" by the leader, especially at this early stage. Yet even their internal awareness of how needy they feel is too threatening and potentially exposing. Whatever their initial "success" is at outdoing all the competitors, they begin to feel exposed and unsuccessful in their attempts to find either a safe haven or a "special" place. They use their tried and trusted means. Frequently this takes the form of pairing up and off with women in the group or with other men. Inevitably, however, they begin to feel too much. Often this is experienced first as confusion and then as boredom in the face of overstimulation. Overwhelmed by the intensity of the group and feeling increasingly inadequate in the face of its demands, male members feel flooded by their own affect and ashamed of their yearning.

Counterdependent Defenses

During the initial dependent phase (and later as this phase is repeated during the life of the group), the awareness men have of their dependent wishes is heightened by the presence of the women, by the experience of the group itself as "mother" (Scheidlinger 1974), and by the parental transference to the leader. In response, counterdependent defenses become prominent: with Mr. G, angry distance; with Mr. H, compulsive helpfulness; with Mr. I, intimidating machismo; and with Mr. J, aloofness and, when that fails, flight.

Flight, withholding and withdrawal, and distancing are common responses to the growing pressure on the male patient's deep hunger for caretaking and profound fear of being humiliated should he acknowledge such wishes. As the men threaten to leave the group, plan business trips to take them away, or disappear into passive-dependent silence, both male and female members will begin to recognize parallel moments in other important relationships when a man responded to emotional demands in just these ways (Fine 1988).

The Role of Women and Its Impact on the Men in the Group

The tendency of many men to invoke counterdependent and distancing defenses is exacerbated by the behavior of the women. More comfortable with sharing affect as the coin of communication and attachment and more aware of their own unmet dependent needs, the female members flood the group with feelings of all kinds. Important among these feelings are a host of resentments and painful memories associated with or suffered at the hands of men. The general display of affect activates male defenses against vulnerability and contact, as well as against intrusion and engulfment. The particular charges generate an atmosphere of defensiveness and unsafety in the group itself. The women are typically more comfortable with open displays of affect than the men are. Not only are the men now uncomfortable with the rising affect in themselves and in the room and with their identification with the men "out there" who have hurt these women, but they are also losing in what increasingly seems to be a hostile competition with women (Gans 1990b). In the face of the rising affective pressure men are likely to try to "solve the problem" by "doing something." The following case example illustrates men's inclination to respond to negative feelings with problem-oriented solutions:

Case 9

Mr. L exemplified the dilemma that men experience. He explained: "If I can fix what makes you feel bad, then I won't have to feel so inadequate around all these bad feelings." Several women responded, "This is just like what happens with my husband/boyfriend. All I want him to do is listen to how I feel." Mr. L agreed, "My wife says exactly what you're saying. But I feel this way—if she's got a problem we can fix, let's fix it. If she doesn't want to fix it, then she should stop talking about it."

The women, seeking empathy, not solutions, experienced the men's latent hostility and felt unmet, invalidated, and angry. We recognized in this group sequence a repetition of the very same dynamic interpersonal process that leads to problems of intimacy in the world beyond the group.

However, when Mr. L said, "I feel this way about it," he told us about something personal, something to which he was quite committed. His problem-solving orientation and his view of how life should be handled reflected both an adaptive, often successful, response and an emotionally avoidant and interpersonally controlling one (Meth and Pasick 1990). His resistance to acknowledging the threat of the intimate pull as he shared her feelingful experience was high and was likely to remain so for some time.

Men often experience substantial risk because of the highly stimulating demands of the heterosexual group environment. These demands quickly evoke dependent yearnings to be taken care of, primitive fears of being engulfed or disintegrated, and grandiose wishes to be the admired center of everyone's attention.

Formation of the Male Subgroup

It is important for the leader to pay attention to the relational process taking place among the men. Wishes for male approval are high, though typically unacknowledged. Dyadic and triangular competition among the men at times seems pro forma, as if the men were expected to compete with one another. Oftentimes, they are more concerned with feeling safe and accepted. The process of male-male bonding is complex and takes overt as well as covert forms. Male-male pairing is common. Competitive joking creates a bond that also exclude others in a hostile way: sexualized humor is an obvious example. Also, sharing a particular male interest with another group member may serve a similar purpose.

Some observers believe that an important male response to the pressure of the group is to form subgroups with other men. This tendency can provide the therapist with an opportunity to acknowledge and affirm the adaptive value of the male stance. It also may bring to the fore male anxieties about closeness with other men. MacNab (1990) suggested that men will bond with each other in an effort to protect themselves from the demands of women and the group leader. Male themes such as sports, work, cars, and women serve to link the men in the group to one another. Men will talk to one another in "displacement," both to avoid direct acknowledgment of an important matter and to decrease the intensity of the affect. Often, in response to the rising feeling evoked by a woman's painful tale, a man will change the affect level by changing the subject, as illustrated in the following example:

Case 10

In Mr. I's group, an important female member had given birth. Other women went on at some length recalling their own tales of labor and delivery. During a pause another man, Mr. M, offered, "I wanted to share something good about myself with the group. I just bought a new car." The women were outraged. "I'm talking about my insides spilling out and it makes Mr. M want to tell us about his new car—give me a break!" One man joined in, "How insensitive can you be?" Several others, including Mr. I, sided with Mr. M. The group seemed split for some time over who was right. Was Mr. M simply insensitive or was he doing something on behalf of himself, the other men, and the group as a whole by signalling that he could not tolerate the level of material being discussed? Perhaps he, along with other members of the male subgroup, needed to feel more connected with one another before exposing themselves fully to the graphic, boundary-less experience of birth.

As the men rally to rebut charges of insensitivity, capitulation of latency and preadolescent rejection of girls and feminine interests can be observed. Subgrouping reactivates the early peer group. Male group members find reassurance in their membership in the male subgroup (Blos 1985). This base-building is seen as a way of connecting with and affirming one's maleness and masculine identity. Securing male-male connections either by pairing or by subgrouping is a process that occurs and reoccurs during the life of the group. It often prefigures working directly on parental transference toward the therapist.

The Mature Group

Having made a place for themselves in the group, male members, individually and as a subgroup, are more able to explore their issues with the group leader (Yalom 1975). The freedom to explore transferential concerns about power and authority and the risks of becoming dependent on the group and its leader(s) are now increasingly present. For many men, in group as in life, true self-disclosure requires the knowledge that one can withstand rejection and protect oneself from aggression. Only then is it possible to openly express in the group one's genuine response to other members and to the leader. With increased safety comes trust. Gradually the male members are able to recognize their transferential projections onto, and distortions of, the group process, its members, and it leader(s). Increasingly, feedback from group members and interpretations from the leader can be heard and worked with, rather than defensively contested. In the course of time, members are increasingly able to diminish their reactivity toward one another and learn to use their experience of the other, as in the case of Mr. G:

Case 5 (*continued*)

Mr. G came to see Ms. K more clearly as a stand-in for his mother. He feared and hated her but also wanted and needed her. As he came to own both aspects of his ambivalence toward her, his responses to her intrusiveness became less charged. More and more he was able to use their relationship in the group as a way to explore his relationships with women in life outside.

Like Mr. G, Mr. H began integrating disowned parts of himself:

Case 6 (*continued*)

Mr. H slowly came to recognize just how secretly competitive he really was being with the other men. His passivity was the "sweet and gentle" disposition his overburdened mother valued. Along with his solicitousness, it was his way of winning the hearts of the women and a place in the family.

The mature group is more able to work actively with the latent relationships (Horowitz 1983). Collusive deals and alliances can now be revealed. Strong attractions and repulsions toward male and female members, as well as toward the leader, become accessible during this phase of increased differentiation. Fears and wishes around engulfment, sadistic impulses, and wishes for phallic prominence are openly acknowledged.

With the growing freedom to acknowledge more and more of their actual experience comes both enchantment with the group and its leader and, in turn, disenchantment (Agazarian 1981). For many men the group has become a unique experience in which they have been able to bring forth their true selves, perhaps for the first and only time in their lives. In the face of their shame and fear, they have shown themselves. They have begun to say what it is they need. And throughout this process, they have been contained and accepted in the group. For many men this acceptance gives rise to great surges of sadness, anger, and grief. They begin to feel the unfelt losses of a lifetime. They begin to mourn the parenting they never received, the opportunities for love and support they were blind to or turned away from, and the injuries to others they are responsible for. Anger often covers the sadness and grief, as occurred with Mr. I:

Case 7 (*continued*)

After 5 years, Mr. I began to talk about leaving the group: "I never knew why I used to cry. Sometimes it would come over me like a wave and I would sob for no reason. Now I know. I learned in this group. I thought you were a bunch of jerks when I started—I knew I could beat the shit out of any of you. That only lasted for a year or so. After a while I saw what people were saying to me. It hurt so much. Then I knew why I cried. I had missed so much. I had to be so tough. It wasn't fair. I was just a little kid. Everybody in here seemed more together than me. You knew what you felt—worse, you knew what I felt. I didn't know shit. Especially you, Doctor. I thought you knew everything. I wanted to be like you, to be your son. I don't feel that way anymore. I'm all right now. I kind of like who I am. I love this group. But now that I can say this to you and really mean it I know I can leave here and be okay."

Treatment Considerations

Several technical issues should be kept in mind.

Conjoint Therapy: Individual and Group

Given the kind of resistance men bring to the therapeutic process, individual therapy plays an important role in the development of readiness for group therapy and in making group work for the resistant or reluctant male patient (Gans 1990a). Although all potential group members should be carefully evaluated and prepared for entering group therapy, particular care is warranted where male patients are concerned. Men frequently have a difficult time saying either to themselves or to anyone else, "I'm not sure I'm ready; I'm scared and don't want to do it."

A therapy group can be a strange and challenging milieu. Male patients need directed assistance in exploring their anticipatory anxiety in emotional terms rather than in situational terms (e.g., parking is going to be a problem). Inquiry into a man's previous experience (informal and formal) in groups will yield a great deal of highly relevant material. Who he was and what his experiences were on sports teams, in military units, and in clubs, as well as in his own family group, will reveal important data for discussion and allow the therapist to anticipate certain core dilemmas and characterological responses.

Many new male group members find the immersion in the affect-laden process of group to be threatening and silencing. A strong therapeutic alliance with the group leader will bridge the transition from individual to group treatment.

Ongoing conjoint treatment heightens the utility of the group and individual work, particularly with male patients who have a hard time understanding why the world responds to them as it does. At times, shame-laden material will be stimulated by the group process. Primitive states and the affects associated with them stimulate characterological defenses against engulfment (in various forms), rage, and loss of self-esteem.

Given the propensity of some males to become highly defensive in the face of shame as well as other powerful affects, the individual session may provide a safe harbor to work through some of the more disorganizing and shameful feelings before having to deal with the whole group. To the extent that the therapist and the group can recognize these states and the defenses they trigger, the male patient's rising discomfort may be contained. To the degree that the male patient's characterological response can be understood in its adaptive aspects (as a strength that has served him well while limiting him), he, other male patients, and the group as a whole will benefit. This is particularly so in relation to distancing and intellectualizing defenses.

Many patients, male and female, lack effective means for regulating interpersonal closeness. How to set effective boundaries and maintain them in the face of emotional pressure and threat is a critical lesson to be learned in the group. Given the right milieu, men can become less guarded by learning to tolerate rejection on the one hand and learning to say no on the other:

Case 5 (*continued*)

After considerable prodding Mr. B. erupted: "Damn it! I'm doing the best I can. I'm not happy about how I'm handling this but stop pushing me. There is some standard here that I'm not living up to. It's a thin line between being pushed to change and being judged as inadequate. Just back off."

Although there are wide divergences in actual clinical practice, male candidates for an ongoing dynamic group are, in our view, best served by having had a significant therapeutic experience before joining the group. Treating such men for a year or more before thinking about referral to a group will lessen the likelihood of premature dropouts and other forms of acting out.

Dynamic Conflicts

Male patients bring gender-linked issues and dynamics into group. Successful group work with male patients (either in a mixed group or an all-male group) depends on the therapist's sensitivity to these concerns, as well as a willingness to explore their special meaning in the lives of men.

Male Sex-Role Ideals and Feelings of Shame

The spectrum of male-specific experiences includes concerns related to having a male body, being socialized as a male, and sharing in activities such as combat, sports, and being the primary breadwinner. In all of these areas, sex-role stereotypes, along with ego ideals, exert powerful pressure on a man's self-image and self-esteem. In contrast to the ideals associated with each of these domains is the experience of each individual who fails to fulfill one ideal or another. Being physically small, fat, fearful, unathletic, impotent or infertile, or unemployed is potentially stigmatizing. Powerful feelings of inadequacy and insufficiency accompany these experiences. In a sense, the shame of these shortcomings is as painful as the shortcoming itself (Morrison 1989).

The leader needs to be sensitive to the shame struggles underlying much common male behavior. Much male silence and withholding may be understood in terms of a reluctance to share shame-laden experience. Premature dropouts and frequent absences may also be understood in this light. Some men become enraged and physically threatening or assaultive when overwhelmed by shameful feelings.

The leader can take an active role in creating a group atmosphere that is relatively free from the threat of humiliation (Alonso and Rutan 1988). The leader's interest in emotional safety highlights this important issue for male patients.

Concerns About Homosexuality

Another powerful force that inhibits men's lives and their reactions to other men is concern about homosexuality. Some men experience the warmth and support of the group in ways that leave them feeling too dependent and too close to other male members and the male leader. Heterosexual men learn to defend both their public presentations of self as well as their internal sense of self from the implication that they are homosexual. Men may confuse feelings of tenderness and yearning for support with feelings that they identify as homosexual. Feeling passive, too connected, moved, or revealed may stimulate homophobic avoidance and withdrawal. Disdain and ridicule may cover men's emotional retreat and mask fears of being taken advantage of.

Yet most men have deeply frustrated and suppressed yearnings for protection, support, and guidance from paternal and sibling figures. Indeed, it is their inability to tolerate and integrate passive longings that gets split off and becomes the foundation of their impulsive and compulsive behavior. Some men are extremely homophobic and may not be able to tolerate much direct affect among men. Most men are reassured by the therapist's normalizing of passive and dependent feelings as they arise in the group. In group, men can discover their capacity to be nurturant and to explore what it is like to care for and to be cared for by another man in a nonerotic way. Given the volatility of this issue, sensitivity toward these concerns is warranted (Friedman 1988).

Problems With Aggression

Overtly or covertly all men wrestle with concerns around the management of aggression: their own and that of others. It is important for the leader to pay attention to the group's fears that aggression will get out of control and that someone will get hurt. Men are brought up to fear other men and to fear being vulnerable to men or to women. Their fear of being hurt physically or emotionally often conceals their anxiety over being too aggressive and sadistic. At the same time, men are often unable to acknowledge their own vulnerability unless they feel reassured that they will not be attacked (Lansky 1984). Women frequently serve to diffuse and buffer male aggression. The group provides an opportunity for men to explore and learn to modulate these feelings. Until men feel comfortable vis-à-vis aggression around other men, it is difficult for the group process to continue on its developmental course.

Role of the Leader

As the person who makes all formative decisions about the group's structure and membership, the leader is an authority figure and the focus of the group's wishes and fears. The leader becomes a stand-in or surrogate for parental and other authority figures. This projective process is the essence of the transferential process as it occurs in the group context. The competitive wish for the leader's attention drives the development of the group; anxiety over competition among the members, and with the leader, sets up the defensive character of the group dynamics. For men with intense conflicts in the areas of control and dependence, the leader's tasks can be particularly complex.

Male Expectations

There is a traditional cultural stereotype wherein the leadership qualities of authority, power, and control are deemed masculine attributes. By contrast, being empathic, supportive, or providing for emotional safety are attributes associated with the feminine position (Broverman et al. 1972). These are not generally recognized as leadership qualities.

This stereotypic but pervasive orientation toward leadership sets the ground for important and revealing work with male clients. Men overrely on sex-role stereotypes to assist in the emergent masculine identification. Their internal imagery may be further complicated by a family of origin where a strong and dominant mother was the center of the household and a weak or absent father was a more peripheral member.

To be effective, group therapists must demonstrate both a reasonable degree of authoritative control and considerable capacity for empathy and support. On the surface the male patient's difficulty with the leadership style of his group therapist may reflect certain gender-related beliefs about how a leader should behave and who should lead. But with any persistence these attitudes soon enough reveal themselves to be dynamically linked to the male patient's historical experience with parental figures, fathers in particular, and others who have occupied positions of emotional power in the patient's life (Lanksy 1989). One brash and blustery lawyer put it this way:

> I like it when I see you [the male leader] as critical and harsh. I understand that: that's how I see men. I know what to do, how to take care of myself. Lately I've been letting myself see that you have a gentle and caring side that other people here appreciate and get something from. I know I'm drawn to that in you, but it makes me anxious and confused. It's weird.

The Contract and the Frame

It is the leader's task to build a group that is well defined contractually. This promotes a well-functioning group while supporting obsessional defenses in the face of a new and highly ambiguous situation. A limit-setting group contract (e.g., no physical violence, no outside group contacts, and no uninvited touching in the group), coupled with an attitude of containment, also helps men who are concerned about aggression: that of others as well as their own. When men are anxious about being shamed as they reveal secret fears and inadequacies, the leader who manages to keep the group relatively free of humiliation is seen as a trustworthy ally. Finally, men will respond in the group to the degree that the leader recognizes well-learned adaptive skills in their defensive distancing, intellectualizing, and avoidance. By affirming the strengths that have served thus far, albeit with increasingly serious limitations, prideful and shame-prone men will find it easier to embrace alternative modes of coping and relating.

Modeling Authority

A leader who communicates that his or her authority is not simply structural (i.e., "I'm the professional, it's my group") but is based on confidence in his or her professional experience and in the group role offers the anxious male patient a sense of reassurance and safety, even in an alien situation. Men, faced with insecurity and felt inadequacy, often turn to structure and rules for reassurance.

Case 11

Mr. N lost his father to divorce and death before he was 12 years old. His dry, obsessive-compulsive defenses protected him from feeling out of control but isolated him at the same time. In the group he was the rule keeper. When members paired up for a ride home after the session, or when there was talk of a member's upcoming wedding, Mr. N would become indignant. "That's a violation of the rules—a break in the contract. Are you going to let them get away with that, Doctor?"

One of the crucial decisions the leader must make concerns the affect-behavior continuum. Many men are stylistically and characterologically more comfortable focusing on behavioral problems and solutions than they are on addressing underlying feelings. This tension is vital and must be acknowledged. The question to be addressed is to what extent the leader gratifies the group's wish for concrete problem-oriented solutions and to what extent he or she holds the position that the demand for answers and exercises serves to avoid important feelings. Some therapists working with male clients or running all-male groups find it useful to provide anxiety-binding structures that limit initial competition and prevent premature confrontation. Others attempt to integrate cognitive-behavioral exercises aimed at anger control, stress management, or assertiveness. Although it is possible to do integrative group work that combines cognitive-behavioral approaches with affective-uncovering approaches, it is difficult to strike a balance that feels containing and consistent. Some men will not be able to tolerate exploration through experience of feeling when the more gratifying, problem-oriented solution is within reach. A clear stance with respect to this tension helps to set the group's expectations in a realistic way.

When the leader is female, issues of authority are compounded in particular ways. In the experience of most men, female authority is either maternal or unfamiliar. The conflict for men over their regressive yearnings for maternal guidance and direction often leads men to deny their wishes and adopt postures of pseudomaturity and control. The wish to be (and the shame of being) a "mama's boy" leaves male members in a quandary in the face of female leadership. How does a man relate to a powerful woman, and how does he feel in her presence? These and other questions become part of the opportunity to explore the gender bias.

Countertransference and Projective Identification

Men often bring a "phallocentric bias" (Ross 1975) to male-male encounters, especially when there is a status and power differential. When this bias is active, the group leader will be forced to struggle with a hostile, competitive oedipal rival on the one hand and a dependent, needy, and easily wounded pre-oedipal character on the other. In the face of the multiple transferences, counterdependent defenses, and confusing interpersonal stances, the male group leader must do the delicate work of making room on his lap while encouraging separation and disidentification.

When the leader is a woman, these same issues take on a different spin. A female leader will have to work with the propensity of men to transform dependent feelings into sexual ones. A female leader may also contend with becoming the object of sexualized competition among male members. A female leader may also serve as a replacement object for men, thereby muting the intensity of their yearning.

Strong countertransference experiences are evoked as male members struggle to find a working stance within the group space and in relation to the leader. Counterdependent behaviors and attitudes challenge and provoke, particularly early on in the life of the group. These can be seen as tests of the limits of the group's contract and of the leader's capacity to contain without retaliation. Competitive and retaliatory impulses in the therapist are not uncommon. Awareness of shame and the potential for humiliation is also a frequent aspect of countertransference. Shame-related feelings may arise as men struggle to acknowledge their own dependent needs and indirectly express wishes to cuddle up in the therapist's lap. As the bravura gives way, the therapist may feel called on to be more nurturant, the facilitating pre-oedipal father. The countertransferential pull toward overcompensating for the paternal deprivation many men share can be quite compelling.

In group work with men who have been sadistic or malignantly narcissistic toward women and children, the therapist is likely to feel whipsawed by the countertransference reactions. Contempt and revulsion are evoked by the some of the acts one hears about, whereas the perpetrators themselves often seem terribly deprived and in need. The leader faces an internal dilemma of how to offer empathic contact on the one hand while wishing for distance on the other. Female leaders may find the material so anxiety arousing that they may have difficulty feeling safe and allowing a full airing of what must be shared.

As the group moves into a mature phase, other countertransference pulls emerge. When men in the group engage in honest self-examination, the leader must contend with strong wishes to be included (as one of the boys) and perhaps taken care of. Along with these wishes come complementary feelings of being left out and excluded. When men are actively exploring new role expectations while struggling to moderate traditional male entitlements, the leader may find his or her own values and choices under pressure.

Group work with male clients places intense demands on the group leader. Men are often aggressive but not tough. They are defensive but injure easily. An effective leader must offer considerable containment while being willing to come out and meet the anxious male patient at the boundary of his self-protection. Inevitably, male and female leaders fail to live up to the idealized expectations (and their negative counterparts) that male clients bring to treatment. Male hurt and disappointment in the face of the failure of the idealized leader are poignant and potent, as is the fury that sometimes overlies the felt vulnerability. Tolerating the expression of these feelings and the accompanying attitudes often requires real fortitude and maturity.

Supervision or consultation that enables the therapist to acknowledge and expose the countertransference pressure that is produced by group work with men is an invaluable tool. The shameful, rageful, fearful feelings that sometimes arise can be managed only by acknowledgment and working through. This process then leads to a richer and safer group environment.

Contraindications

Group therapy is not for all men. Several categories of male patients should not be referred to a mixed psychodynamic group. Actively psychotic men will find the format and the material too stimulating and disorganizing. However, once the individual has compensated to an adequate degree, a mixed ongoing group with other patients of a similar developmental level can provide important support and life direction. In such cases a long-term group is often the treatment of choice.

Men expressly seeking to control addictive, obsessive-compulsive behaviors (such as drinking, gambling, and drug abuse) should be referred to appropriate programs. This is particularly true when impulse control problems are involved. Rage responses, including battering, sexual assault, and criminal violence, along with substance abuse, are among the most prominent presenting complaints specific to male patients (see Chapters 5 and 15).

Difficult Male Patients in Group Therapy

Narcissistic character disorders represent a special challenge to the long-term mixed group. For many patients with brittle defenses, the demands of the group will prove intolerable. Mr. J., for example, seemed to function quite well until the group began to threaten his account of himself and his "solutions." At that point he took issue with a misunderstanding and used it as a pretext to flee the group.

The affective intensity, degree of self-exposure, demand for commitment, and accountability all fly in the face of the narcissistic male character defense. Such men are at risk of leaving with little or no warning. Although this repetition of their basic life stance may or may not affect them adversely, the sudden loss of a group member can be quite disruptive to an ongoing group. There is also a small group of narcissistically vulnerable men whose response to the inevitable injuries sustained in the group is to decompensate either into a rage reaction or into paranoid ideation. Careful screening and thorough knowledge of one's patient constitute the only bulwark against an unfortunate placement of this nature.

Problems can be anticipated even among the great range of male patients for whom a mixed ongoing psychotherapy group represents a treatment of choice. Many men respond to demands for intimacy with distance and to the threat of exposure with narcissistic defenses. Male group members often experience these demands and threats in the context of the group. They are prone to act out around issues of commitment to the group and the contract. They may attempt to regulate their exposure to the group by planned and unplanned absences and by periodic threats to leave the group. All of this, although problematic, represents nothing other than the working through of male character defense.

Conclusions

Group therapy provides men in need of character change with a uniquely suited milieu in which to grow. It supports their efforts by building on gender-linked experiences and strengths. It challenges them by asking that they expose their fears and vulnerabilities and that they try on new behaviors. It does so in a context where the group provides both active modeling and support for experimentation. The particular mix of structural and dynamic factors makes ongoing psychodynamic psychotherapy groups an important treatment modality for the contemporary male patient.

References

Agazarian YM: Phases of group development, in The Visible and Invisible Group. Edited by Agazarian YM, Peters R. London, Routledge & Kegan Paul, 1981, pp 124–147

Alonso A, Rutan S: The experience of shame and the restoration of self respect in group psychotherapy. Int J Group Psychother 38:3–14, 1988

Balswick J, Peek C: The inexpressive male: a tragedy of American society. The Family Coordinator 20:363–368, 1971

Bem SL: Gender schema theory: a cognitive account of sex typing. Psychol Rev 88:354–364, 1981

Blos P: Son and Father: Before and Beyond the Oedipus Complex. New York, Free Press, 1985

Broverman IK, Vogel SR, Broverman DM, et al: Sex role stereotypes: a current reappraisal. Journal of Social Issues 28:59–92, 1972

Chodorow N: Feminism and Psychoanalytic Theory. New Haven, CT, Yale University Press, 1989

Erikson E: Childhood and Society. New York, WW Norton Company, 1950

Fine R: Understanding men's emotional problems, in Troubled Men. Edited by Fine R. San Francisco, CA, Jossey-Bass, 1988, pp 1–24

Friedman EC: Male Homosexuality. New Haven, CT, Yale University Press, 1988

Gans J: Broaching and exploring the question of combined group and individual therapy. Int J Group Psychother 40:123–137, 1990a

Gans J: On the use of hostility in groups. Int J Group Psychother 39:499–516, 1990b

Jacklin CN: Female and male: issues of gender. Am Psychol 44:127–133, 1989

Horwitz L: Projective identification in dyads and groups. Int J Group Psychother 33:259–279, 1983

Komarovsky M: Patterns of self-disclosure of male undergraduates. J Marriage Fam 36:677–686, 1974

Lansky MR: Violence, shame, and the family. International Journal of Family Psychiatry 5:21–40, 1984

Lansky MR: The paternal imago, in Fathers and Their Families. Edited by Cath SH, Gurwit A, Gunsberg L. Hillsdale, NJ, Analytic Press, 1989, pp 27–47

Levinson D: The Seasons of a Man's Life. New York, Knopf, 1978

Lewis RA: Emotional intimacy among men, in The Gender Gap in Psychotherapy. Edited by Reiker PP, Carmen E. New York, Plenum, 1984, pp 181–193

MacKenzie KR: Time-Limited Group Psychotherapy. Washington, DC, American Psychiatric Press, 1990

MacNab T: What do men want? Male rituals of initiation in group psychotherapy. Int J Group Psychother 40:139–154, 1990

Meth RL, Pasick RS: Men in Therapy. New York, Guilford, 1990

Morrison A: Shame: The Underside of Narcissism. Hillsdale, NJ, Analytic Press, 1989

Osherson S: Finding Our Fathers. New York, Free Press, 1986

Osherson S, Krugman S: Men, shame and psychotherapy. Journal of Psychotherapy 27 (Spring):327–337, 1991

Rice C: The "we" of the beholder. Paper presented at the 44th American Group Psychotherapy Conference, New Orleans, LA, February 1987

Ross JM: Beyond the phallic illusion: notes on man's heterosexuality, in The Psychology of Men: New Psychoanalytic Perspectives. Edited by Fogel G, Lane G, Liebert R. New York, Basic Books, 1986, pp 49–70

Rutan JS, Stone WN: Psychodynamic Group Psychotherapy. New York, Macmillan, 1984

Scheidlinger S: On the concept of the mother-group. Int J Group Psychother 244:17, 1974

Sternbach, J: The men's seminar: an educational and support group for men. Paper presented at 9th Annual Symposium for the Advancement of Social Work in Groups, Boston, MA, October 30, 1987

Wright F: Men, shame and antisocial behavior: a psychodynamic perspective. Group 11:238–246, 1987

Yalom ID: The Theory and Practice of Group Psychotherapy. New York, Basic Books, 1975

PART VI

New Applications of Group Theory and Technique

CHAPTER 22

Time-Limited Group Theory and Technique

K. Roy MacKenzie, M.D., F.R.C.P.C.

Introduction

The idea of setting a time limit for psychotherapy is not new. Early psychotherapeutic work was conducted in a structure that today would be termed brief psychotherapy. As analytic work became increasingly concerned with ideas of characterological change, assumptions arose concerning the importance of selection for suitability and the need for a lengthened course of therapy. Briefer approaches were derided as being of necessity superficial and at best suited to facilitating recompensation after stress. These views were challenged by Alexander and French (1946/1980), but broader acceptance of shorter time limits did not occur until the 1970s. Marmar's review paper (1979) stands as a marker of that shift. An introduction to contemporary time-limited individual psychotherapy was provided by the following authors, most of whom began their work in the 1960s: Balint et al. (1972), Davanloo (1980), Malan (1979), Mann and Goldman (1982), and Sifneos (1987). This material was integrated and expanded by Budman and Gurman (1988) and MacKenzie (1988).

The application of time-limited techniques accelerated during the 1980s because of concern regarding cost containment in the provision of mental health services. Systematic application of the principles of time-limited psychotherapy has been found particularly in managed care systems, where the mental health professional must function in part as a service administrator. This interest has been reinforced by the demonstration of significant reduction in general medical care costs after brief psychiatric intervention (Mumford et al. 1984). So, perhaps for the wrong reasons, the mental health service delivery system is now in a position where there are demands for the justification of longer-term therapeutic strategies, rather than criticism of time-limited approaches.

Interest in the use of time-limited group psychotherapy has developed in parallel with developments in individual psychotherapeutic work, although with a lag time of several years. Descriptive articles involving groups with preset time limits appeared in the late 1970s (Bernard and Klein 1977; Waxer 1977). Imber et al. (1979) provided a comprehensive review of the preceding literature. This literature dealt primarily with the use of time-limited group psychotherapy for patients in crisis or in acute situational stress. Budman et al. (1980) reported the use of 15- to 20session groups that had more ambitious therapeutic goals. A theory of group development and social role functioning of particular interest in the context of time-limited groups was described in the first American Group Psychotherapy Association monograph by MacKenzie and Livesley (1983) and Livesley and MacKenzie (1983). Other articles have dealt with specific target populations and delineated therapeutic strategies for maximizing effect (Dies 1985; Goldberg et al. 1983; Klein 1985; MacKenzie et al. 1986; Poey 1985; Rosenbaum 1983). Several studies have shown that in randomized clinical trials, patients in group therapy achieve similar improvement to those in individual treatment (Budman et al. 1988; Pilkonis et al 1984; piper et al 1984; Toseland and Siporin 1986). Piper et al. (1992) reviewed the application of psychoanalytically oriented theory and technique to the context of a time-limited group. A recent basic text was devoted to time-limited group psychotherapy (MacKenzie 1990).

A discrete body of literature has developed regarding the use of groups in inpatient settings (Kibel 1981; Leszcz 1986; Maxmen 1984; Rice and Rutan 1987; Yalom 1983). A set of articles in the *International Journal of Group Psychotherapy* in 1988 reviewed various approaches to inpatient group work (Beeber 1988; Brabender 1988; Kanas 1988). The inpatient literature places greater emphasis on the characteristics of the setting than on the issue of brief treatment, per se. Inpatients place high value on this component of their treatment programs, although it is difficult to translate this into specific outcome effects because of the multimodal nature of the inpatient treatment milieu.

As an introductory summary, the following eight basic features are presented; all are common to both individual and group time-limited psychotherapy:

1. There is an expectation that the time limit will increase the tempo of psychotherapeutic work and encourage rapid application to real-life circumstances.
2. Careful assessment and selection are used to rule out patients who might be at risk for harm from an active approach.
3. An explicit verbal agreement regarding circumscribed goals is openly negotiated between the patient and the therapist.
4. The therapist will intervene actively to develop and maintain a therapeutic climate and maintain a working focus on the identified goals.
5. From an early point in therapy, there is an expectation that ideas will be actively applied to outside circumstances.
6. The therapist will expect the patient to assume responsibility for initiating therapy tasks and will encourage him or her to do so.
7. There will be encouragement to mobilize the use of outside resources that can reinforce positive changes.
8. It is anticipated that the change process will continue after therapy terminates and, therefore, that the full range of problematic issues need not be addressed within the therapy context.

Throughout this chapter a distinction is drawn between groups that have limited goals of psychoeducation, crisis management, or support and groups that are designed for active intrusive interpersonal work. Both approaches have their place, but they require a markedly different emphasis in terms of therapeutic strategy. It is essential that the therapist clearly acknowledges this distinction and uses it as a guide in clinical application.

The challenge in brief group psychotherapy is to adapt usual clinical practices to the restraints of limited time. Strategies for achieving this adaptation lie in three major areas: pregroup preparation, maximum utilization of the group system, and modification of therapeutic technique. By attending to each of these areas, the group psychotherapy experience can be "packaged" to achieve optimum results. Failure to focus on these three areas may result in a group that either fails to coalesce at all or that terminates with the patients suspended in mid-process.

Pregroup Preparation

The first opportunity to maximize the effectiveness of time-limited group psychotherapy occurs before the group begins. The pregroup tasks of the therapist can be divided into several categories:

- Defining a set of objectives for the group
- Assessing potential members to exclude those unlikely to benefit
- Making group composition decisions
- Preparing patients for the group experience

By sequentially addressing these tasks, the therapist lays the groundwork for the group to have a successful beginning.

Defining the Group Objectives

A careful consideration of the objectives chosen for a group will influence assessment decisions, composition issues, time structures, and therapeutic activity.

Group objectives are developed primarily in regard to the needs of a particular target population. For example, one may think of a group for young adult women with bulimia nervosa, or a group focused on adaptation to a specific stress such as the loss of a spouse. The characteristics of the diagnostic category or stress situation will have a major impact on the sort of patient likely to be in the group. A second type of group objective deals with the nature of the interactional climate that can be realistically attained and that would be of most value to the participants. These objectives need to be carefully considered because they will later serve as guidelines to the therapist in monitoring the progress of the group and in determining therapeutic priorities.

The group interaction can be usefully conceptualized as lying along a continuum that at one end deals with the provision of practical support and at the other end deals with expectations of intensive introspection. Groups at one end will relieve anxiety, and groups at the other end will stimulate anxiety. All groups will use the interpersonal events of the sessions as a vehicle for therapeutic effect, but at one end this is limited to general mechanisms of encouragement, reinforcement, and modeling, whereas at the other end, the nature of the interactional patterns among the members will be the specific focus of therapeutic attention. Groups may be located at a few characteristic points along this continuum.

Social skills.   Such groups are suitable for patients with major deficiencies in basic social functioning. Often these deficiencies are associated with long-term medical or psychiatric morbidity. These groups make substantial use of the support available among the group members. The leader will have a higher profile, both modeling support and encouragement and directing group interaction. Specific homework tasks are often used. There may be a purposeful extension of the group activities into the community. Members may be asked to plan activities together between sessions or to try out specific social skills in their supervised accommodations or sheltered workshops. These groups are usually one part of a general range of rehabilitative efforts, but they may be designed as specific time-limited activities that focus on particular social skills.

Educational and cognitive focus. Groups with a psychoeducational objective provide the support of a cohesive group along with specific information or techniques. These ingredients may be quite effective in producing a greater sense of mastery for the members. The focus of the group is centered on the material to be covered, and general group mechanisms of support and reinforcement are important. Such groups can be very useful for dealing with adaptation to specific diseases such as diabetes mellitus or renal dialysis or in coming to terms with specific stress issues such as adapting to a new college environment. Cognitive-behavioral strategies may be effectively applied in such an interactional context. For example, group approaches to phobic problems or to the self-defeating thought patterns typical of some depressed states have been described. Groups at this level may have high morale and much enthusiasm and may be composed of quite psychologically competent members, but the actual group work is purposefully of a general nature and targeted quite specifically to the externally defined objective. The interactions amongst the members are maintained in a positive valence and are not themselves the subject of intrusive questions.

Interpersonal-restitutive. Many time-limited groups are designed to deal in more depth with adaptation to a specific stress. The goal of such groups is to work through the personal implications of that stress. Attendant changes in basic self-concept or interpersonal style may occur during this process, but these are not seen as the principal task of the group. This distinction is important to both the therapist and the members. If a group is set up to deal with acute situations and has a predefined short time span, then allowing the group to stray into more intrusive interactional work may create a demand for longer treatment accompanied by a sense of dissatisfaction and abandonment when the time limit is imposed. In this sort of brief group there may be expectations for quite active individual psychotherapeutic work, whereas the group context is used more as a background facilitator than as the main focus for inquiry.

Relationships among group members may be used to identify patterns, but the emphasis is quickly turned to the external circumstances and adaptation to them.

Interpersonal-explorative.   In these groups there is an expectation that the participants will actively explore internal states with a view to identifying areas of conflict or ambivalence, isolated or denied ideas, and patterns in relationships perhaps connected with early life experiences. In such groups the role of the leader is less active and is particularly concerned with interpretative interventions that will tend to increase anxiety. There is active use of the interpersonal relationships within the group as a model for understanding the self and relationship difficulties.

This seemingly mundane topic of group objectives is described in some detail because the goals chosen will form the basis on which the group will be constructed. Groups begin as an idea held by a therapist, or perhaps by a supervisor or program manager. This idea must become the guiding principle in all subsequent steps of implementing a time-limited group. If there is lack of clarity regarding the purpose of a group, it may lose the focus and intensity required for effective use of the limited time available.

Exclusion Criteria

A few criteria preclude the likelihood of an individual benefiting from a group therapy environment. The same criteria may also identify individuals who will seriously disrupt the process. These criteria lie along a spectrum of intensity. When they are present to a strong degree, they should be used to exclude patients from even the less ambitious levels of group therapy. Group treatment is contraindicated for people who are overstimulated in the group, patients with serious sociopathic traits, and patients who are too psychotically disorganized to tolerate the ambiguity.

These exclusion criteria are pertinent to any therapy group. However, they are particularly important for time-limited groups. Because of the need to move rapidly into group work, the inclusion of patients with the qualities outlined above may seriously hinder the effectiveness of the group for other members.

Group Composition

Structure and composition will be easier to address if the objectives of the group have been carefully considered. The value of diagnostic evaluations will increase as the goals of the group become more ambitious. In contrast, in groups with supportive or psychoeducational objectives, only the more extreme exclusion criteria need be applied.

Group size.   As the group size increases, there will be less personal interaction among the members and the process will become more leader centered. Smaller groups encourage more self-disclosure and less subgrouping. There are some natural division points. For groups intending to utilize high levels of intermember interaction, a size of 5 to 10 members seems a reasonable range. If the group is designed to work at the level of developing social skills or with educational and cognitive-behavioral objectives, then the size could be somewhat larger. Above the 15- to 20-member level, the group will develop a classroom atmosphere. This may be quite appropriate for some objectives, but that decision needs to be explicitly defended.

Closed or open groups.   There are advantages in using a closed-group format for time-limited psychotherapy. Certainly for groups that meet for 8 to 12 sessions, the advantages of a closed format outweigh the disadvantages of asking new members to wait until the beginning of the next group. An obvious exception to these guidelines are those groups that take place in intensive treatment settings such as day hospitals or inpatient units. In these settings, rapid patient turnover is inevitable, but the opportunities for reinforcing group cohesion extend beyond the group setting itself and are embodied in the total program milieu. Indeed, the presence of group members at a later stage of treatment may be an asset.

Duration of the group.   Enough time must be allowed to develop a cohesive group atmosphere; otherwise, the advantages of a group context are lost. Six sessions are probably a minimum. Most time-limited group programs operate over a longer duration than that. There are examples of 8-session programs, but most are in the 12- to 20-session range. The idea of time-limited psychotherapy is most clearly implemented in a brief closed group. With that format, the group must deal with the implications of the time limit collectively. If the group is open, it is more difficult to adhere to the time limit for any given member, except through a general manner of expectation. In practice, the questions of duration and an open or closed format are intertwined. Clearly these decisions depend on the objectives chosen.

Pretherapy Preparation

The final pregroup task is to prepare the members for the experience. Studies indicate that systematic preparation results in fewer early dropouts and faster development of group cohesion (Piper and Perrault 1989). It is to be expected that the effects of pretherapy preparation will wash out after the first six to eight sessions as the actual group experience becomes the predominant factor.

The preparation itself may be done either in a group or in individual sessions. A group context provides greater reality and a controlled entry into the experience of being in a group. The clinician running the group may also note the level at which patients are functioning and use this to make final decisions regarding group suitability or composition.

This pretherapy material is straightforward. The important thing is that its presentation be seen as a specific task before the group begins. Many programs use a simple handout that explains these matters. The therapist goes over it point by point to reinforce the material and answer additional questions. The potential group member can then enter the first session with some knowledge of how groups operate and a reasonable cognitive orientation regarding what is expected of a group member.

In summary, there are important tasks to be undertaken before the group begins. The leader should have a clear understanding of the objectives and the implications of these objectives for selection and composition decisions. Patients should be excluded if they are unlikely to benefit from the group experience. Some dimension of homogeneity in group composition is useful. Pretherapy preparation will prevent early dropouts and enhance early group cohesion. These matters apply to all therapy groups, but they are particularly relevant to time-limited ones. It is critical that the group master early group tasks quickly. Careful attention to these preliminary details will facilitate that process.

Utilizing the Group System

Efforts to create a working group system must take precedence in the early sessions. If the group does not coalesce promptly around its common tasks, dropouts are inevitable and a gradually sagging morale will sap the group of its potential for useful effects. If the group is not showing a rising curve of group identity and commitment by the fourth or fifth session, it is in difficulty. This is particularly critical for a time-limited group, where the number of sessions available for active group work will rapidly diminish if the introductory phase is protracted. Most group dropouts occur in the first six sessions. Generally, members drop out for one of two reasons. The individual member may feel out of place in the group or apprehensive about tackling personal issues. The second major factor is at a group level. If the group fails to come together, a sagging sense of pessimism and hopelessness may develop. This section discusses useful ways of conceptualizing and using the power inherent in the group system.

Group Cohesion

One of the important basic features of the whole group is group cohesion. Some terms used to describe highly cohesive groups are "high morale," "lots of commitment," and "group energy." High levels of group cohesion are usually easy to detect. This feeling of "groupness" is directed at the group itself and does not reside in the relationships among specific group members, although these may enhance cohesion. If there are specific ties, they are more likely to be with the group leader. These are some of the specific indicators of group cohesion:

1. The members attend regularly and are punctual.
2. There are few premature terminations.
3. Members are vocal about their enthusiasm to remain in the group and have no regrets about joining.
4. There is a warm feeling among the members and they are attracted to each other.
5. There are high levels of active participation.
6. There are high levels of self-disclosure, indicating that the members are beginning to trust each other.
7. There is a shared belief system about the goals of the group and how it should operate.
8. There is a high level of investment in the work of the group.

Group Developmental Stages

Another way of conceptualizing the group is with the language of group developmental stages. There are various systems for describing group stages, most of them in substantial agreement (Beck 1974; MacKenzie and Livesley 1983; Tuckman 1965). For the purposes of time-limited groups, it is adequate to think particularly in terms of how the group negotiates the early stages. In this simplified schema the relevant stages are engagement, differentiation, interpersonal work, and termination. Virtually all studies confirm the importance of an initial stage of group formation, followed by a stage of testing and conflict, before the group gets down to more personalized interactional tasks. After the group has achieved a working atmosphere, the boundaries between stages become less precise and more variable in their timing. The speed at which a given group moves through its developmental tasks will vary according to the objectives of the group, the psychological level of the members, and the techniques used by the therapist.

Engagement stage.   The tasks of the engagement stage are closely related to group cohesion. This involves the development of an identification between each member and the group and a commitment to the tasks of the group. The process is carried out through relatively superficial self-disclosures that reflect the emergence of trust among the members. The process of initial self-revelation is generally accompanied by both anxiety and relief. The information revealed is usually accepted by the other group members in a supportive and uncritical fashion. A powerful mechanism at work during the engagement stage is universality. The group members begin to realize that they have had similar experiences, reactions, or symptoms. The awareness of similarities pulls the members together. The therapeutic task during this stage is to encourage and support participation, and a reasonable degree of therapist activity is appropriate during this stage.

During the engagement stage, themes of confrontation, criticism, and conflict need to be dampened. The group must develop a sense of strength in its own resources and trust among the members before more conflictual material can be effectively handled. It may seem quite clear to the leader that the material being presented is not being adequately explored or tested. The members may seem content with global statements and the ready acceptance of self-justifying comments. At the same time they appear to be increasingly involved in the work. The therapist should ensure that all of the members participate in some fashion as evidenced by personal contributions and participation in the group interaction. At that point, a watch can be kept for evidence of emerging conflict.

Differentiation stage.   The next component of group development is the differentiation stage. The function of this second stage is to appreciate and learn to deal with the uniqueness of the individual and diverse points of view. This identification of differences also brings a confrontational atmosphere often accompanied by reactions of irritation or anger. In the engagement stage, statements are uncritically accepted, and the emphasis is on support more than understanding. Thus the work of the differentiation stage addresses the danger of complacency and lack of challenge. One manifestation of this stage may be group criticism of the leader.

The time of appearance of challenge and assertion will depend on the level of psychological maturity of the members, the development of group cohesion, and the style of leadership. In weekly outpatient groups such material usually begins to surface somewhere between the fourth and eighth session. Earlier emergence carries the danger of conflict before cohesion has developed. Delayed appearance may reflect a group, or perhaps a leader, that is having difficulty with negative affect and is stuck in early universalization material beyond the point of productivity.

The more conflictual atmosphere of the differentiation stage forces members to look more seriously at themselves and the nature of their group involvement. The process is accompanied by a marked increase in the information the members have about each other. Indeed, members often blurt out information to justify their positions that reveals underlying important attitudinal positions. The therapist's task during this stage is to allow these processes without interfering with them.

The therapist must attend to the professional responsibility of ensuring that no particular member is ignored if he or she is hurt through these confrontational events. The more divergent group members may elicit negative reactions from others that can result in persistent attacks. The therapist may need to support the scapegoat or control the attacking process if it threatens to get out of hand. Group cohesion will inevitably slump during this type of work, and the leader may need to bolster group morale or remind the members that they have a history of getting along positively. The differentiation stage pushes the group to more advanced work. It can be seen to be coming to an end when the group is able to manage conflict resolution through a cooperative style. Members may agree to disagree but nonetheless to keep working on the issues.

A decision to allow the group to move into differentiation stage issues also entails a commitment to see these matters through. It is unwise to terminate a group while it is struggling with how to handle confrontational material, because termination is by its very nature tinged with negative affect. As members look back on a group experience, they see it through the terminal experiences. If these are composed of unresolved conflictual issues, the image retained of the group may be unpleasant, and this can discolor and perhaps undo useful experiences that occurred during earlier sessions.

Interactional work stage.   During the foregoing early period, the leader assesses group behavior in terms of its appropriateness to group needs. As the group moves into a more advanced working stage, the therapist's priorities shift. The important learning experiences will now deal to a much greater extent with understanding the individual member. This does not mean that the needs of the individual are forgotten during the first two stages, nor that maintaining a therapeutic group culture is unimportant in the working stages, but the sense of orientation appropriately alters.

Termination stage.   Systematic management of termination issues is an important component of all psychotherapeutic work. It centers around the adaptation to loss. Members may find that their sadness at termination becomes associated with past situations of grief. Elements of anger are also to be expected. Disengagement usually involves a review of the events of therapy, a process that helps to internalize the experience. The strength of the termination process will vary with the degree of commitment and involvement of the individual. In brief psychoeducational groups, the termination process will be modest. In intensive time-limited groups, it may become a major part of the therapeutic experience.

An important aspect of time-limited approaches is the expectation that patients will rapidly apply the learning from therapy to outside circumstances. This implies a dimension of patient initiative and activity that, although present in all therapies, is particularly prominent in the time-limited approaches. The degree of dependency on the therapist or the therapeutic setting must be kept limited. The imposition of a time limit automatically throws into focus the question of personal responsibility and autonomy. Termination brings this to a head. Mann and Goldman (1982) expressed the issue particularly effectively:

> The major plague of human beings is a simultaneous wish to merge with another and the absolute necessity of learning to tolerate separation and loss without undue damage to feelings about oneself. (p. 42)

MacKenzie (1988) described three methods for establishing a time limit in individual psychotherapy. The first of these is the "Procrustean alternative." Therapy has an established duration and the patient is bound by it. Mann and Goldman (1984), for example, used a 12-session format for brief individual therapy. A second approach is the "sporting alternative." A specific date of termination is set in advance, but the pace may vary. Sessions may be held more frequently to begin with and then less frequently towards the end, as in an educational learning paradigm. The third approach is the "elastic alternative." No set time limit is established, but there is constant pressure to keep the process as short as possible. If the earlier recommendation of using a closed format for time-limited groups is adopted, then the Procrustean alternative is automatically applied.

For closed groups, the ending date needs to be set well in advance. Generally it is established at the beginning, and there is a contract between the members and the therapist that commits all to participate to the end. It is useful early in the group's life to reinforce the date of termination so that it is clearly understood. During the assessment process it is also helpful to review each patient's calendar to ensure that he or she will be available throughout the proposed duration of the group. As the group nears termination, perhaps during the last four to six sessions, the theme of termination needs to be reintroduced. Members may spontaneously bring this subject up, but if they do not, it is clearly the responsibility of the therapist to do so.

It is possible to offer time-limited group psychotherapy in an open group format. Here the "elastic alternative" can be used without setting predetermined dates of termination for an individual member. Often the departure date for a given member coincides with other group events, such as a break for vacations. It is helpful for the group to deal with terminations and then have one or two sessions with the remaining group members or a short break before introducing new members. This clarifies the shifting membership boundary and makes it is easier to address the need for the group to become reconstituted as a system. In open groups the contributions of longer-standing members as they approach termination are often quite helpful for newer members.

In time-limited approaches it is not uncommon for termination to be associated with the feeling that insufficient therapy has been received. This is a disguised plea of helplessness that must be addressed thoroughly and promptly. The termination work will then bring into perspective existential themes of personal responsibility. When worked through, this awareness reinforces the members' sense of self-esteem and self-efficacy.

Patients remember the group experience through the filter of the ending. If that ending is left in a suspended state, it may color the perception of the entire experience and undo useful learning. It is possible that some of the members may indeed need more therapy. When this is the case, it is useful to interpose a brief "treatment holiday." The new therapy can then be seen as a second phase, not simply as an unhappy necessity connected with the ending of the group.

In planning time-limited groups there are some clear advantages to carefully working out the entire sequence—from assessment through preparation to the establishment of the number of sessions and the date of termination. This is somewhat like scheduling an academic course, and that analogy is not out of place. This attention to the "frame" of therapy encourages a purposeful use of termination stress to focus on important psychological work.

Therapeutic Technique

A fundamental assumption in all of the brief therapies is that a specific task will be addressed and kept in focus throughout the therapy. The therapist has a responsibility for developing with the patient a suitable set of target goals and for ensuring that the therapy process does not stray too far from these goals. Rather than encouraging undirected associative flow, the therapist and the patient must limit their consideration to those issues that are relevant to the therapeutic task. Simultaneously, this will serve to keep dependence on the therapeutic process to a minimum. This stringent approach is based on the assumption that if the target task is well chosen, a significant change regarding it be amplified throughout other areas of functioning. It is left up to the patient to manage these extended effects. There is empirical evidence that indeed these effects routinely occur. The trend for improvement that begins in therapy customarily continues to increase in the 6 months after termination and gradually flattens after a period of about 2 years. This trend is in keeping with the idea that the patient actively applies therapeutic learning after the formal therapy has ceased.

By insisting on maintaining a therapeutic focus, the therapist may precipitate stresses within the therapeutic alliance that are rooted in patient resistance to dealing with an important area. The rationale for a defined and restricted therapeutic zone of activity is equally applicable to individual and group time-limited therapies.

Attention to a therapeutic focus begins during the assessment period. However, a passive application of the idea of specific targets, or problem orientation, may result in the development of superficial goals primarily dealing with the relief of symptoms. If the therapy is designed to deal with underlying mechanisms, such clinically inappropriate goals may trivialize the intent of the therapeutic effort. The literature on time-limited psychotherapy has emphasized two ways of addressing this problem.

The first way is a dialogue between clinician and patient to develop a reasonable set of therapeutic goals. This dialogue usually evolves over several sessions. The intent of this important process is to stimulate a thoughtful assessment of underlying patterns that might be recurrently problematic. This collaboration generally results in a more useful therapeutic focus.

The second major way to establish a therapeutic focus is by the selective use of interpersonal language rather than intrapsychic concepts. This is not to deny the importance of internal mechanisms, but rather to focus on the implications of these mechanisms for specific, real relationship situations. Establishing a therapeutic focus entails a careful probing of specific relationships in the present and in the past with a particular interest in the meaning that the patient places on these relationships and on important events involving them. This focus on interpersonal construing patterns provides descriptive material that is understandable to the patient and easier to track in the therapeutic process.

A specific work focus at an early point in the clinical process has an additional important advantage. During the first few sessions, the patient is likely to be anxious and uncertain about the processes of therapy. This is a time when customary defenses such as denial, isolation of affect, and rationalization may be less in evidence. As the patient becomes familiar with the therapeutic setting, typical defenses may be reconstituted. Thus an early and direct probing of important interpersonal mechanisms can be productive in helping to establish the direction in which therapy might most usefully be oriented. Alexander and French (1946/1980) likened the early assessment period to an observer standing on a hill able to see the larger features of the landscape. As therapy progresses, the therapist and patient descend into the valley, where local features can obscure the larger picture.

Establishing an Interpersonal Focus

The current time-limited literature contains several methods for establishing an interpersonal focus. Five of these methods are reviewed to give an idea of the clinical nature of the methodology.

Core conflictual relationship theme.   Luborsky (1984) translated interpersonal vignettes into the following standard format:

> I (the patient) wish/need/intend _____
> from _____ (the other), BUT
> _____. (p. 199)

The first part of the statement reflects a central issue in the relationship
with the other person. The "BUT" represents attempted solutions to the
satisfaction of that interpersonal wish. Answers to the "BUT" may be sub-
divided into those that focus on the response of others, such as "BUT he
will reject me if I express my affection," and those that focus on the response of self, such as "BUT I may lose control if I begin to show my anger."
This approach encourages the clinician to think of the material in a psychotherapy session in terms of a succession of specific interpersonal "short
stories" and to probe the meanings given to these events by the patient.

Configurational analysis.   Horowitz (1988) similarly dealt with the
attitude or expectation that lies behind different specific relationships.
Horowitz described the overt behavior shown, the emotional qualities,
the level of control, and the defensive arrangements. He related them to
issues of self-concept, role relationship models, and conflictual-relation-
ships schemata. This work is particularly interesting because of its emphasis on trying to identify several such typical models for a given patient.
The research was particularly focused on those points in a therapy session
when the patient shifted relationships models, phenomena Horowitz
called "states of mind."

Structural analysis of social behavior.   Benjamin (1974) developed a
system for assessing personality and interpersonal behavior based on a
two-dimensional model of interpersonal functioning. The first dimension is that of positive to negative affiliation (love and acceptance to hate
and rejection). The second dimension is one extending from independence and autonomy to interdependence and enmeshment. These two
dimensions are applied in terms of how the individual acts on others
(transitive focus) and how the individual reacts to others (intransitive
focus). Also important is how the individual acts toward himself or herself
(introspection). This model provides a useful space in which to plot interpersonal relationships and is particularly helpful in the process of defining a therapeutic focus.

Thematic content. A system has been developed (Klerman et al. 1984) for the time-limited psychotherapy of depressed patients that is also applicable to a broader range of nonpsychotic presentations. This system consists of four thematic categories: grief and loss, interpersonal disputes, role transitions, and interpersonal deficits. Each category carries with it a set of anticipated issues that form the basis of therapeutic work when linked to specific intervention strategies.

Adult life developmental stages. This viewpoint is particularly helpful because it implies a positive orientation in which the role of therapy is seen as helping to remove blocks that stand in the way of a natural maturational process. This is in keeping with the earlier observation that progress continues after therapy ends. Budman et al. (1980) utilized this approach as a method for achieving group homogeneity.

These five methods offer different ways of establishing a central therapeutic focus using interpersonal terminology. They all have the advantage of having been tested in the crucible of empirical research projects where interrater reliability and the relationship between process and outcome were central concerns. The references provided will guide the reader to more detail regarding these techniques.

The Two Triangles

The above assessment techniques have a common recognition of the importance of internal tension reflected in ambivalence or conflictual responses to a situation or relationship (Malan 1979). This idea of opposing reactions to a specific stress is captured with the idea of the "triangle of conflict." This triangle is shown in Figure 22–1 in its most generic form. The problematic issue (P) stimulates a negative response characterized by anxiety associated with an anticipated negative consequence (A). This tension results in attempts to find a solution (S) that will modulate between the underlying wish and the feared consequences. The model can be usefully applied to the therapeutic focus chosen for an individual and may serve to clarify the meaning of dysfunctional responses.

The triangle of conflict may be placed within the larger "triangle of person," as shown in Figure 22–1. The triangle of person simply identifies the importance of trying to understand the application of conflictual issues in major areas of the patient's life. At the bottom lies the area of the past (P), usually family of origin and early developmental experiences.

Along the right margin is a line of important relationships culminating in those that are currently active (C). The top left corner represents the therapeutic relationship (T). Efforts made to define a focus using the triangle of conflict will alert the clinician to its recurrence in the various corners of the triangle of person.

Group therapy is primarily concerned with relationship issues. In this regard, it offers an arena of greater variability and complexity than individual therapy. Groups offer the individual member an opportunity to establish different types of relationships among the various participants, including the leader. Thus the effort to establish an interpersonal thera-

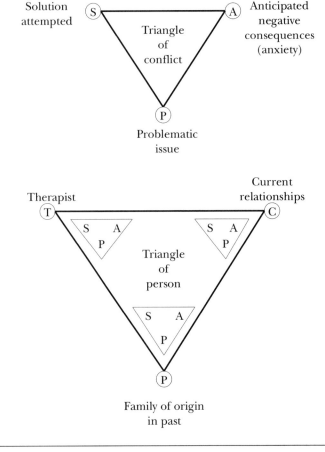

Figure 22–1. Triangle of conflict and triangle of person.

peutic focus is particularly relevant to group work. By undertaking this assessment in a careful and systematic manner, the therapist is better prepared to accurately identify phenomena in the group interactional process that are pertinent to a given patient's area of greatest need. Similarly, the patient is alerted through the assessment process to the sorts of issues that are most likely to need his or her attention during the therapy.

It is helpful to make sure that these issues are attended to at an early point. One technique is to ask each member during the first session to discuss the sorts of relationship matters that need to be understood better during the course of therapy. Opening statements can be used as a point of reference later in the group's life. Using Alexander's imagery, the therapist is able to remind the individual of the main features of the valley that may have been obscured by the underbrush of group events. The therapist should systematically encourage each group member to maintain an awareness of the central issues of each of the other members. Thus the responsibility for accurate interventions can be increasingly transferred to the group members. This not only results in an enhanced sense of interpersonal competency on the part of each member, but also helps to develop a more sophisticated appreciation of interpersonal behavior.

Therapists may wish to monitor their own behavior in this regard. Any statement that does not reinforce a specific dimension relevant to a group developmental-stage task or that does not deal with an individual's focal issue is extraneous. In brief therapy there is limited scope for extraneous interventions.

Composing groups with some dimension of homogeneity will assist the focusing process. If members share common concerns, they are in a better position to understand the concerns of others. This idea of "it takes one to know one" has been usefully applied to groups with target diagnoses such as substance abuse or bulimia nervosa. In homogeneous groups, it is also possible to find group collusion in maintaining common defensive positions. Thus time taken during the assessment to acknowledge problematic defenses is time well spent.

If the therapeutic focus has been accurately assessed, then it is bound to apply to outside circumstances as well. More centrally in time-limited psychotherapy, a major task of the therapist is to systematically encourage the members to consider how they can best apply in-group learning to current real-life situations. This encouragement may need to be done cautiously or with some preplanning within the group so that errors based on naiveté or excessive enthusiasm can be forestalled. Nonetheless, there is clear evidence that patients who quickly begin to apply what they are learning in therapy to their current relationships tend to have better outcomes. The therapist can reinforce this process by encouraging specific planning for the period after termination.

Critical Incidents

Therapy groups are complex interactional fields. It is easy for the therapist to lose a clear sense of the thematic relevance of group events. One useful technique is to think of a group session as a series of "critical incidents." A critical incident constitutes a few minutes of group interaction that focuses on a common theme, often with a common emotional tone. Sometimes it involves the entire group and sometimes only a subset of members. It is particularly helpful if the therapist can identify the initiating event because it often contains the kernel of importance that makes the critical incident understandable. The initiating event is often a specific interaction between two members or between the members and the leader that generates an affective response that gives psychological power to the event. Typically this sense of aroused interaction builds in intensity and then plateaus. The point at which the intensity is beginning to fade is an opportune time for an intervention. Conceptualizing the ongoing group process into discrete critical incidents will help the therapist to focus on the group process as well as content.

The "two triangles" model of conflictual focal themes can be usefully applied. This simple schematic approach provides a shorthand method for tracking major themes as they emerge within the group. Working through the application of the model at regular intervals will enable the therapist to sharpen his or her ability to detect and monitor such events.

Therapist Control

It has been emphasized that the therapist must be prepared for active participation to ensure that the group-stage tasks are addressed properly and that the individual maintains a focus on target therapeutic areas. These types of therapist activity are primarily directed at the group process. It is easy to confuse them with high levels of therapist control. However, this is not the intent. Most of the phenomena described in this chapter will emerge spontaneously within the group interaction. The therapist can augment this natural progression by reinforcing those aspects that meet the identified goals, while ignoring or dampening those that are extraneous. Indeed, the therapist may feel comfortable in sharing with the group the reasons for his or her process-structuring activities. Within this framework of process expectations there is plenty of room for patient initiative and autonomy, and these should be expected and encouraged. As long as the group is reasonably addressing the appropriate tasks, the therapist may remain relatively inactive, stepping in only as required to reorient the group to its major task. A high degree of therapist control will actively work against the objective of enhanced patient responsibility for applied learning. By primarily using operant conditioning techniques, the therapist can effectively mold the nature of the group experience without tightly controlling it.

The Future of Time-Limited Group Psychotherapy

The current literature supports the importance of general group-therapeutic factors in promoting a positive outcome. The challenge now facing the field concerns the extent to which time-limited formats can be effectively used for more active psychotherapeutic work. This chapter has emphasized the need to carefully design a brief group approach to take maximum advantage of known factors. This is an essentially conservative position that views time-limited group psychotherapy as a compressed version of longer-term approaches with limited goals. There are a number of questions regarding therapeutic technique that remain unanswered (McCallum and Piper 1988): selection criteria for specific types of groups, the advantages and disadvantages of various ways of creating group homogeneity, the role of group normative persuasion versus specific genetic interpretations, the use of group versus individual interpretations, and the vigor with which the leader controls the group process. These issues and others await further exploration with the outer limits of a brief format. It seems likely that goals to date have been overly restrictive.

The role of time-limited psychotherapy is likely to grow with the increasing impact of managed health care systems. Groups offer a methodology for providing psychotherapy more efficiently. Studies comparing individual and group approaches indicate no differences in outcome. Despite this empirical evidence, the professional community tends to show a profound preference for individual work. (See Chapter 25 for a discussion of training impediments for preparing group leaders.)

A major factor hindering the development of group modalities lies in the simple logistics of putting a group together. It is much easier to make arrangements with one patient than with several. For that reason, groups tend to proliferate in health care systems where there is a larger flow of patients from which to compose groups. It is useful to have staff members trained to deliver both individual and group psychotherapy. This helps to diminish prejudicial biases and may enhance the appropriateness of group referrals. A larger system also offers the opportunity for composing groups in creative ways to meet the needs of the population being served.

There has been a strange history of assigning group therapy tasks to those least equipped to manage them. This seems to be rooted in the unusual belief that managing several people is in some way easier than managing one. Perhaps this belief is a distortion of the idea that much of the therapeutic impact of groups is produced through the interaction among members. It is then concluded that the role of the group leader is less central. Nothing could be further from the truth. Groups have the potential to harm as well as help, a phenomenon well documented in the literature. The type of focused group work discussed in this chapter requires a high degree of therapeutic sophistication and management skill.

There are well-documented grounds for claiming that time-limited group psychotherapy can provide a satisfactory and sufficient therapeutic approach for a great many, probably most, patients seen in outpatient settings. This is true only if the service system and the staff employed within it make a commitment to the provision of quality services. Group programs used as an unsupervised resource to accommodate the unwanted patients of an overburdened system cannot live up to the potential of the modality. With planning and careful development, however, time-limited groups can produce effective therapy. Moreover, such programs tend to have a high level of staff enthusiasm and are fun to be in. It is likely that longer-term and even individual approaches will come under increasing pressure for justification when groups might be used as an alternative. These developments are predictable and can be met with entrenched resistance or treated as an opportunity to enhance the development of time-limited group therapy skills.

References

Alexander F, French TM: Psychoanalytic Therapy: Principles and Application (1946). Lincoln, NE, University of Nebraska Press, 1980

Balint M, Ornstein P, Balint E: Focal Psychotherapy: An Example of Applied Psychoanalysis. London, Tavistock, 1972

Beck AP: Phases in the development of structure in therapy and encounter groups, in Innovations in Client-Centered Therapy. Edited by Wexler DA, Rice LN. New York, John Wiley, 1974, pp 421–463

Beeber AR: A systems model for short-term, open-ended group therapy. Hosp Community Psychiatry 39:537–542, 1988

Benjamin LS: Structural analysis of social behavior. Psychol Rev 81:392–425, 1974

Bernard HS, Klein RH: Some perspectives on time-limited group psychotherapy. Compr Psychiatry 18:579–584, 1977

Brabender V: A closed model of short-term inpatient group psychotherapy. Hosp Community Psychiatry 39:542–545, 1988

Budman SH, Gurman AS: Theory and Practice of Brief Therapy. New York, Guilford, 1988

Budman SH, Bennett MJ, Wisnecki MJ: Short-term group psychotherapy: an adult developmental model. Int J Group Psychother 30:63–76, 1980

Budman SH, Demby A, Redondo JP, et al: Comparative outcome in time-limited individual and group psychotherapy. Int J Group Psychother 38:63–86, 1988

Davanloo H (ed): Short-Term Dynamic Psychotherapy. New York, Jason Aronson, 1980

Dies RR: Leadership in short-term group therapy: Manipulation or facilitation? Int J Group Psychother 35:435–455, 1985

Goldberg DA, Schuyler WR, Bransfield D, et al: Focal group psychotherapy: a dynamic approach. Int J Group Psychother 33:413–431, 1983

Horowitz MJ: Introduction to Psychodynamics: A New Synthesis. New York, Basic Books, 1988

Imber SD, Lewis PM, Loiselle RH: Uses and abuses of the brief intervention group. Int J Group Psychother 29:39–49, 1979

Kanas N: Group therapy with schizophrenics: a review of controlled studies. Int J Group Psychother 36:339–351, 1988

Kibel HD: A conceptual model for short-term inpatient group psychotherapy. Am J Psychiatry 138:74–80, 1981

Klein RH: Some principles of short-term group therapy. Int J Group Psychother 35:309–329, 1985

Klerman GL, Weissman MM, Rousaville BJ, et al: Interpersonal Psychotherapy of Depression. New York, Basic Books, 1984

Leszcz M: Inpatient groups, in Psychiatry Update: The American Psychiatric Association Annual Review, Vol 5. Edited by Frances AJ, Hales RE. Washington, DC, American Psychiatric Press, 1986, pp 729–743

Livesley WJ, MacKenzie KR: Social roles in psychotherapy groups, in Advances in Group Psychotherapy: Integrating Research and Practice. Edited by Dies RR, MacKenzie KR. New York, International Universities Press, 1983, pp 117–135

Luborsky L: Principles of Psychoanalytic Psychotherapy: A Manual for Supportive-Expressive Treatment. New York, Basic Books, 1984

MacKenzie KR: Recent developments in brief psychotherapy. Hosp Community
Psychiatry 39:742–752, 1988

MacKenzie KR: Introduction to Time-Limited Group Psychotherapy. Washington, DC, American Psychiatric Press, 1990

MacKenzie KR, Livesley WJ: A developmental model for brief group therapy, in
Advances in Group Psychotherapy: Integrating Research and Practice. Edited
by Dies RR, MacKenzie KR. New York, International Universities Press, 1983,
pp 101–116

MacKenzie KR, Livesley WJ, Coleman M, et al: Short-term group psychotherapy
for bulimia nervosa. Psychiatric Annals 16:699–708, 1986

Malan DH: Individual Psychotherapy and the Science of Psychodynamics, 2nd
Edition. London, Butterworth, 1979

Mann J, Goldman R: A Casebook in Time-Limited Psychotherapy. Washington,
DC, American Psychiatric Press, 1982

Marmar J: Short-term dynamic psychotherapy. Am J Psychiatry 136:149–155,
1979

Maxmen JS: Helping patients survive theories: the practice of an educative
model. Int J Group Psychother 34:355–368, 1984

McCallum M, Piper WE: Psychoanalytically oriented short-term groups for outpatients: unsettled issues. Group 12:21–32, 1988

Mumford E, Schlesinger HJ, Glass GV, et al: A new look at evidence about reduced cost of medical utilization following mental health treatment. Am J
Psychiatry 141:1145–1158, 1984

Pilkonis PA, Imber SD, Lewis P, et al: A comparative outcome study of individual,
group, and conjoint psychotherapy. Arch Gen Psychiatry 41:431–437, 1984

Piper WE, Perrault EL: Pretherapy preparation for group members. Int J Group
Psychother 39:17–23, 1989

Piper WE, Debbane EG, Bienvenu JP, et al: A comparative study of four forms of
psychotherapy. J Consult Clin Psychol 52:268–279, 1984

Piper WE, McCallum M, Azim HFA: Adaptation to Loss Through Short-Term
Group Psychotherapy. New York, Guilford, 1992

Poey K: Guidelines for the practice of brief, dynamic group therapy. Int J Group
Psychother 35:331–354, 1985

Rice CA, Rutan JS: Inpatient Group Psychotherapy: A Dynamic Perspective. New
York, Macmillan, 1987

Rosenbaum M: Handbook of Short-Term Therapy Groups. New York, McGraw-
Hill, 1983

Sifneos PE: Short-Term Dynamic Psychotherapy, 2nd Edition. New York, Plenum,
1987

Toseland RW, Siporin M: When to recommend group treatment: a review of the
clinical and group literature. Int J Group Psychother 36:171–201, 1986

Tuckman BW: Developmental sequence in small groups. Psychol Bull 63:384–399, 1965

Waxer PH: Short-term group psychotherapy: some principles and techniques. Int J Group Psychother 27:33–42, 1977

Yalom ID: Inpatient Group Psychotherapy. New York, Basic Books, 1983

CHAPTER 23

Cognitive-Behavior Group Therapy

Allen Fay, M.D.
Arnold A. Lazarus, Ph.D.

Introduction

Lazarus (1958) introduced the term *behavior therapy* into the literature to describe the discipline that attempted to apply the findings and methods of experimental psychology (especially theories of learning) to disorders of human behavior. Subsequently, the proliferation of clinical and experimental studies in this area proved to be so extensive that contemporary behavior therapy now embodies a diversity of views and a broad range of procedures (Franks et al. 1990; Lazarus and Fay 1984a). In fact, a compendium of behavior therapy techniques described some 200 interventions in the practitioner's armamentarium (Bellack and Hersen 1985).

One major change in the 1970s was a growing acceptance that cognitive processes may play a significant role in generating and maintaining dysphoric affects and dysfunctional behaviors (e.g., Lazarus 1971; Mahoney 1974; Meichenbaum 1977). Hence the term *cognitive-behavior therapy* has become standard nomenclature. The reciprocal effects of behavior, cognition, and affect are stressed, and maladaptive response patterns in each domain are evaluated and modified. When we use the term "behavior" or "behavior therapy," we do so in the broadest sense, encompassing a methodology and an array of techniques that have a direct impact on each of these domains. The most comprehensive application of what is referred to as social learning theory is found in the concept of multimodal therapy (Lazarus 1976, 1989), in which behavior, affect, sensory experience, imagery, cognition, interpersonal relationships, and biological processes are assessed and approached therapeutically in a direct and systematic manner. The acronym BASIC ID encompasses these seven dimensions of personality. (In the interest of euphony, D [drugs] is substituted for B [biology].)

Before discussing the application of behavioral techniques to group therapy settings, we present a brief discussion of the basic assumptions of this orientation. Behavior therapy rests on a set of fundamental assertions about the nature of human beings and their problems. Among them are the following (Lazarus and Fay 1984a):

1. Psychological disorders represent some combination of biological determinants and learning factors. Examples of the latter would be trial-and-error learning and vicarious learning.
2. Abnormal behavior that is a product of learning factors is acquired and maintained according to the same principles as normal behavior.
3. Dysfunctions attributable to faulty or inadequate learning, and even many disturbances with strong biological inputs, may be alleviated by the application of techniques derived from learning principles. Examples of problems with major biological determinants whose manifestations have responded in some degree to behavioral interventions include obsessive-compulsive disorders, depression, anorexia nervosa, and even catatonia, autism, and dementia. The field of endeavor encompassed by the term "behavioral medicine" addresses a variety of medical problems that may be partly or substantially ameliorated or prevented (risk reduction) by cognitive-behavioral methods. Patient adherence to prescribed therapeutic regimens is a major focus of attention in behavioral medicine.
4. Presenting problems are viewed as real problems and are investigated on their own merits, rather than being regarded as symptoms of some underlying problem or process.
5. The focus is on the present rather than on remote antecedents or unconscious processes. Immediate antecedents and current factors maintaining behavior are emphasized. This in no way gainsays the significance of early life experience or the operation of mental processes outside of conscious awareness. The behavioral view merely asserts that for the successful treatment of most psychological problems, extensive exploration into these areas is unnecessary, and it questions the necessity or the desirability of invoking psychodynamic explanatory models or interventions.

6. Notwithstanding items 4 and 5, assessment involves investigation of *all* areas of behavioral, cognitive, and interpersonal functioning to discover problems or deficits that are not immediately presented.

7. Simple behavioral descriptions are preferred to diagnostic labels. Thus instead of (or in addition to) referring to patients as "borderline," a precise description of the individual's behavioral, cognitive, and affective responses and the contexts in which these responses are manifested would be specified.

8. Although recognizing that to some extent therapy involves transmission of values, behavior therapists tend to minimize value *statements*. Rather than behavior, per se, being labeled as good or bad or healthy or sick, its consequences are specified.

9. The therapist is active and interactive, often assuming the role of a teacher and serving as a model.

10. The locus of resistance is considered to be primarily in the therapy and in the therapist, rather than in the patient. This is not intended as a dogmatic assertion, but simply as a way of placing the fullest possible responsibility on the therapist for finding appropriate interventions, rather than attributing failure to the patient and to his or her pathology.

11. Emphasis is on self-management. Patients are taught specific self-management techniques so that the likelihood of autonomous functioning in problem areas is maximized, and dependency on the therapist is reduced. Assigned homework is an essential part of the behavioral approach (e.g., Shelton and Ackerman 1974).

12. Involvement of the patient's social network is desirable and often necessary. It permits the therapist to structure an optimal reinforcement environment and to resolve interpersonal conflicts through such approaches as communication training and contracting (e.g., Gurney 1977; Patterson et al. 1975; Stuart 1980).

Behavioral clinicians address social and psychiatric problems within a testable conceptual framework; they employ treatments that are open to objective measurement; they apply outcome criteria that can be validated; and they emphasize the need to assess the effectiveness of specific methods applied to particular problems.

Cognitive therapy specifically deals with identifying and challenging maladaptive beliefs, values, perceptions, attributions, and self-talk. These are either reported by the patients or inferred from the patients' verbal statements or from other overt behavior. Often semantic restructuring is useful. This involves suggesting alternative ways of referring to or expressing feelings or cognitions.

Group cognitive-behavior therapy can be discussed in terms of skills that are taught, problems that are addressed, or specific behavioral techniques that are used. There are several critical skills that are taught to groups of people who may or may not have psychiatric-psychological dysfunction or impairment but who are suffering from the consequences of skills deficits and may experience an increase in well-being and gratification from the acquisition of such skills. Examples of skills that may be taught in a group therapy context are job-seeking skills, negotiating skills, parenting skills, and communication skills. Some of these skills are partly subsumed under others, and there is clearly a degree of overlap. These skills have wide applicability, and their acquisition may be helpful in a variety of psychiatric conditions, particularly depression and anxiety disorders.

In group behavior therapy, an attempt is made by a person or persons to modify the maladaptive behaviors of two or more unrelated individuals through the systematic application of empirically validated processes and procedures. Data are typically gathered to assess the impact of these procedures on the members of the group. Initially, behavioral principles and techniques that had been developed in individual settings were applied to groups (Lazarus 1961, 1968; Paul and Shannon 1966); whereas later, the group, per se, was regarded as a useful context for modifying behaviors that either might not occur or would be difficult to modify in a one-to-one relationship (Lazarus 1974; Rose 1977; Upper and Ross 1979).

The distinction has been made between therapy *in* a group and therapy *through* a group. In the former case, the group leader administers the same therapy, either simultaneously or seriatim, to the entire group as that administered to individual patients. In therapy through the group, members play a critical role in the therapy, particularly through modeling and reinforcement procedures and other elements of group dynamics.

Group therapy in general developed because it can make more efficient use of the clinician's time and effort and fosters therapeutic contact with a greater number of people in need of assistance. In cognitive-behavioral groups, the members are given a learning set appropriate to a didactic model of behavior change, and the group context is employed so as to maximize the development of adaptive interpersonal skills. Behaviors are sampled in a manner that is more veridical than in a one-to-one situation, and the group members learn and practice new behaviors in a supportive context that provides appropriate feedback and reinforcement. As we show, many behavioral groups have emphasized the acquisition of social and assertive skills because they are viewed as important to successful living. The behavioral group format provides an immediate arena for change and practice. Goldstein et al. (1976) identified a series of 37 specific skills and showed that they are not isolated behaviors but form the basis of an entire repertoire of responses necessary to cope with many daily demands. Thus various *skills training* procedures are an integral part of group behavior therapy.

Behavior therapists are interested in the mechanisms by which dysfunctional patterns are acquired and maintained, as well as the most facilitative ways of unlearning maladaptive responses and acquiring more adaptive ones. Several mechanisms are postulated to explain learned behavior. One of these is the *classical conditioning* (Pavlovian) model, wherein intrinsically neutral stimuli (for example, words) are temporally associated with intrinsically noxious stimuli (physical punishment or shouting) and are then able to elicit such maladaptive responses as fear or depressive responses by themselves. These responses are then often perpetuated by other mechanisms.

The fundamental proposition of the *operant conditioning* (Skinnerian) model is that behavior is a function of its consequences. Behavior that is followed closely by pleasant consequences will tend to be strengthened and that which is followed by aversive consequences or no consequences will be attenuated or eliminated. *Observational learning* involves the acquisition or inhibition of a response by watching others perform or fail to perform certain behaviors and observing the consequences to that person. Learning tends to be facilitated when the "model" is admired by the patient (subject) and shares certain characteristics (race, sex, age, etc.).

As the conceptual framework of behavior therapy was broadened and the technical armamentarium expanded, an ever-increasing number of problems became amenable to these methods. Whereas Marks (1981) felt that the range of applications was limited, others (Daitzman, 1980) proposed behavioral approaches to the entire DSM spectrum. It was not long after the modern development of behavior therapy that reports began to appear about its application in group, couple, and family contexts as well as in such diverse settings as the inpatient and outpatient hospital and other mental health facilities, classrooms, the workplace, prisons, and patients' homes.

The application of behavior therapy to groups of patients has in fact become almost a separate area of specialization, several volumes on the subject having appeared in recent years (e.g. Rose 1977, 1989; Upper and

Ross 1979, 1980, 1981, 1985). The group format has particular importance and relevance to behavior therapy because of the pivotal role of social influence in generating and maintaining maladaptive responses and the use of modeling and reinforcement in their remediation.

Although the cognitive-behavioral techniques used in individual and group therapy are essentially the same, there are important advantages to group behavioral work. The powerful effects of modeling as a mechanism of behavior change have been abundantly demonstrated (Bandura 1986). Often, the therapist is not a suitable model for the acquisition, augmentation, diminution, or elimination of specific responses. This may be because the therapist's life experience is limited or because of differences in age, sex, race, educational background, or economic status. Therapists who are less disclosing are apt to be seen as "mastery" models rather than as "coping" models. The former perform desired behavior flawlessly and without anxiety, whereas the latter muddle through with a bit more proficiency than the patient. Mastery models are often intimidating and may inhibit the acquisition of new skills. The variety of patients' behavioral skills, levels of competence, cognitive styles, affective responses, and life experiences offers increased opportunities for effecting change.

Another advantage of group cognitive-behavior therapy is that the group provides greater opportunities for actually *practicing* the learning and unlearning of various responses. It has become clear within the past decade that performance-based approaches to therapy are more effective than purely cognitive approaches. Role-playing exercises in a group have advantages over similar exercises in one-to-one therapy because they more realistically approximate the social experiences of the individual members. Encouragement to modify cognitive or behavior patterns and the reinforcement of change often have a greater effect coming from different individuals than they would coming from an individual therapist. Also, desensitization to feared social situations is greatly facilitated in many individuals by exposure to group members, and the likelihood of generalization of the adaptive responses to extratherapy contexts is increased.

Behavioral methods have been applied in groups to constellations of problem behaviors and skills deficits encompassed by various diagnostic categories such as the range of anxiety disorders, some mood disorders, eating disorders, substance abuse, stress management, couples and family communication problems, personality disorders including borderline and antisocial personalities, habit disorders, sexual dysfunction, paraphilias, and a variety of problems subsumed under the rubric of behavioral medicine, such as coronary prevention and pain management.

Similar issues exist in behavioral group therapy as in other orientations—the size of groups, matching with respect to the nature and severity of the problems (heterogeneous or homogeneous), age of the patients, open ended or time limited, single leader or coleaders, concurrent individual treatment for group members, issues of confidentiality, and rules of conduct within the group and outside of the group. Because of the short-term, problem-focused nature of behavior therapy, most groups are conducted at weekly intervals for 8–12 sessions of 1.5–2 hours' duration. A greater number of fixed-session groups or open-ended groups are used for patients with multiple or complex problems requiring more extensive work. With regard to other policies, practice varies widely.

Most groups that utilize behavior therapy techniques are led by laypersons rather than professional therapists. The most popular of these address problems of obesity, cigarette smoking, alcohol and other substance abuse, and compulsive gambling. Because of the didactic nature of much of behavior therapy, there is often a blurred boundary between educational classes and group therapy. For example, groups are conducted in which parents of children with a variety of behavior disorders are taught cognitive-behavioral skills, which they then apply to their children.

In the "traditional" behavioral group, directed by a professional leader, there is an initial discussion of the purpose of the group, which is to promote the relief of distress, the enhancement of satisfaction, and the sharing of experience, information, and feedback with one another in order to accomplish these goals for all of the group members. To the extent that there are rules and other constraints, they are often specified. These may take the form of interdicting smoking, discouraging interruptions, the expressed expectation of regular attendance, and discouraging social interaction outside of the group. It is our feeling that the fewer rules there are, the better. For example, we do not interdict extragroup socializing but rather feel that most experience is grist for the therapeutic mill. Often, it is easier for patients to carry out in vivo behavioral assignments in pairs or larger groups than individually. With such flexibility, there is certainly a risk that people who are looking for companionship, affection, or love will find it within the group and drop out of the group without having learned the requisite skills for meeting such needs independently. In our experience, however, the benefits of being relatively nonrestrictive outweigh the risks. Nevertheless, there is significant diversity among practitioners, and many cognitive-behavior therapists tend to discourage "socializing" except when specific therapeutic assignments are made. Clearly, as in other orientations, physical violence is not tolerated, and floridly psychotic individuals or patients who manifest severely destructive behavior or gross affect instability are not considered suitable candidates for group therapy. The issue of confidentiality is stressed in the sense that patients are expected to agree that there will be no disclosures about other members of the group without their explicit consent, although self-disclosure is often strongly recommended, provided that it serves the purpose of promoting social facility and is not compulsive and overwhelming to the recipient.

As in any other form of therapy, there is an assessment process, an intervention process, and an evaluation process. Most of the patients are interviewed before the first group session. In some cases, after discussion with the referring therapist and a brief phone contact with the patient, admission to the group is arranged. In the first group meeting, patients are asked to state the presenting problem and their goals with respect to that problem. Other life areas are explored as well for maladaptive patterns or skills deficits that may be interfering with satisfaction and fulfillment. Measures previously used by the patient to cope with the problem, either in or out of therapy, successfully or unsuccessfully, are reviewed. Target behaviors are identified and characterized with respect to frequency, intensity, duration, and context. An essential part of the behavioral evaluation process is the determination of eliciting stimuli, behavioral (affective, cognitive) responses, and the consequences of those responses. Eliciting stimuli may be external environmental events or internal (cognitive or sensory) experiences.

Members are asked to relate incidents in their lives that may be relevant to the problem under discussion. Although it is possible to devote most of a single session to the problems of one patient, it is particularly important at the beginning for each person to be able to state his or her problems and goals. In any event, it is most important in the behavioral approach for patients to give a great deal of support as well as spontaneous reactions and corrective feedback. The importance of practicing techniques and skills within the group cannot be overestimated. In fact, the most essential element in learning a skill is the practicing of adaptive, facilitative responses. The group is a laboratory for trying out new behaviors in a supportive context. Reinforcement is provided by other members of the group to encourage practicing, per se, and also to support successive approximations to the desired level of proficiency. Even in "homogeneous" groups, in which all patients have a similar problem (e.g., agoraphobia and ethanol abuse), there are significant individual differences requiring special attention, such as deficient parenting skills, sexual dysfunction, job-related assertiveness issues, and time management problems. Strategies to promote *generalization* of results to extratherapy contexts and *maintenance* of therapeutic improvement over time are developed and implemented (Lazarus and Fay 1984b). Relapse prevention strategies (Marlatt 1985) are built in to the therapy. Involving significant others in the patient's environment, intermittent phone contact with the therapist, and follow-up group sessions perhaps 1 and 6 months after "termination" may contribute to this end. Above all, we want to avoid a major trap of group therapy, namely, that of developing a group of individuals who are simply good at group therapy.

Techniques

As already indicated, the technical armamentarium of behavior therapists is vast, but in general many of the specific techniques can be grouped according to the learning model from which they are derived

The classical conditioning model has spawned a number of techniques, the best known and most studied of which is *systematic desensitization*. It is clear from many studies that irrational fear can be overcome in most patients through their progressive exposure to the anxiety-eliciting stimuli (Wolpe 1958, 1991). This exposure may be accomplished *behaviorally* (i.e., through actual in vivo exposure to the stimuli) or *imaginally* (i.e., by using mental imagery to visualize being in the threatening situation). *Flooding* (in vivo or imaginal) refers to exposure to massive doses of the fear-eliciting stimuli rather than exposure in progressively increasing doses.

One of the most important techniques, which serves an assessment function as well as a therapeutic function, is *self-monitoring*. The observation of one's own behavior (maladaptive and adaptive) and the recording of these observations constitute one of the cornerstones of the behavioral approach. This technique gives more precise information about the frequency, intensity, and duration of a problem than do subjective impressions. It provides a baseline against which to measure progress. In addition, the mere monitoring of a process often influences that process. Thus by recording in a notebook each time one has the impulse to smoke a cigarette, one tends to make the habit less automatic and therefore usually reduce the frequency of its occurrence. On the other hand, focusing on depressed feelings may serve to maintain them or intensify them. In such cases it would be more useful to monitor the number of times one challenges negative cognitions or engages in activities that under normal circumstances would be pleasurable. In general, it is more effective to monitor therapeutic efforts rather than dysfunctional behavior.

Numerous techniques have been generated by the operant conditioning model, which views behavior as a function of its consequences. The organism acts, and the environment responds in a way that influences future behavior. If the consequences increase the probability of future occurrences of the behavior, they are considered to be *reinforcing*. This process is accomplished by the application of a positive stimulus (*positive reinforcement*) or by the withdrawal of a negative stimulus (*negative reinforcement*), contingent on the occurrence of a particular behavior. The systematic application of such consequence conditions to modify behavior is known as *contingency management.* That is, when these consequences are applied, contingent on the occurrence of a behavior, the behavior will be modified in the desired direction. The other consequence conditions are *nonreinforcement,* in which the behavior is followed by no consequence, leading to its attenuation or extinction, and *punishment,* in which an aversive consequence follows the particular behavior, leading to suppression of the behavior. *Differential reinforcement* refers to the application of positive consequences for desired behavior and the ignoring of maladaptive or undesired behavior. Punishment procedures are used relatively infrequently, except as a self-management tool. An example is the wearing of a rubber band on the wrist and snapping it hard when an impulse to do something damaging occurs. Behavior therapists have been severely criticized for the use of punishment procedures. Punishment is used only with the full consent of the patient and, in rare cases, of a legal guardian (e.g., treatment of severely autistic or self-mutilating children.) Punishment is, of course, the major mechanism used in societies to control deviant behavior. *Self-reinforcement* (e.g., self-praise, purchase of a treat, or deliberately engaging in an unscheduled pleasurable activity) is used commonly for improvements in adaptive functioning or for therapeutic steps that are taken, such as resisting destructive impulses.

One of the techniques derived from the contingency management approach is *contracting,* which has been used extensively in a number of contexts, particularly in institutional settings and in parent-child and spousal relationships. Here the operant techniques are incorporated in a formal contract in which a specified behavior performed to a certain standard is associated with a specific positive or negative consequence. In group therapy with people who may not be highly motivated, a refundable deposit may be required at the beginning of therapy, with a percentage to be refunded each time patients attend the group. The refundable deposit also has been used successfully, at least on a short-term basis, in weight management groups, where paybacks are given contingent on attendance and/or weight loss. The *token economy* is usually applied in closed institutional systems and in families, where tokens are given to patients, children, or inmates when adaptive behaviors are performed. They are withdrawn (*response cost*) when maladaptive behaviors are manifested. The tokens are exchangeable at some future time for "backup" reinforcers, which may take the form of material rewards or permission to engage in highly desired activities.

Observational or *vicarious* learning or *zero trial* learning utilizes the technique of *modeling*. The observation of another person engaging in or avoiding a behavior will often lead to imitation or inhibition of that behavior in the subject or patient, depending on whether the behavior is desired and whether the consequences to the model are positive or negative. Groups of teenage first offenders may be addressed by individuals with life sentences, or they may benefit by observing films in which prosocial behavior is rewarded and antisocial behavior is punished. Frequently, desensitization, positive reinforcement, and modeling are combined to produce powerful therapeutic changes.

In the discussion that follows, several representative skills, problem "symptoms," and techniques are discussed in order to acquaint nonbehavioral therapists with cognitive-behavioral approaches to common clinical problems.

Assertiveness Training

We use assertiveness as an example of a set of skills that has universal relevance to the adaptive functioning of human beings in social contexts. Possibly it is the most important set of skills for promoting need satisfaction.

The term *assertiveness* encompasses a variety of skills that lead to the behavior of asking for what one wants, resisting unwelcome requests or exploitation by others, initiating conversations and relationships, and engaging in these behaviors without shame, guilt, or undue anxiety and without compromising other peoples' feelings or acting in an exploitative manner. In the behavior therapy group, this concept is articulated and examples are given of assertive behavior, unassertive behavior, and aggressive behavior. Patients are asked to describe themselves in terms of their overall style and their context-related behaviors. For example, some individuals are assertive (or aggressive) at home but unassertive in the workplace. Patients are told that everyone has deficits in assertiveness and that problems relate to the degree and context. They are asked to provide examples from their daily interactions and to relate incidents observed involving others in their social environment. One or more members of the group are asked to present a problematic situation they have experienced recently, be it with a spouse, employer, employee, neighbor, friend, lover, or someone else.

Although the biological modality is not emphasized in behavioral groups, patients are told that there is a biological component to personality and that some people are less assertive partly because of the biological structure of their nervous systems, but that assertiveness is for the most part a learned skill. Because assertiveness skills are not taught in any systematic fashion in the school system, and because most extramural modeling experiences vary from suboptimal to disastrous, most of us come by our assertiveness deficits quite understandably.

Among the techniques used in assertiveness training groups are modeling (the therapist or group members share anecdotes about their own experiences and display the desired behavior in the group), positive reinforcement of a given patient's successive approximations to the desired behavior (called *shaping*), and the prescription of self-monitoring outside of the group. Rehearsal of various examples from real life and rehearsal within the group with members playing significant others in the identified patient's social network are often employed. Patients bring in episodes from their life experiences between sessions. They are assigned the task of writing a revised script each time they are less assertive than they might have been. In this exercise the patient composes an alternative scenario to the one that actually occurred. This "homework" is shared with the group. Problem-solving skills are taught and applied to difficult situations confronting the patient (content issues).

Clinical Example

An example that is often presented is a woman in the role of domestic drudge who asks her husband to share in the chores. He may decline, pleasantly or unpleasantly, he may agree but procrastinate or fail to comply with the request, he may participate to a limited but unsatisfactory degree, or he may participate fully but act as if he is doing his wife a great favor, for which he deserves eternal gratitude. In this seemingly simple, common interaction, we are dealing with a whole range of cognitions, affects, and behaviors that need to be addressed.

Among the important cognitions that govern the patient's behavior in her relationship are her definition of marriage, her expectations, her views about parity of marital partners, her views about parity of the sexes, her view of housework as a shared function or as her job, and attributions about her spouse's behavior (he acts as he does because he's a sexist, or because he has never learned that it is reasonable to be a full partner in domestic chores). Other cognitions may include any of the following: he treats me like dirt; it's his fault; it's my fault; I stay with him because I'm afraid of rejection; I might lose him; I can't stand the idea of being alone; I'd never be able to find someone else. The woman's assessment of the perceived overall contributions of each spouse and her assessment of the overall reinforcement economy (perceived benefits derived by each) are important. Assessment of her view as to whether she has the right to ask, her style of asking (words, nonverbal communication such as posture, gestures, and voice tone), and associated affect are also important. The cognitive appraisal of potential consequences, risk-reward characteristics of assertive behavior, and the evaluation of the marriage as a whole and of her husband's overall treatment of her are further considerations. Although expression of anger can be enormously cathartic and is practiced in the group with other members playing the part of the patient's husband, the teaching of assertive responses and behavior modification techniques to use with her spouse is more fundamental to the behavioral approach. Desensitization to rejection, behavior rehearsal, role reversal, reinforced practice, shaping, and extragroup behavioral assignments (such as monitoring, rewriting the script, practicing with a tape recorder, practicing with an empty chair, and practicing with friends) are also used.

Dating Skills

In a dating skills group, the behavioral objective is defined. Is the criterion of success to greet another person? Is it asking the other person for a date? Is it a sexual encounter? Is it an ongoing relationship? Marriage? What is the level of skill of the members? How do they meet prospective dates? On their own, through friends, or through dating services? Do they go to parties, bars, lectures, concerts, sporting events, museums, or churches? Do they go alone or with a friend? How are they dressed? Groomed? How is their personal hygiene? The self-confidence and social life of a male patient increased considerably after he responded to encouragement to have a large and unsightly facial cyst removed.

How does the patient approach others? What are the words, tone of voice, degree of eye contact, posture, and gestures? Are these behaviors likely to inhibit or facilitate dating? What is the quality of the associated affect? What is the patient's cognitive matrix associated with dating? Does the patient feel that he or she has the right to ask for a date? Does he or she feel guilty or anxious about making such a request? Is the patient unduly concerned about rejection? Is the patient worried about what will happen if the request is accepted? For example, is there anxiety about sexual performance or about the other person's expectation of a commitment?

A variety of dysfunctional cognitions may interfere with date-seeking behavior. Included among these are the following: I don't have confidence in myself; the other person will see my inadequacies and reject me; rejection is terrible; I am not good enough for this person; it won't lead anywhere anyway so what's the use; even if I get a date I won't know how to conduct myself; even if I get a date I won't be able to satisfy the other person sexually; it is considered pushy for women to ask men for dates; the other person might laugh at my inadequacies or idiosyncrasies; the other person may tell friends, relatives, or a therapist about my inadequacies; I'm not intelligent enough, interesting enough, or sexy enough; when he or she finds out XYZ about me or my family or my past, it will be over. . . .

The belief that one has the right to be happy and to ask for what one wants as long as one is not compromising anybody else's rights is a cornerstone of the cognitive approach to assertiveness training and the teaching of dating skills. Dysfunctional cognitions are actively challenged in the group by the leader and by other patients as well.

Imagery is a powerful component of dysfunctional cognitive schemata. In addition to the beliefs, there often are fantasies of failure, rejection, unsatisfactory performance, and so forth. A number of imagery procedures are used in addition to challenging irrational and dysfunctional cognitions (Lazarus 1984). Two basic prescriptions are *coping imagery* and *imaginal flooding*. In the former, the patient pictures asking someone for a date, being rejected or accepted, and remaining calm. Flooding involves massive exposure to the circumstance that is feared, so that the patient pictures asking for a date and being deluged with a barrage of bizarre criticisms. One would picture the rejector saying, "You are disgusting, revolting, grotesque, and stupid, and I wouldn't go out with you if you were the last person on earth." In most instances repeated practice of this imagery exercise leads to a desensitization to the feared situation. As a parallel exercise, picturing oneself succeeding repeatedly will make it more likely that one can effect the desired behavior in reality.

A self-monitoring technique we described many years ago in a self-help manual (Lazarus and Fay 1992) is used as well. Patients are asked to record in a notebook every instance in which they are in geographic proximity to someone they find appealing. They then record the behavioral outcome of that juxtaposition. If they say nothing to the person they find attractive, they mark a *0* (zero) in the notebook. If they simply greet the other person ("Hi") or make a simple comment ("Isn't it a beautiful day?"), they record a *1*. If there is further conversation, with some give and take, then a *2* is entered in the notebook. If the patient requests a phone number or a future contact, a *3* is recorded. It doesn't matter whether the prospect's response is positive or negative. The *3* is awarded for making a request for a future date or asking for a phone number, regardless of how the prospect responds. The measure of success is asking, not acceptance. People with deficits in dating skills often find that after a week or two of using this monitoring exercise, there are fewer *0*'s and *1*'s and more *2*'s and occasional *3*'s. Notebooks are brought into the subsequent group sessions, and episodes are shared with the group. Bibliotherapy is prescribed (Alberti and Emmons 1986; Fay 1990; Jakubowski and Lange 1978).

For anxiety associated with anticipated dating, relaxation exercises are recommended, either in association with imagery exposure to the situation or in vivo practice in the group. Using behavior rehearsal, patients ask other patients in the group for a date and the participants respond in a variety of ways, including enthusiastic acceptance, bland indifference, reluctant acceptance, tactful rejection, and abusive rejection. All members have the opportunity to practice, and any attempt at assertive behavior receives considerable positive reinforcement from other group members.

In addition, a paradoxical exercise (Fay 1978) is prescribed in which people are encouraged to collect at least three rejections during the course of the week between sessions. Acceptances are permissible, but the specific assignment is to get rejected at least three times. This "reframing" reduces performance pressure and tends to facilitate the desired outcome. In most of the groups, patients are exposed to the BASIC ID multimodal concept referred to earlier (Lazarus 1989). Although medication is usually not prescribed in cognitive-behavioral groups, people with severe dating anxiety that precludes social contact (social phobia) are informed that the use of either a monoamine oxidase inhibitor for a period of time until the requisite skills can be practiced sufficiently or a beta blocker taken shortly before any planned dating initiative or actual social engagement may be of great benefit.

Anxiety Disorders

The cornerstone of the behavioral management of anxiety disorders comprises a variety of techniques designed to dampen central nervous system arousal. In using such techniques, the presumption is made that "nonpsychiatric" disorders (e.g., caffeinism and hyperthyroidism) have been excluded or treated. Most of the anxiety disorders, including general anxiety disorder, obsessive-compulsive disorder, and posttraumatic stress disorder, are amenable to group intervention. Techniques such as progressive muscle relaxation, meditation, and self-hypnosis are frequently taught in behavioral groups. Again, adopting the individual customized therapy model, patients who find that muscle relaxation techniques or meditation lead to *increased* tension are given alternative methods that promote reduction of anxiety for them. Audiotapes that describe the technique and take patients through the procedures are given to the members for home use, after the technique is demonstrated and practiced in the group.

The cognitive-behavioral treatment of anxiety disorders has been the subject of enormous research activity for more than 20 years (Barlow 1988; Beck and Emery 1985). The core of this approach involves relaxation training, exposure to feared stimuli (in vivo and/or through imagery, either graded or massive), cognitive restructuring (identifying and challenging irrational, self-defeating cognitions and substituting benign, noncatastrophic self-talk for anxiety-generating internal statements), response prevention (blocking avoidance behavior), assertiveness training, problem solving, and positive reinforcement and nonreinforcement for adaptive and maladaptive responses, respectively. For example, if some patients in a group for people with obsessive-compulsive disorders are excessively concerned about contamination or have washing rituals, the entire group may practice rubbing their hands on the floor or the bottom of their shoes and then shaking hands with one another. Field trips outside the office involve touching garbage or other contaminated objects and refraining from hand washing for the duration of the session. Thus we have the three-pronged behavioral approach to obsessive-compulsive disorders—exposure, response prevention, and participant modeling. Again, all areas of functioning are assessed, and other interventions are used when indicated, especially assertiveness training and relationship therapy.

Mood Disorders

The cognitive-behavioral approach to mood disorders has been applied widely to patients with nonbipolar depression. Although several studies have shown cognitive-behavior therapy to be equally effective and even superior to pharmacotherapy in these individuals, it is important to emphasize the critical role that biological intervention plays in the management of mood disorders, especially those of severe intensity. In general, the more flexible the therapeutic repertoire, the greater the number of favorable outcomes.

Because one of the hallmarks of the behavioral approach is the reinforcement of adaptive behavior and the nonreinforcement of maladaptive responses, group members are told at the outset that the focus will be on promoting facilitative behaviors rather than on the repetitious expression of negative feelings and references to their remote sources, historical or unconscious. To the extent that environmental triggers can be identified (for example, comments from a critical spouse), patients are desensitized to the stimuli by exposure in the group through role playing by other group members and by practicing various coping strategies, including relaxation, imagery exercises, and assertive responses. In the management of depression, assertiveness training is often an essential component. Although, as we have already underscored, there are groups devoted entirely to assertiveness training, it is a major element in most behavioral groups. As indicated earlier, suboptimal proficiency in this area is widespread in the population because of the lack of formal training and highly imperfect role models.

One of the often-expressed behavioral formulations of depression involves the notion of insufficient positive reinforcement. People who lack the skill to make assertive overtures or to deny others' exploitative or unwelcome requests have a more difficult time having their needs met and maintaining high self-regard.

Patients are often asked to identify worthwhile qualities in themselves and are assigned homework involving recitation of positive qualities from a list composed in the group. Although this recitation is often as labored as the proverbial dental extraction, repeated recitation, especially with simulated positive affect, is associated with therapeutic gains in some patients. Alternatively, sometimes group members will enthusiastically agree with a depressed individual's self-denigrative statements. If the intragroup relationships are seen as supportive and the intervention is made benevolently, such paradoxical comments are often facilitative and lead to a smile or laughter on the part of the patient under scrutiny.

Although there are many cognitive-behavioral formulations of the etiology and treatment of depression, the most well known are reflected in the work of Beck and Lewinsohn. Regardless of the correctness of etiological theories of depression in terms of a paucity of reinforcement or the relevance of dysfunctional cognitions, the cognitive-behavioral *approach* has been demonstrated to be effective (e.g., Beck et al. 1979; Lewinsohn 1974). Bibliotherapy assignments usually include *Feeling Good* by Burns (1980) and *Control Your Depression* by Lewinsohn et al. (1978). Patients are urged to identify and engage in activities that were highly pleasurable to them in the nondepressed state (e.g., walking, going to movies, and bowling). Relaxation techniques are also often a part of the therapeutic management of depression.

Patients are urged to share these techniques with family members and friends and to attempt to enlist their aid in avoiding reinforcement of "depressive behavior," in exhorting the patient to engage in pleasurable activities, and in responding positively to desirable changes in overt behavior and verbal statements about themselves or about their problem.

Although there are many behavioral techniques that can be applied to a variety of disorders, one of the major objectives of effective therapy in groups as well as in individual work is to fit the therapy to the individual patient's needs. Sometimes patients are referred for vocational skill training or to a peer-directed group such as Gamblers Anonymous or Alcoholics Anonymous. Substance abuse may have a major impact on depression. Some patients need couples therapy. Some need more work with assertiveness than others. Some need specific instructions about the cognitive-behavioral approaches to sleep disorders. These include relaxation exercises, avoidance of stressful events before bedtime, the challenging of damaging beliefs about sleep (if I don't sleep, it's terrible; I must sleep or I'll get sick), and a variety of *stimulus control* techniques. These consist of getting out of bed after 15 or 20 minutes of not sleeping and not returning until somnolence is experienced, eliminating naps, and avoiding reading, eating, or watching television in bed. In the management of depression it may be helpful to use a stimulus control approach wherein the patient's time is structured so that he or she spends fewer hours in the location that has been most associated with depression.

Conclusions

In presenting this succinct overview of group behavior therapy, we have endeavored to underscore the systematic, comprehensive, and flexible nature of the enterprise. The psychoeducational thrust of behavioral groups helps patients acquire many skills and habits that relieve psychological distress, promote well-being, enable a higher level of adaptive functioning, and foster more effective interpersonal dealings. Once viewed as a passing fad, the behavioral orientation has great potential for augmenting the therapeutic repertoire of psychiatric clinicians. Although some may regard behavioral methods as ancillary to the focus of resolving intrapsychic conflicts, it is abundantly clear that the cognitive-behavioral approach has emerged as a major force in mainstream psychotherapy.

References

Alberti R, Emmons M: Your Perfect Right. San Luis Obispo, CA, Impact Publishers, 1986

Bandura A: Social Foundations of Thought and Action. Englewood Cliffs, NJ, Prentice-Hall, 1986

Barlow DH: Anxiety and Its Disorders. New York, Guilford, 1988

Beck AT, Emery G: Anxiety Disorders and Phobias: A Cognitive Perspective. New York, Basic Books, 1985

Beck AT, Rush AJ, Shaw BF, et al: Cognitive Therapy of Depression. New York, Guilford, 1979

Bellack AS, Hersen M: Dictionary of Behavior Techniques. Elmsford, NY, Pergamon, 1985

Burns D: Feeling Good. New York, New American Library, 1980

Daitzman RJ: Clinical Behavior Therapy and Behavior Modification. New York, Garland STPM Press, 1980

Fay A: Making Things Better by Making Them Worse. New York, Hawthorn, 1978

Fay A: PQR: Prescription for a Quality Relationship. New York, Simon & Schuster, 1990

Franks CM, Wilson GT, Kendal PC, et al: Review of Behavior Therapy: Theory and Practice, Vol 12. New York, Guilford, 1990

Goldstein AP, Sprafkin RP, Gershaw NJ: Skill Training for Community Living. New York, Pergamon, 1976

Gurney BG: Relationship Enhancement: Skill Training Programs for Therapy, Problem Prevention and Enrichment. San Francisco, CA, Jossey-Bass, 1977

Jakubowski P, Lange AJ: The Assertive Option. Champaign, IL, Research Press, 1978

Lazarus AA: New methods in psychotherapy: a case study. South African Medical Journal 32:660–664, 1958

Lazarus AA: Group therapy of phobic disorders by systematic desensitization. Journal of Abnormal and Social Psychology 63:505–510, 1961

Lazarus AA: Behavior therapy in groups, in Basic Approaches to Group Psychotherapy and Group Counseling. Edited by Gazda GM. Springfield, IL, Charles C Thomas, 1968, pp 149–175

Lazarus AA: Behavior Therapy and Beyond. New York, McGraw-Hill, 1971

Lazarus AA: Understanding and modifying aggression in behavioral groups, in The Group as Agent of Change. Edited by Jacobs A, Spradlin W. New York, Behavioral Publications, 1974, pp 87–99

Lazarus AA: Multimodal Behavior Therapy. New York, Springer, 1976

Lazarus AA: In the Mind's Eye. New York, Guilford, 1984

Lazarus AA: The Practice of Multimodal Therapy. Baltimore, MD, Johns Hopkins University Press, 1989

Lazarus AA, Fay A: Behavior therapy, in The Psychiatric Therapies. Edited by Karasu TB. Washington, DC, American Psychiatric Association, 1984a, pp 485–538

Lazarus AA, Fay A: Some strategies for promoting generalization and maintenance. The Cognitive Behaviorist 6:7–9, 1984b

Lazarus AA, Fay A: I Can If I Want To. New York, Morrow 1992

Lewinsohn PM: A behavioral approach to depression, in The Psychology of Depression: Contemporary Theory and Research. Edited by Friedman RM, Katz MM. New York, John Wiley, 1974, pp 157–178

Lewinsohn PM, Munoz RF, Youngren MA, et al: Control Your Depression. Englewood Cliffs, NJ, Prentice-Hall, 1978

Mahoney MJ: Cognition and Behavior Modification. Cambridge, MA, Ballinger, 1974

Marks IM: Review of behavioral psychotherapy, 1: obsessive compulsive disorders. Am J Psychiatry 138:584–592, 1981

Marlatt GA: Relapse prevention: theoretical rationale and overview of the model, in Relapse Prevention: Maintenance Strategies in The Treatment of Addictive Behaviors. Edited by Marlatt GA, Gordon JR. New York, Guilford, 1985, pp 3–70

Meichenbaum D: Cognitive Behavior Modification. New York, Plenum, 1977

Patterson GR, Reid JB, Jones RR, et al: A Social Learning Approach to Family Intervention. Eugene, OR, Castalia Publishing, 1975

Paul GL, Shannon DT: Treatment of anxiety through systematic desensitization in therapy groups. J Abnorm Psychol 71:124–132, 1966

Rose S: Group therapy: A Behavioral Approach. Englewood Cliffs, NJ, Prentice-Hall, 1977

Rose S: Working With Adults in Groups. San Francisco, CA, Jossey-Bass, 1989

Shelton JL, Ackerman JM: Homework in Counseling and Psychotherapy. Springfield, IL, Charles C Thomas, 1974

Stuart RB: Helping Couples Change: A Social Learning Approach to Marriage Therapy. New York, Guilford, 1980

Upper D, Ross SM (eds): Behavioral Group Therapy, 1979: An Annual Review. Champaign, IL, Research Press, 1979

Upper D, Ross SM (eds): Behavioral Group Therapy, 1980: An Annual Review. Champaign, IL, Research Press, 1980

Upper D, Ross SM (eds): Behavioral Group Therapy, 1981: An Annual Review. Champaign, IL, Research Press, 1981

Upper D, Ross SM (eds): Handbook of Behavioral Group Therapy. New York, Plenum, 1985

Wolpe J: Psychotherapy by Reciprocal Inhibition. Stanford, CA, Stanford University Press, 1958

Wolpe J: The Practice of Behavior Therapy. New York, Pergamon, 1991

PART VII

Research

CHAPTER 24

Research on Group Psychotherapy: Overview and Clinical Applications

Robert R. Dies, Ph.D.

Introduction

There is growing awareness by practitioners that research on group treatments has clear implications for clinical practice. The quality of empirical investigation has increased significantly in recent years, and the conclusions drawn by investigators have become more directly and concretely applicable. Perhaps more important, however, is the fact that pressures from insurance companies, legislators, and patient-consumers to document the efficacy, safety, and cost-effectiveness of treatment have made it clear that it is no longer feasible to ignore the potential scientific foundations of group interventions (Dies 1983a, 1986, 1990a).

There is accumulating evidence of improved communication between researchers and clinicians. This improved communication is reflected, for example, in more reviews of research literature offering pragmatic suggestions for the practitioner (Dies 1989a), specially designed group treatment manuals based on empirical findings (Lewinsohn and Clarke 1984), a greater number of publications on how to integrate research measures into clinical practice (Corcoran and Fischer 1987; Lambert et al. 1986; MacKenzie and Dies 1982) and how to design research projects within mental health settings (Robison et al. 1989), and even demands by editors of group psychotherapy journals for investigators to make their results relevant to the clinician (Dies and Emery 1985). Thus there are promising signs of greater rapprochement between therapists and researchers within the field.

The purpose of this chapter is provide an overview of major research findings on group treatments that have distinct applications for clinical practice. The first two sections present a review of broad patterns evident within the literature and highlight results of a recent international survey of prominent researchers within the field (Dies and Cohen: International perspectives on group psychotherapy research. Unpublished manuscript, 1992). The remainder of the chapter is devoted to an integration of research findings into a general framework for group interventions with suggestions on how to optimize therapeutic gain.

Reflections on Four Decades of Research

A little over 10 years ago, I published a critique of developmental patterns in the empirical investigation of group psychotherapy covering a 30-year period (Dies 1979). The first trend noted in that report was the rapid growth of the group literature. A more recent analysis shows that this proliferation of theoretical, technical, and empirical work on group interventions has not attenuated in the least (Dies 1986, 1990a). There has been a shift, however, in the nature of the group experiences that have become the primary focus of research investigation. Surveys of various facets of group treatments in both inpatient and outpatient settings have continued (Kanas 1986; Kaul and Bednar 1986; Leszcz 1986), but reviews of research on personal growth groups and T-groups, once popular in the mid-1960s and early 1970s, have been replaced by the "new group movements" of the current decade, namely, short-term psychotherapy groups (Burlingame and Fuhriman 1990; Dies 1985a; MacKenzie 1990) and self-help groups (Jacobs and Goodman 1989; Lieberman 1985, 1990).

Several other trends in the literature were previously identified (Dies 1979):

1. Heightened confidence in the efficacy of group treatments
2. Greater specificity about outcome and process variables
3. More pragmatic and personalized approaches to empirical investigation
4. A growing recognition of the need for improved communication within the field

These additional trends will be highlighted briefly.

Greater Confidence About Group Therapeutic Outcome

In a prior review (Dies 1979), I noted that investigators had become increasingly optimistic about the efficacy of group methods and that their research techniques had become increasingly sophisticated. Thus the tentative conclusions about group therapeutic outcome published 15 or 20 years ago (Bednar and Lawlis 1971; Bednar and Kaul 1978) have been supplanted by significantly more confident statements. Indeed, contemporary surveys (Dies 1986; Kaul and Bednar 1986; Orlinsky and Howard 1986) indicate widespread endorsement of group psychotherapy as a viable and vital treatment modality. The issue of the therapeutic efficacy of group treatments has been explored by using a variety of methods. Smith et al. (1980), for example, applied a quantitative technique called "meta-analysis" (based on average change scores on dependent measures) in their comprehensive examination of psychotherapy outcomes in hundreds of studies conducted across a wide range of clinical settings. These authors concluded that group psychotherapy was as effective as individual treatments in the alleviation of psychological disorders. A subsequent application of the meta-analytic approach found that although individual therapy was slightly more successful, it was certainly not consistently superior to group interventions (Shapiro and Shapiro 1982).

Toseland and Siporin (1986) warned that conclusions derived from meta-analysis are based on separate studies using different therapeutic modalities rather than on investigations making direct comparisons between treatment types. Consequently, they scanned the literature for reports in which individual and group treatments were directly contrasted. They discovered that in three-fourths of the investigations, no significant differences in effectiveness were identified. In the remaining studies, group psychotherapy was established as more efficacious. Tillitski's subsequent meta-analysis (1990) of the same investigations generally confirmed these conclusions.

In their comprehensive review, Orlinsky and Howard (1986) also scrutinized studies that directly compared individual and group interventions. Interestingly, only one-third of the investigations evaluated by these authors overlapped with those reported by Toseland and Siporin (1986). Nonetheless, the observation of relatively little differential outcome of individual and group treatments was essentially the same.

On the whole, the conclusions from several major meta-analytic reviews, as well as independent surveys of the outcome literature (Bednar and Kaul 1978; Kaul and Bednar 1986), uniformly support the generalization that group psychotherapy is an effective form of treatment intervention. Although the evidence relating treatment outcome to particular patient diagnoses must be regarded as tentative, the number of empirical reviews documenting the unique advantages of group methods for patients suffering from alcoholism (Solomon 1982), anxiety disorders (Galloucis and Kaufman 1988), bereavement (Lieberman 1990), bulimia (Oesterheld et al. 1987), depression (Lewinsohn and Clarke 1984), schizophrenia (Kanas 1986), sexual abuse (Kitchur and Bell 1989), and other conditions has increased dramatically. Moreover, several literature surveys have shown that the risk of harmful effects from group treatments is generally quite negligible (Dies and Teleska 1985; Erickson 1987; Orlinsky and Howard 1986).

In their review of comparative studies, Toseland and Siporin (1986) also addressed the issue of the relative efficiency of treatments, and they demonstrated that group therapy was more cost-effective in more than 80% of the investigations they analyzed. They argued that "given the increasing emphasis on cost containment and efficiency in the human services, as well as the tremendous need and the competing demands for scarce public funds, the issue of efficiency deserves more attention" (p. 196). Undoubtedly, practical considerations such as staff flexibility and cost-effectiveness have contributed to the popularity of group interventions. Winick and Weiner (1986), for example, have shown that even though the typical fees charged for group psychotherapy have gone up substantially in recent years, the rates are still significantly below those assessed for individual therapy.

Given the mounting pressures to justify the expense of psychotherapy (Beigel and Sharfstein 1984), it is conceivable that clinicians may face even greater challenges to explain why the treatment of choice for most patients is not group psychotherapy. Indeed, if group interventions are comparably effective and potentially more cost-efficient, this question should not be too surprising. However, because the limited number of studies on cost-effectiveness precludes any firm generalization, this challenge may be premature. Besides, factors other than expediency, staff efficiency, and reduced fees, such as sound clinical judgment based on a thorough understanding of particular patient needs and specific treatment offerings, should guide the assignment to appropriate therapeutic modalities (Dies 1986).

At the very least, it should be quite evident that group treatments represent a demonstrably efficacious and arguably cost-efficient form of intervention. These factors must certainly contribute to the finding that literally millions of people spend portions of their time in group therapy or counseling each week to overcome a broad spectrum of personal and interpersonal difficulties (Dies 1986).

Greater Specificity About Outcome and Process

In my review of trends in the empirical literature (Dies 1979), I indicated that investigators had moved away from the generic question, "Does group therapy work?" to an exploration of the particular dimensions of group process that foster therapeutic change. This shift was reflected in the emergence of increasingly specialized reviews of empirical literature and in greater efforts by researchers to investigate the association between specific group processes and clinical improvement.

The publication of specialized reviews has continued. Outcome surveys have focused more on particular patient groups (e.g., anxiety disorders, depression, bulimia, and schizophrenia), as well as on group interventions for a range of nonpatients, including women (Huston 1986), the elderly (Leszcz 1990), individuals in mid-life career change (Zimpfer and Carr 1989), visually impaired people (Johnson 1989), and family caregivers (Toseland and Rossiter 1989). Similarly, reviews of process and therapist variables have appeared with greater frequency on topics such as cohesion (Drescher et al. 1985), composition (Waltman and Zimpfer 1988), feedback (Kivlighan 1985), leadership (Dies 1983b), norms (Bond 1983), pregroup contracting (Piper and Perrault 1989), roles (Livesley and MacKenzie 1983), therapeutic factors (MacKenzie 1987), and so on. In each of these reviews the authors attempt to link specific group processes to particular therapeutic gains.

The substantial growth of research on various psychotherapeutic modalities has made it possible for reviewers to search for common and distinctive factors contributing to clinical change. Thus Orlinsky and Howard (1986) offered a broad range of conclusions about critical therapeutic parameters common to various forms of psychological intervention. Fuhriman and Burlingame (1990), on the other hand, concluded from their comparative analysis that although many parallels exist among treatment modalities, there are properties inherent in group interventions that create a uniquely therapeutic learning environment:

> Factors common to both formats are those experienced by oneself (e.g., insight, catharsis), with the therapist (e.g., hope, disclosure), or with others

(e.g., reality testing, identification). Factors unique to group are those experienced only in the presence of others (e.g., vicarious learning, universality) or engaged with others (e.g., altruism, family reenactment). (p. 55)

The clear challenge to clinicians and researchers is how to understand and apply these unique interpersonal processes within the group setting to enhance treatment effectiveness and to circumvent therapeutic casualties (Dies and Teleska 1985). Recent research has underscored the complexity of this task by demonstrating that the role of these therapeutic factors may depend, for instance, on the phase of group development, the duration and type of group experience, and the leadership style implemented by the clinician (Dies 1988).

More Pragmatic and Personalized Approaches to Investigation

A trend toward greater pragmatism, that is, a shift from "what to look at" in group research to "how to look at it," was outlined in my former survey (Dies 1979). This practical view was apparent primarily in recommendations for overcoming common methodological and design problems. More recently, this trend is documented by an increasing number of articles and books on how practitioners can incorporate research instruments into their clinical work, not only to improve their objective understanding of diagnostic (Wetzler 1989) and treatment issues (Barlow et al. 1984), but also to enhance the quality of their group therapeutic interventions (Dies 1983a, 1987, 1990a; MacKenzie and Dies 1982). For example, Corcoran and Fischer (1987) stressed the mounting pressures on practitioners for accountability in their clinical activities and recommended that careful measurement of therapeutic interventions would be a principal way to fulfill this commitment. They provided suggestions on how to introduce simple and systematic measures into clinical practice to evaluate how well treatment is progressing and to ascertain whether interventions have actually facilitated therapeutic gain. Many authors (e.g., Corcoran and Fischer 1987; MacKenzie and Dies 1982) have furnished detailed lists of "rapid assessment instruments" that are not only manageable within a busy practice, but also sufficiently reliable and valid to meet the requirements of third-party payers to document the efficacy of treatment interventions. These authors have also offered concrete guidelines on how to implement measures into clinical work without confronting significant patient resistance.

The introduction of empirical measures into practice may accomplish another goal, which is to "personalize" treatment interventions. Regrettably, clinicians have typically looked askance at instruments as an unwelcome invasion into their treatment domain because patients are generally used as "subjects" in the research. Ironically, however, the personal and individualized advantages of instrumentation include clarification of goals and contract issues, encouragement of patient and therapist involvement in and communication about treatment, and the capacity for interventions to be tailored more sensitively to the unique needs of the individual patient (MacKenzie and Dies 1982).

Recognition of the Need for Improved Communication

In an earlier report (Dies 1979), I indicated that one of the central dilemmas within the field was the failure of researchers and clinicians to communicate, a factor that presumably played a principal role in forestalling notable progress in the understanding of group treatments. Other reviewers (e.g., Bednar et al. 1987; Bennis 1960; Hartmann 1979) have reached similar conclusions over the years.

A careful reconsideration of this issue, however, suggests that there is substantial evidence to refute that allegation (Dies 1990a). Although there are certainly many practitioners who are neither consumers nor purveyors of research, their disinterest does not hamper progress within the field if other clinicians and researchers are actively exchanging ideas and collaborating in their efforts to understand group treatments. At least three lines of evidence contradict the "myth of noncommunication":

1. The observation that the dichotomy of clinician versus researcher is a fallacy, given that the preponderance of the published research is promulgated by investigators who spend extensive portions of their time actually conducting group treatments
2. Documentation of substantial scientist-clinician dialogue within the field through symposia at professional conferences, numerous special journal issues devoted to this topic, and hundreds of published studies and empirical reviews that attempt to integrate research and practice
3. Reinterpretation of the presumed "attitude problems" of clinicians and researchers by demonstrating their shared commitment to patient welfare (i.e., the apparent reciprocal negativism stems from uneasiness experienced by both clinicians and researchers about participating in a scientific endeavor that may conflict with moment-

by-moment patient needs or the natural evolution of the therapeutic group process)

I have proposed that rather than denigrating the practitioner as being "antiresearcher," or the investigator as "anticlinician," it is more profitable to regard both of their positions as "propatient" or "protreatment." Such an interpretation is far less likely to maintain the unhealthy clinician-versus-researcher tension that overshadows the profession (Dies 1990a).

Overall, the general trends in the literature showing ample empirical confirmation that group treatments represent a uniquely powerful form of therapeutic intervention, the increased ability of investigators to address more pragmatic, personalized, and specific group processes and outcomes, and the growing recognition that practitioners and researchers share much in common suggest that significant progress is being made. One way to evaluate this conclusion is to survey those who are most intimately involved in the investigation of group treatments. In the next section of this chapter, therefore, I consider findings from a recent inquiry of internationally recognized group psychotherapy researchers.

International Perspectives on Group Therapy Research

Recently, 156 group psychotherapy investigators representing 29 different countries responded to a detailed questionnaire on group treatment research (Dies and Cohen 1992). The sample was divided into three subgroups to examine international patterns in the results. The North American respondents consisted of 56 clinician-researchers who are major contributors to the group literature. The other two subgroups were a sample of 63 West European and 37 East European or Asian experts in group psychotherapy research. The findings from this survey revealed a number of interesting international differences. These differences are highlighted briefly to provide a foundation for an exploration of the clinical implications of research in the final section of this chapter on the implications of research for optimizing therapeutic gain.

General Observations About Research Methods

One general finding from this international project was that North American researchers had very limited awareness of empirical investigations of group treatments in other countries. This parochialism is reflected in the observation that very few articles appearing in our journals cite papers published in other segments of the world, despite the existence of scores of international group psychotherapy journals; many of our American colleagues are not even cognizant of the fact that there are at least 9 major journals devoted almost exclusively to group interventions in the United States and nearly 400 different journals that contain reports on various aspects of group treatments (Dies 1986).

A second general trend in the international data showed that North Americans were much more inclined to favor large-scale correlational or experimental studies, whereas Europeans placed more importance on the intensive qualitative study of single clinical groups. This pattern is clearly congruent with prevailing theoretical orientations espoused in different regions of the world, with proportionately more North Americans disposed toward empirically based models (e.g., cognitive-behavioral and social learning theory approaches) and Europeans and Asians being partial to experientially grounded or phenomenological positions. The international opinions on the types of measures that are most valuable for studying groups were generally consistent with these findings. Thus there was consensus that multimethod and multiperspective procedures should be applied insofar as feasible to evaluate clinical improvement, but the North Americans were much more outspoken about this issue.

Although these international trends reflect clear philosophical differences in how group psychotherapy research should be conducted, with North Americans generally favoring the "big is better" approach and Europeans and Asians espousing the "qualitative validity" position, there is evidence in the literature of a growing alliance between these perspectives (Dies 1983a; Kaul and Bednar 1986; MacKenzie and Dies 1982). Indeed, it has become increasingly clear that these two research ideologies are fundamentally isomorphic in their commitment to understanding complicated group phenomena and even in their hypothesis-testing operations (Dies 1990a). Thus the integration of both ideographic (e.g., clinical) and nomothetic (e.g., empirical) approaches is now more widely accepted.

Our international researchers indicated that practical problems due to the sheer complexity of group therapy represented the principal roadblock hindering progress in the comprehensive understanding of treatment process and outcome. Other important obstacles were related to limited funding to support research, heavy service demands preventing research involvement, and potential loss of income from time devoted to research. These factors were stressed more by the North Americans. On other factors, such as limited training in research methods, lack of appropriate measures, conflicting role demands (as clinician versus researcher), and lack of both administrative and staff support, there was considerable consensus among the international investigators. By and large, these researchers agreed that a host of factors pose serious barriers to the potential investigator of group treatments.

There was agreement among our international investigators about the types of problems characterizing studies on group treatments. Criticisms of the research included the failure to link group process and outcomes, lack of follow-up evaluations, disregard of outside factors influencing therapeutic progress, use of inadequate measures, insufficient description of group treatments, limitations of experimental design, and unrepresentative patient samples and clinical settings. These factors are commonly cited by critics of group research (Bednar et al. 1987; Kaul and Bednar 1986).

Types of Groups and Patients Most Commonly Investigated

The international experts were requested to indicate the type of therapy groups and patients most frequently studied in their countries. Overall, short-term group treatments with primarily adult patients, using a closed-group model in an agency-based, outpatient setting, were most typically mentioned. Undoubtedly, this relates to research expediency, that is, to the opportunity to conduct relatively simple investigations unencumbered by uncontrolled complications such as patient attrition, frequently changing group membership, and inability to disentangle contextual factors from treatment-related variables (e.g., in hospital settings patients are exposed to multiple therapeutic interventions, so it is difficult to attribute clinical improvements exclusively to group treatments). Research in private practice settings, where patients are providing reimbursement for services and where clinicians may have precious little time or external support for involvement in research, is understandably less common (Dies 1990a). Similarly, empirical investigation of group treatments for children is less frequently undertaken, perhaps due to the need for parental permission, the rapid developmental changes in youngsters, the significant impact of other nontreatment factors on children's adjustment, or the greater difficulty of using selfreport measures with younger populations (Dies and Riester 1986).

Despite general agreement about the types of groups most often inves-tigated, there were some international differences, with Europeans more likely to conduct research with longer-term, open-ended, and diagnosti-cally mixed groups. The questionnaire requested the international re-searchers to list three types of patients who were studied most often in their countries; no other guidelines were furnished. Although a prepon-derance of the investigators identified various diagnostic groups, other researchers listed either developmental criteria (e.g., children, adoles-cents, and elderly) or general dimensions (e.g., inpatient-outpatient and acute-chronic). The findings demonstrated that the majority of patients who serve as subjects in group psychotherapy research carry some form of nonpsychotic diagnosis (e.g., "neurotic," personality disordered, sub-stance abusing, eating disordered, bereaved, and situationally dis-tressed). Although there are certainly reports in the literature of research on group treatment of schizophrenic patients (Kanas 1986), more of the published reports address less symptomatically dysfunctional patients (e.g., Brandsma and Pattison 1985; Leszcz 1989; Lewinsohn and Clarke 1984; Oesterheld et al. 1987).

Two other international differences were noteworthy. One was the finding that the North American researchers were much more inclined to list students or trainees as frequent participants in group research. This finding is consistent with reviews in the literature criticizing American investigators for overutilizing nonpatient samples in their empirical stud-ies. Indeed, this is one of the factors contributing to the impression that research may not be pertinent to clinical practice (Dies 1983a, 1990a). The second difference was that the Europeans were more likely to iden-tify "neurotic" or "psychosomatic" patients. This finding is probably un-reliable, however, because the official criteria outlined in DSM-III-R (American Psychiatric Association 1987) no longer contain these labels, so Americans would be unlikely to use them; instead Americans more often cited depression, anxiety, or situationally distraught patients.

International Perspectives on Outcomes and Process

The international researchers were invited to judge the extensiveness of their own knowledge about outcome variables, and Table 24–1 presents these results.

The first finding that should be noted is that the average ratings are generally quite low across the entire sample on the 4-point scale. Thus all of the variables fall below 3 on the rating continuum, which was only "a

Table 24–1. Outcome and process variables researchers know most about

Variables (rank ordered)	Means			
	North America	Western Europe	Eastern Europe/Asia	Total
Outcome				
Symptomatic changes	2.79	2.83	2.95	2.84
Social adaptation	2.48	2.70	2.49	2.57
Attitude changes	2.45	2.63	2.57	2.55
Dropouts or casualties	2.63	2.44	2.54	2.53
Self-concept	2.48	2.60	2.38	2.51
Work/school adjustment	2.30	2.52	2.28	2.41
Cognitive changes	2.38	2.33	2.46	2.38
Family adjustment	1.82	2.21	2.14	2.05[a]
Physiological changes	1.57	1.59	1.84	1.64
Process				
Cohesion	3.02	2.98	2.92	2.98
Group climate	2.70	2.79	2.65	2.72
Communication patterns	2.52	2.84	2.76	2.71[b]
Therapeutic factors	2.77	2.71	2.51	2.69
Stages	2.71	2.54	2.81	2.67
Self-disclosure	2.70	2.63	2.65	2.66
Structure	2.64	2.56	2.78	2.64
Patient roles	2.55	2.51	2.92	2.62[c]
Feedback	2.54	2.70	2.59	2.62
Therapist technique	2.38	2.70	2.70	2.58[d]
Selection	2.29	2.59	2.73	2.51[e]
Pregroup contracting	2.77	2.38	2.27	2.49[f]
Composition	2.32	2.57	2.62	2.49
Norm development	2.48	2.44	2.46	2.46
Underlying dynamics	2.18	2.56	2.32	2.37[g]
Therapist personality	2.20	2.38	2.38	2.31

Note. Ratings were on a 4-point scale: 1 = almost nothing; 2 = very little; 3 = a fair amount; 4 = very much. Abbreviations: N = North America; W = Western Europe; E = Eastern Europe/Asia.

[a]One-way analysis of variance (ANOVA) ($F = 5.95$, df = 2,153, $P < .01$): N < W and E.
[b]One-way ANOVA ($F = 3.57$, df = 2,153, $P < .05$): N < W.
[c]One-way ANOVA ($F = 4.35$, df = 2,153, $P < .05$): N and W > E.
[d]One-way ANOVA ($F = 3.22$, df = 2,153, $P < .05$): N < W.
[e]One-way ANOVA ($F = 4.76$, df = 2,153, $P < .01$): N < W and E.
[f]One-way ANOVA ($F = 5.57$, df = 2,153, $P < .01$): N > W and E.
[g]One-way ANOVA ($F = 3.74$, df = 2,153, $P < .05$): N < W

fair amount," and many approached 2 or "very little." There were almost no international variations, but rather there was widespread agreement that researchers are most aware of symptomatic alleviation and to a lesser extent social adaptation, attitude and self-concept changes, and therapeutic dropouts and casualties. There was also reasonable consensus that researchers know comparatively little about the impact of group treatments on the daily lives of patients (i.e., on their family, work, or school adjustment). Undoubtedly, the international consensus is largely due to the fact that most researchers rely quite heavily on self-report measures of change and have rarely sought evaluations from significant others in their patients' lives, such as family members, employers, teachers, or friends (Dies 1983b; Dies and Riester 1986). The primary concentration on symptomatic amelioration by researchers is perhaps understandable, given the goals of most patients seeking therapeutic relief in short-term treatments and given the greater ease and availability of self-report, symptom-oriented measures.

The international investigators were also instructed to evaluate levels of knowledge about various dimensions of group process, and these results are summarized in Table 24–1 as well. Once again, the first notable observation is that none of the variables average above 3, or "a fair amount," on the rating continuum. Apparently, the international experts believe that there is still much to learn about the complex processes that influence treatment outcomes. That cohesion ranked first is no surprise because of the longstanding history of research on this phenomenon in both the group dynamics and group treatment literature. The other top-ranked factors in Table 24–1 have not received nearly as much attention.

It would appear that our international experts believe that researchers understand more about general dimensions of group atmosphere (e.g., cohesion and climate) than they do about such critical topics as selection, composition, therapist techniques, and underlying group dynamics. Certainly, our perceived failure to know more about suitable selection criteria and how to properly combine patients in our treatment groups (i.e., composition) must be viewed as quite disappointing. The statistically significant international differences shown in Table 24–1 probably relate to unique trends in respective regions of the world. For example, North Americans have been exposed to several reviews of the pregroup contracting literature (e.g., Kivlighan et al. 1985; Mayerson 1984; Piper and Perrault 1989) but very little recent empirical work on selection (Woods and Melnick 1979) or underlying group dynamics. This is undoubtedly related to the emphasis on "big is better" research in the United States, as opposed to the more experientially based investigation by Europeans, which is more likely to address subtle undercurrents of group process.

Overall, the results of the international survey provide a broad perspective on the types of groups and patients evaluated in research. These results suggest that empirical investigation has contributed only modestly to our understanding of general group process and outcome. The findings are certainly consistent with opinions offered in major reviews of the empirical literature (e.g., Bednar and Kaul 1978; Kaul and Bednar 1986; Parloff and Dies 1977).

In the remainder of this chapter, I evaluate more specifically the group process variables that have been linked to clinical improvement. The discussion is organized into pregroup, early group, and working-group phases. Although the international data imply that we still have much to learn about group treatments, certain interpretations may be warranted. The following review is not designed to be exhaustive, but rather to represent the types of findings that are available for practitioners to guide their clinical interventions.

Implications of Research for Optimizing Therapeutic Gain

From our international survey we have found that most of the empirical investigation of group psychotherapy has focused on moderately disturbed, adult outpatient groups. These findings are consistent with general publication patterns in major group therapy journals (Dies 1989b) and with results of a recent survey of clinicians, who commonly favor such an emphasis in the literature (Dies 1990b). Therefore, in the following sections, which offer generalizations based on research, I focus on these types of patient groups.

It is apparent that highly specific extrapolations may not be justified given the current state of development of the literature. Our international findings certainly suggest this conclusion, as do most of the empirical reviews on the principal aspects of group intervention, including pregroup contracting (Piper and Perrault 1989), group process variables such as cohesion (Drescher et al. 1985) and therapeutic factors (Bloch 1986), leadership (Dies 1983b), and outcome (Kaul and Bednar 1986). Virtually every prescription about group psychotherapy must be qualified in terms of the type of patient, duration of treatment, phase of group development, leadership style, and therapeutic context. Nevertheless, it is possible to offer general guidelines based on the research literature that can be applied across a broad spectrum of clinical settings.

Pretreatment Considerations

The three major issues that clinicians face in their preliminary negotiations with patients for group psychotherapy include selection, composition, and contracting. The bottom-line issue, of course, is establishing the optimal therapeutic "fit" among the patient, the therapist(s), and the group system. This requires substantial sensitivity, perceptiveness, and skill on the part of the clinician, especially in the midst of enormous obstacles that restrict the therapist's flexibility. These encumbrances include limited case loads or referral sources for private practitioners and administrative pressures for agency-based clinicians, who are not always able to control which patients have access to particular treatment groups. Thus the exigencies of time and context may preclude proper selection, assignment, and contracting. Although the findings from the international survey revealed that selection, composition, and pregroup training all rank in the lower one-third of the process variables "we know most about" (Table 24–1), the literature does contain some very useful recommendations under each of these categories.

Selection.   In their comprehensive review of the empirical literature on selection criteria published over a decade ago, Woods and Melnick (1979) indicated that traditional diagnostic interviews were most prevalent, despite the fact that behavioral and interpersonal approaches held more promise. More recent contributions show increasing emphasis on interactive terminology, due in large part to the recognition that conventional diagnoses are not especially useful (Corazzini and Heppner 1982; Unger 1989; Vinogradov and Yalom 1990). Clearly, patients carrying the full range of diagnostic labels have been successfully treated with group methods. The central issue is whether or not a particular treatment group is suitable for a specific patient at a given point in the manifestation of that patient's symptomatology and the group's current level of development. Thus, although some authors have argued that paranoid, drug-addicted, acutely psychotic, antisocial, or organically impaired individuals are poor candidates for group treatment, others have taken the opposite stance (Unger 1989); this position is based, for example, on the assumption that homogeneous groups could be designed to work effectively with such patients.

It has become evident that therapists do not actually select patients for group psychotherapy, but rather deselect, that is, exclude patients who seem to be inappropriate candidates. Vinogradov and Yalom (1990), for example, offered pragmatic guidelines that are not based on traditional diagnostic criteria. Their standards for exclusion of a patient included inability to tolerate the group treatment situation, likelihood of assuming a deviant role within the group, extreme agitation, potential noncompliance with group norms, and marked incompatibility with one or more of the other group members. Their inclusion indices comprised capacity to perform the group task, motivation to participate in treatment, commitment to attend group sessions regularly, and congruence of the patient's problems with the goals of the group. Klein (1985) also noted that patients who have circumscribed complaints, acute-onset symptoms, and a history of good premorbid adjustment will generally benefit most from treatment.

Unfortunately, procedures for predicting how patients will behave in the group setting are not highly developed. Typical psychometric methods have not demonstrated adequate utility, nor is there sufficient research on interpersonal diagnostic techniques and direct sampling of group-relevant behavior to warrant much enthusiasm for these procedures (Woods and Melnick 1979). There has been increasing emphasis on the construction of interpersonal measures that predict social behavior in group situations (Benjamin 1984; Keisler 1986; Wiggins et al. 1987), and more efforts have been made to employ pretherapy group trials (Mayerson 1984; Yalom 1985); however, the results are just too limited to be of much practical benefit. Thus the recent empirical literature has focused less on screening out the "unsuitable patient" and more on providing pretherapy training to help prepare the individual for effective therapeutic work (Garfield 1986).

In the simplest form, the basic tasks of the selection process include

1. *Intrapersonal diagnosis* to establish that the patient's psychopathology is such that treatment in a group is feasible (i.e, sufficiently distressed but not too agitated, impulsive, or manipulative to disrupt treatment)
2. *Interpersonal assessment* to evaluate willingness to cooperate with others, capacity to conceptualize problems in relationship terms, and compatibility with other group members along interpersonal dimensions, including general level of adjustment

3. *Motivational appraisal* to secure willingness to remain in treatment despite difficulties associated with intensive interpersonal work
4. *Goal setting* to establish realistic and manageable objectives that suit the time frame of group treatment
5. *Evaluation of expectancies* about the therapeutic process and outcome to ensure their reasonableness
6. *Initiation of the therapeutic alliance* (Corazzini and Heppner 1982; Woods and Melnick 1979)

Several of these issues are given additional attention in the following sections.

It is clear that patients who do not possess the requisite emotional, behavioral, and interpersonal resources to participate effectively in group treatment are high risks for either premature termination or therapeutic casualty (Woods and Melnick 1979). A number of reviews of the empirical literature have documented a host of patient, therapist, and treatment variables that contribute to negative outcomes (Dies and Teleska 1985; Erickson 1987; Roback and Smith 1987). Most relevant to the selection process are factors such as characterological defenses that result in major interpersonal deficits. "Included in this category are problems with self-disclosure, difficulties with intimacy, generalized interpersonal distrust, excessive use of denial, and a tendency to be either verbally subdued or hostile" (Roback and Smith 1987, p. 427). Other variables include limited motivation, unrealistic expectations, and diagnostic considerations such as persons in situational crises who are too preoccupied to engage effectively in group therapeutic work (Roback and Smith 1987), as well as borderline, narcissistic, schizoid, or acutely disturbed patients who are placed in group therapy prematurely (Dies and Teleska 1985). Other authors have offered additional research-based recommendations for limiting early attrition and potential negative outcomes (e.g., Bernard 1989; Korda and Pancrazio 1989). The various findings would suggest that patients who rely extensively on *externalizing defenses* (e.g., hypochondriacal, paranoid, or sociopathic individuals), those who do not have sufficient *internal focus* (i.e., psychologically minded, nondefensive, anxious, or distressed), and those who are too embroiled in *external crises* are not good candidates for ongoing group therapy.

Group composition.   One way to conceptualize the relationship between selection and composition is to consider selection as predominantly individually oriented and composition as interaction oriented.

Thus selection addresses factors such as patient motivation, level of distress, goals for treatment, expectations about outcome, and initial therapist-patient bonding, (i.e., the patient's amenability to group treatment in general). In contrast, composition emphasizes interpersonal factors regarding the particular treatment group, such as demographic mix (e.g., age, gender, and race), potential interpersonal harmony, and relative homogeneity or heterogeneity along diagnostic or relationship dimensions. The paramount issue of "fit," then, evaluates the individual's preparedness for group treatment through careful selection criteria and the patient's compatibility with other participants within a unique group system (i.e., composition). As discussed below, pregroup contracting attempts to enhance the therapeutic match by capitalizing on individual strengths and educating patients about group-level parameters.

The factor most commonly cited in the composition literature is that of homogeneity versus heterogeneity. Melnick and Woods (1976) offered the most salient generalization from that body of empirical evidence:

> Homogeneous groups appear to coalesce more quickly, offer more immediate support to members, have better attendance, less conflict, and provide more rapid symptomatic relief. However, they are seen as remaining at more superficial levels of interaction and are less effective in producing more fundamental interpersonal learning. (p. 495)

More recent writers have changed very little in their perspective on this important issue (Unger 1989; Yalom 1985).

From their analysis of the research, Melnick and Woods (1976) suggested that group composition should be guided toward furnishing an optimal balance between conditions maximizing interpersonal learning (heterogeneity) and considerations ensuring group maintenance (homogeneity). They proposed a support-plus-confrontation model favoring moderate diversity in composition:

1. Avoidance of extreme demographic differences and patients with high potential for becoming group misfits
2. Creation of reasonable balance in conflict areas and adaptive patterns
3. Selection of patients who are sufficiently different to "ensure group resources varied enough to generate warm, responsive interactions between some members . . . with sufficient dissonance to provide alternate role models for more effective ways of behaving and coping with stress" (p. 509)

Despite the apparent wisdom of such recommendations, it is obvious that the assertions lack clarity. For example, any group composed for homogeneity on one variable is likely to be quite divergent on many others (Melnick and Woods 1976). Moreover, Unger (1989) has concluded that any treatment group could be viewed as either homogeneous or heterogeneous and that a skilled practitioner would be able to focus on either similarities or differences, depending on the needs of the group at that particular moment in time. A recent critique (Waltman and Zimpfer 1988) of the composition literature demonstrated that structure and duration of treatment served to moderate the effects of group composition. On the basis of their meta-analysis of the pertinent empirical research, the authors concluded that "highly structured groups may suppress composition effects and that there is a minimum exposure time necessary if composition is to be a significant factor in determining group outcome" (pp. 178–179). The authors suggested that the concern about composition is most relevant for unstructured, longer-term treatment groups (more than 12 hours). The current emphasis on short-term, symptom- or theme-centered groups would imply that composition, within limits, is not a critical issue for many groups comprising moderately distressed outpatients. Although research demonstrates that structure may be more important for severely disturbed patients, and at particular moments in the group's development (Dies 1983b), there is little investigation of how these considerations relate to group composition.

The assessment of interpersonal compatibility to provide optimal balance within the group system has received minimal attention from researchers. Earlier work with Schutz's self-report measure (1961) of concerns about inclusion, control, and affection showed initial promise, but such research has not been substantially continued. Nor have investigators sufficiently employed the newer interpersonal measures to explore their capacity to compose groups according to prominent dimensions of interpersonal functioning (Benjamin 1984; Kiesler 1986; Wiggins et al. 1987). The absence of composition research on objective indices of interpersonal style means that practitioners must rely on their clinical judgment. Although guidelines have been published by other research-oriented clinicians (Corazzini and Heppner 1982; MacKenzie 1990; Yalom 1985), more attention needs to be devoted to the development of standardized procedures for determining group composition.

Yalom (1985), on the other hand, contended that the preoccupation of many clinicians with problems of group integrity and survival, based on the difficulties in accumulating sufficient numbers of patients to form and maintain groups, leads them to place composition low in their list of priorities. He noted that "the time and energy spent on delicately casting and balancing a group is not justified given our current state of knowledge; you do better to invest that time and energy in careful selection of patients for group therapy and in pre-therapy preparation" (p. 274).

Pregroup contracting.   Although our international survey showed that pregroup contracting ranked quite low overall, the North American researchers placed it rather high on their roster of process variables "we know most about" (Table 24–1). Undoubtedly, this high placement is due to the publication of several major reviews on this topic in our journals (e.g., Kaul and Bednar 1986; Kivlighan et al. 1985; Mayerson 1984; Piper and Perrault 1989; Tinsley et al. 1988). A variety of models of pregroup preparation have been evaluated, and opinions vary as to their relative merits. The most positive endorsement came from Orlinsky and Howard (1986), who reviewed studies examining both individual and group treatments. These authors concluded that a majority of the investigations strongly favor role preparation procedures; findings show significantly better outcomes in terms of reports from patients, therapists, independent raters, and psychological tests for patients who received some form of early preparation compared with patients who did not.

In contrast, Piper and Perrault (1989) were more cautious in their conclusion from the group therapy literature that the empirical evidence is not particularly impressive. Although research does reflect immediate changes in terms of improved knowledge about material covered in pre-training, increased motivation, reduced dropout rates, and to a lesser extent certain aspects of group functioning (e.g., enhanced feedback and heightened self-disclosure), the findings concerning treatment outcome often seem disappointing. Despite their rather guarded position on the value of pregroup training, however, Piper and Perrault (1989) asserted that

> While the gains associated with PGT [pregroup training] may be modest, for example, likely benefit for attendance and possible benefit for remaining and some process variables, the costs are relatively small (one hour or less). Thus, on purely economic grounds PGT may be regarded as worth the effort. (p. 30)

I have reasoned that pregroup contracting can be conceptualized as a way to facilitate the match between the individual patient and the particular treatment group. This facilitation is generally accomplished by attempting to mollify negative anticipations regarding treatment while instilling positive role and outcome expectations, and by educating patients about constructive interpersonal behaviors, group developmental issues, and helpful therapeutic factors. Researchers have explored the efficacy of various methods to implement these facets of the contract, including audiotape and videotape interventions, verbal instructions, printed materials, interviews, trial groups, and combinations of these procedures. The literature suggests that multiple strategies yield better results than single methods (Kivlighan et al. 1985) and that more realistic interventions (e.g., videotapes or practice sessions as opposed to instructions or written handouts) are more productive (Tinsley et al. 1988). Because investigators have rarely devoted more than an hour to the pretraining process, some reviewers have expressed their surprise that any impact has been identified (Piper and Perrault 1989). The positive effect of the pretraining process is especially surprising given the host of other conditions that might affect patients' involvement in and benefit from treatment. Obviously, the patient's actual experiences in the early developmental phases and in the working stages of group psychotherapy would be expected to exert a much more powerful influence on both involvement and outcome than any brief pretherapy manipulation would.

In a recent overview of the research literature (Dies 1988), I summarized a number of studies documenting the general preference of patients for individual therapy over group modalities, both before and after treatment, despite comparable outcomes. Indeed, investigators (e.g., Slocum 1987; Subich and Coursol 1985) have demonstrated that a significant percentage of patients have a range of *negative expectations* regarding group interventions: fears of attack, embarrassment, emotional contagion or coercion, and actual harmful effects. Most clinicians are well aware of these pervasive concerns and therefore attempt to alleviate the discomfort by emphasizing the safe and supportive nature of the group experience (Vinogradov and Yalom 1990). Similarly, efforts are introduced to enhance *positive expectations* regarding group treatment, particularly those associated with self-efficacy (i.e., the belief that the patient can adequately engage in the necessary interpersonal behaviors) and therapeutic outcome (Mayerson 1984). The literature suggests that quelling apprehensions and fears, disabusing patients of misconceptions about their own behaviors and the group's functioning, and establishing optimistic attitudes can significantly influence treatment process and outcome (Beutler et al. 1986).

In addition to their efforts to modify pretreatment expectations, researchers have also evaluated the effects of providing information to patients about role behaviors and group process. Kivlighan and his colleagues (1985), for instance, summarized empirical findings on specific skills such as self-disclosure, interpersonal feedback, anxiety management, and here-and-now interaction. The literature generally supports the effectiveness of teaching patients about these important role behaviors in terms of both group process and outcome. In the same vein, the value of educating patients about various dimensions of the group process has been reasonably well documented (Kivlighan et al. 1985; Mayerson 1984; Yalom 1985). Most critical, of course, given patients' diffuse anxieties about group interventions, is the need to furnish a solid rationale for treatment in the group format. Mayerson (1984), for example, noted that patients are informed that the "group therapy setting is one which provides a special opportunity to interact with others so as to gain insight into one's current interactional patterns and to experiment with new ones" (p. 194). The interpersonal nature of psychopathology is emphasized, if not in its etiology, at least in its manifestation and resolution. Also highlighted in pregroup training are general ground rules (e.g., confidentiality and regular attendance), developmental trends (i.e., information to prepare patients for inevitable group hurdles or potential stumbling blocks), and a general description of therapeutic factors or central interpersonal processes that foster individual gain. These pretreatment interventions are designed to provide a coherent framework for comprehending individual experiences and events within the group and to minimize the likelihood of premature attrition and therapeutic casualties (Dies 1983b; Dies and Teleska 1985).

Early Developmental Issues

Careful selection of individual patients, proper assignment to appropriate treatment groups, and pregroup training provide the foundation for effective group intervention. Nevertheless, these initial negotiations with patients represent only a small portion of the preliminary therapeutic work that must be accomplished. The experiences of patients in the earliest phases of group development undeniably play an even more fundamental role in determining the ultimate impact of group treatments.

In fact, Bednar et al. (1974) concluded from their review of the literature that clarifying role expectations, furnishing a conceptual scheme for patients to anticipate group evolution, and modeling effective behavior should be regarded as continuing treatment factors and not just as pretherapy training exercises. Indeed, they proposed that the absence of ample structure in early sessions "not only fails to facilitate early group development but actually feeds client distortions, interpersonal fears, and subjective distress, which interfere with group development and contribute to premature client dropouts" (p. 31).

These observations lead to questions about the type of structure, developmental focus, therapeutic factors, group cohesion, and leadership style that are essential for productive group treatment. The findings from the international survey (Table 24—1) suggest that we know a fair amount about these topics, because they generally rank in the top one-third of the process variables evaluated. In the following sections, I address these important dimensions of group treatment.

Structure.   A survey (Dies 1983b) of research conducted on group leadership during the 1970s prompted the conclusion that the type of structure or therapist activity that seems most beneficial in the group setting is that which adds meaning and significance to the group therapeutic enterprise. In other words, patients appear to be most satisfied with group sessions when they feel that task-oriented or therapeutic events have occurred. A recent update of this review (Dies 1988) confirmed that generalization. Indeed, the vast majority of studies on therapeutic structure demonstrate the superiority of more directive treatments; I found that in over 85% of the investigations comparing structured and more ambiguous group interventions, the former were more likely to generate constructive group processes and/or to foster more favorable therapeutic outcomes. It should be noted, however, that most of the research has focused on short-term group interventions. Hence, the empirical foundation for distilling conclusions about longer-term group treatments has not been sufficiently established.

The literature demonstrates that it is not therapist activity, per se, that is critical, but rather interventions that define the nature of the task (Dies 1983b). Lieberman et al. (1973) found that structure offered by leaders in terms of "meaning attribution" (i.e., providing concepts that help patients comprehend behavior and group experiences) was highly conducive to client improvement. On the other hand, structure in terms of the "executive function" (e.g., setting limits, suggesting rules, and managing time) was curvilinearly related to outcome; either too much or too little direction was counterproductive. Similarly, group treatments with contrasting (but equally active) structures may facilitate different outcomes for individual patients. Thus there is some evidence to suggest that directive treatments that are tailored to individual personality styles or particular psychological conditions might produce larger and more enduring gains (Dies 1988) than treatments that are not. For example, Beutler et al. (1986) demonstrated that a preponderance of clinical studies found positive interactions between therapist directiveness and patient attributional styles.

Bednar et al. (1974) proposed that structure tends to reduce patient responsibility and increase risk taking and cohesion in early group sessions, that is, the leader assumes more of the responsibility for promoting behavior that might leave members feeling vulnerable and threatened without some form of guidance. Later, a helpful group climate provides feelings of security that reduce the risk of self-revelation and augment personal responsibility. Other reviewers have corroborated this position (e.g., Stockton and Morran 1982). One implication from this literature is that therapists should gradually reduce their level of activity and the focus of their structuring as group members improve in their understanding of the therapeutic task and their role in helping each other to accomplish individual goals (Dies 1983b, 1986).

Group structure that builds supportive norms and highlights positive member interactions is generally most effective. Initially, the leader's interventions are predominantly group centered and focus on "culture building" (Yalom 1985), establishing clear norms (Bond 1983), and creating the therapeutic potential of the group. For example, premature excursions into intimate revelations or confrontative exchanges before a climate of trust has been established may be detrimental to the individual patient and ultimately to the group system. Research has shown that patients' fears of attack or coercion, either from the therapist or comembers, represent a principal reason for premature attrition (Dies and Teleska 1985; Roback and Smith 1987). Korda and Pancrazio (1989) noted that the patient who withdraws from the group may experience a sense of failure and diminished self-esteem, and "the remaining group members may become preoccupied with the possibility of group disintegration and experience a concomitant decrease in morale and cohesion" (p. 113). Consequently, group therapists should do all they can to prevent dropouts because they inevitably place the integrity of the entire group in jeopardy. Recommendations have been made for how clinicians can monitor the group process to identify potential early terminators (Dies 1983a, 1990a).

Formative stages of group development. MacKenzie (1987) observed that the first task of any treatment group is the issue of member acceptance or engagement. Yalom (1985), on the other hand, emphasized the need for orientation and the search for meaning. In either case, early group structure helps members to share common experiences and reactions and to develop a sense of universality, that is, an appreciation that they have had comparable experiences and can therefore understand each other.

> The individual member contributes to this by relatively superficial self-disclosure . . . this may be experienced as intensely arousing and threatening, since it brings with it the possibility of being found unacceptable. Once accomplished however, it results in a sense of satisfaction and acceptance that contributes strongly to the development of group cohesion. (MacKenzie 1987, p. 29)

According to MacKenzie (1987), the basic task in the second stage is differentiation, that is, the recognition of differences among members. This process is often characterized by polarization, anger, and conflict. Indeed, most theorists highlight issues of control, dominance, and rebellion as members wrestle with questions about how much they must sacrifice as individuals to comply with pressures for group conformity. If patients cannot develop guidelines for the cooperative exploration of such intermember differences, the group is at risk for developmental arrest and loss of the more vulnerable, resistive, or disgruntled members. Yet if the participants are adequately prepared for this systemic tension (e.g., through pretherapy training and clear and supportive norms), they can deal effectively with the confrontational atmosphere and come to realize that conflict is not invariably destructive. MacKenzie and Livesley (1983) claimed that once these two "prework" stages of engagement and differentiation are traversed, the group may advance to the more significant introspection and interpersonal exploration that characterize phases related to individuation, intimacy, and mutuality.

There are multiple models of group development. Although they differ in the specific concepts employed and the actual number of stages articulated, there is consensus that groups progress through a series of developmental hurdles (Burnand 1990; Lacoursiere 1980; Tuckman 1965). Agreement on the first two phases is especially widespread. Much of this research, however, is based on relatively unstructured group experiences. In the face of the initial ambiguity in such groups, it is no wonder that patients first feel confused (stage I: orientation) and then angry (stage II: rebellion), given the leader's failure to structure the therapeutic task. In more actively and positively directed group treatments, however, consternation and hostility are less likely to emerge.

Cissna (1984) reviewed studies presumably contradicting the existence of developmental patterns, but concluded that the negative evidence was not persuasive. He generalized from the research that "every group is like *all* groups in some respects, like *some*—or perhaps even *most*—groups in some respects, and like *no* groups in other respects" (p. 25).

Most critical, perhaps, is the understanding by members that concerns about acceptance, fears of attack or emotional contagion, resistance to urgings for self-disclosure, and interpersonal conflict are natural developmental phenomena in beginning groups. In fact, Kivlighan (1985) proposed a developmental framework for viewing structure and its effects in group therapy. On the basis of his review of the literature, he recommended that the content and timing of training should be geared to the developmental phase of the group. Pregroup contracting would focus on behavioral assessment, anxiety reduction, and patient preparation. Training during the engagement or orientation phase would address general interpersonal and group participation skills. Tolerating and constructively expressing anger would be the focus during the differentiation stage. More advanced helping and communication skills (e.g., expressing intimacy, confrontation, and problem solving) would be highlighted during the working phases. Kivlighan's viewpoint clearly underscores the importance of assisting patients continually to understand the treatment process in order to optimize their therapeutic involvement and to maximize treatment outcome.

Early therapeutic factors.   MacKenzie (1987) tested his developmental perspective by examining results of research on therapeutic factors in brief and long-term treatment groups. He discovered that short-term groups were more inclined to endorse "nonspecific" morale factors such as hope, altruism, universality, and cohesiveness. In contrast, long-term treatment groups favored "psychological work" factors such as catharsis, interpersonal learning, and insight. MacKenzie surmised that "the brief groups may be considered to still be in the process of developing a cohesive nonthreatening atmosphere, while the longer term groups value interpersonal learning and introspection, characteristics of the 'working' phases of group" (1987, p. 30). These conclusions are essentially identical to those of Yalom (1985), who posited that the early group is concerned predominantly with survival, with establishing boundaries, and with maintaining membership. Although cohesion continues to develop and subsequently allows members to engage in more meaningful selfrevelation, confrontation, and feedback, cohesion first is manifested through group support, acceptance, and the encouragement of attendance (Yalom 1985). The research on early therapeutic factors suggests that clinicians should focus a significant portion of their immediate interventions on establishing these general interpersonal resources. Indeed, Lambert et al. (1986) generalized from their extensive review of the literature that these nonspecific or "common factors" (i.e., expectation for improvement, persuasion, warmth and attention, understanding, and encouragement) are paramount in the outcome of most psychological treatments.

Cohesiveness.   Although structure, stages, and therapeutic factors rank high in the list of variables that "we know most about" according to the international researchers (Table 24–1), cohesion is a clear first choice. Unquestionably this relates to the numerous reviews of cohesion that have been published over the years (Bednar and Kaul 1978; Evans and Jarvis 1980; Kaul and Bednar 1986). Nevertheless, most reviewers would concur that "attempts to understand cohesion empirically have been as elusive as attempts to define it" (Drescher et al. 1985).

Probably no other variable illustrates the complexity of group process as readily as the concept of cohesion. In their efforts to bring some coherence to this body of literature, Drescher et al. (1985) proposed a model consisting of four critical dimensions:

1. The *person dimension,* which describes the unit of observation and the unit of analysis (e.g., individual group members, therapists, subgroups, and the total group)
2. The *variable function dimension,* which describes whether cohesion is looked at as an antecedent or response variable
3. The *measurement strategy dimension*
4. The *time dimension*

Briefly, these are called the "who," "what," "how," and "when" dimensions of examining group cohesiveness. In my invited critique of this model (Dies 1985b), I added a fifth dimension, namely, the context of the evaluation (i.e., the "where"). A survey of the research literature shows that the meaning of cohesion varies dramatically as a function of these five dimensions.

From a clinical perspective, however, there is no doubt that the empirical evidence strongly favors efforts to establish positive bonds among group members to enhance both the group process and the outcome. Thus investigators have linked increments in cohesion to factors such as pregroup training, composition and compatibility, and feedback and self-disclosure. Cohesion, in turn, is thought to produce more constructive engagement in therapeutic work (e.g., Yalom [1985] regards it as a precondition for other therapeutic factors) and more meaningful treatment outcomes. Hence it would seem imperative for practitioners to concentrate on maximizing levels of group cohesion, even though researchers cannot agree on its basic definition!

Early leadership interventions.   The research conducted on group leadership over the past two decades indicates that therapists play a central role in fostering group cohesiveness (Dies 1983b, 1986, 1988). For example, there is substantial documentation from studies on relationship variables (i.e., genuineness, empathy, and warmth), valence of therapist-patient interactions (e.g., affection, discomfort, and identification), and therapist self-disclosure to indicate that a favorable relationship between the therapist and group members exerts a potent influence on the development of constructive group norms. That similar conclusions about the value of active therapist involvement (Lambert et al. 1986) and positive engagement (Orlinsky and Howard 1986) are evident in the individual psychotherapy literature serves to bolster this observation. The research shows that group members prefer and apparently benefit more from an actively affirming style of intervention. In fact, as leaders become more vigorously negative, the probability increases that patients will not only be dissatisfied, but also potentially will be harmed by the group experience.

The impact of group leadership is mediated by both *modeling* and *reinforcement.* Overall, therapists who are willing to be open with their group members, especially in terms of here-and-now feelings and their rationale for therapeutic interventions, are more likely to facilitate the development of mutually confirming relationships within their group (Dies 1986). Through modeling, such transparent therapists may promote openness among group members. Nevertheless, even without sharing personal feelings and experiences, group leaders can generate self-disclosure within the group. For example, therapists can reinforce intimate expressions among group members and establish other participants as role models for interpersonal openness (Dies 1977). The astute therapist is the one who knows which members will serve as the most productive resources at critical moments in the group's development. For instance, Bahrey et al. (1991) illustrated how various role behaviors reflect developmental themes and suggested guidelines for how to manage these roles to enhance the quality of group treatment. Other authors have proposed similar recommendations (Dies and Teleska 1985; Livesley and MacKenzie 1983).

Many researchers have demonstrated the powerful effect of therapist reinforcement on a wide range of patient behaviors, including rate of interaction, direction of verbalization, sequence of speakers, hostility toward the therapist, and group cohesiveness. Through the differential application of interest, praise, and warmth, group therapists have been able to modify changes in patients' in-therapy and extra-therapy behaviors (Dies 1983b). Liberman (1971) found, however, that the leader does not serve as the exclusive determiner of group interaction, because patients also prompt and reinforce each other's behaviors. Hence as the group develops, "the group members take over from the therapist some of his influence in shaping behavior. While the therapist initially is important in establishing a group culture, later some of his influence is mediated by the group members themselves" (Liberman 1971, p. 172). These conclusions have been supported by numerous studies in the group literature (Dies 1983b, 1986, 1988).

The Working Group

Once the treatment group has progressed beyond issues of acceptance and differentiation to establish sufficient levels of intermember bonding, patients are prepare to engage in substantially more meaningful therapeutic work. The clinician's efforts to create a positive therapeutic climate and to explain the principal change mechanisms of treatment have undoubtedly facilitated this growth.

Regrettably, there is little empirical examination of more advanced stages of group life. Numerous conceptual models exist to account for the nature of therapeutic activity that transpires in intensive group interactions, but these models are not substantially buttressed by research findings (Cissna 1984; Lacoursiere 1980). Nevertheless, at the level of clinical observation and theoretical construction, there is broad agreement with Yalom's conclusion (1985) that "Much later, the mature work group emerges, which is characterized by high cohesiveness, considerable interpersonal and intrapersonal investigation, and full commitment to the primary task of the group and of each of the members" (p. 300).

Research on therapeutic factors, group process variables (e.g., self-disclosure and feedback), and leadership technique indicate that members in well-established groups are engaged in different types of psychological work; they are less group centered and more likely to be confronting the personal distress and maladaptive interpersonal styles that brought them to treatment in the first place. Certainly these individualized issues have been apparent throughout the group's evolution, but now the therapist and group members have fashioned a supportive and coherent group system to address these deeply personal conflicts in a much more concentrated and effective manner.

Later therapeutic factors.   The international researchers ranked this category fourth in the list of process variables (see Table 24–1), although the average rating was only moderate in terms of empirical understanding. There is a rather extensive body of literature on therapeutic factors, as is evident in reviews by Bloch (1986), Bloch and Crouch (1985), Butler and Fuhriman (1983), MacKenzie (1987), and Yalom (1985). Despite this volume of research, there is a general failure to establish direct links between process variables and clinical improvement. Nevertheless, the concept of therapeutic factors remains popular and clinically significant.

I noted earlier that certain elements are most salient in the formative phases of group treatment. MacKenzie (1987) labeled these the "nonspecific" morale dimensions (e.g., universality, altruism, and hope) because they are mainly important in establishing a safe atmosphere for patients to assume personal risks. In high-turnover inpatient groups, short-term outpatient therapy, and self-help groups, these factors may play a central role in the overall evaluation of treatment (Lieberman 1990; Yalom 1985). However, in most group interventions for moderately distressed individuals, these factors rarely emerge as most salient in judgments about therapeutic efficacy. Quite the contrary, the variables that appear with greatest regularity are interpersonal input (feedback), catharsis, cohesiveness, and self-understanding (Yalom 1985). A fifth factor, interpersonal output (socializing skills), is also mentioned frequently.

There are clearly no universal mechanisms for change, but rather a range of key dimensions that operate across clinical settings, diagnostic compositions, and forms of group therapy. Different patients may benefit from various therapeutic ingredients within the same group (Lieberman 1989), and the availability of multiple sources of learning within sessions may be more important than any limited set of common dimensions (Lieberman 1983). I have suggested that there is a confluence of nonspecific factors (e.g., cohesiveness) working in concert with cognitive, affective, and behavioral ingredients (i.e., self-understanding, catharsis, and interpersonal learning and social skills acquisition, respectively) to facilitate therapeutic gain (Dies 1990a). Thus there is no simple formula for treatment benefit. That behavioral, emotional, and cognitive factors all play a pivotal role should be of little surprise; entire systems of group psychotherapy have been organized around each of these facets of human functioning.

The research literature is also consistent in showing that Yalom's (1985) therapeutic factors of family reenactment, guidance, and identification are seldom viewed as important by group members. It is not especially difficult to figure out why advice and imitation are not foremost in intensive group work, but the failure of family recapitulation to appear as a nuclear therapeutic dimension runs counter to much of the writing about the importance of transference in the treatment context. Conceivably, the short-term nature of most of the group therapies in this body of research may preclude the possibility of establishing this factor as a viable change mechanism. On the other hand, the emotional reliving of earlier family dynamics has been found to be decisive for a group of incest victims (Bonney et al. 1986). It is possible that minor variations across studies often can be accounted for by virtue of the specialized nature of the treatment groups employed. For example, universality was understandably unimportant for a male felony offender group (Long and Cope 1980), whereas "existential awareness" (i.e., responsibility) was regarded as quite significant (MacDevitt and Sanislow 1987).

The fact that patients regard strong affective expression, increased self-awareness, and opportunities to receive interpersonal feedback and to attempt new behaviors as consequential for clinical improvement does not provide much information about the specific interventions that allowed these changes to occur. Notwithstanding, the uniformity of the therapeutic-factors literature on these dimensions, along with comparable reports from the accumulated research on individual psychotherapy (Orlinsky and Howard 1986), certainly testifies to the centrality of these factors. In the following sections, I explore the nature of the therapeutic interventions that facilitate what Orlinsky and Howard (1986) regarded as the "therapeutic realizations" (i.e., insight, catharsis, and interpersonal learning).

One caveat is in order. Most of the research on therapeutic factors is from the patient's point of view, that is, self-report assessments often extracted after the completion of many weeks or months of treatment. Although there is considerable consistency in the findings, the therapeutic factors may be too global a set of conditions to capture adequately the specific learning mechanisms that operate in group psychotherapy (Bloch and Crouch 1985). Ironically, there are many reports of marked discrepancies between patients and clinicians in their evaluation of the importance of therapeutic factors in particular studies. In fact, the abundance of such findings in the literature is one of the chief reasons for recommendations that practitioners incorporate research measures into their treatments to objectify evaluations of process and outcome (Dies 1983a, 1990a).

Self-disclosure and feedback.   The therapeutic factors that emerge as most central in the working group highlight interpersonal processes unique to group therapy that do not necessarily involve direct patient-therapist interactions. Although therapists are certainly instrumental in facilitating the development of an open and supportive atmosphere within the group, it is the interaction among group members that is the most direct mechanism of change in the therapeutic process. Thus in virtually every study comparing the impact of leaders and the impact of comembers on the patient's reported outcome, it is the quality of relationships and certain critical member-to-member interactions that are regarded as most helpful (Dies 1988). The level of self-disclosure and the nature of interpersonal feedback are the two dimensions of group process that are most frequently reported in the literature.

Numerous surveys on the topic of self-disclosure in group treatments have appeared over the years (e.g., Bednar and Kaul 1978; Kaul and Bednar 1986; Morran 1982; Stockton and Morran 1982). Most reviewers are rather critical of this body of literature for its failure to adequately address the multidimensional nature of this phenomenon; frequency, depth, timing, content, valence, and so forth are rarely examined (Dies 1977). Moreover, relatively few investigations have demonstrated unequivocal connections between any of these dimensions and therapeutic outcome. From their extensive review of the psychotherapy literature, however, Orlinsky and Howard (1986) concluded that self-exploration and the willingness to talk about problematic issues in therapy, especially when accompanied by a sense of responsibility about these issues, are related to significant clinical improvement. Similarly, they identified associations between positive outcome and patients' expressiveness and role-investment or engagement and especially between positive outcome and patients' self-relatedness or openness.

Morran (1982) cited studies showing that patients who are willing to reveal themselves are the ones most likely to benefit from group treatment, whereas those who are less open might even experience unfortunate treatment effects. Undoubtedly, the reciprocity of disclosure within the group, the level of available support, the corresponding feedback, the way that the personal material is integrated into a comprehensible framework for the individual, and other considerations will determine the value of therapeutic openness. For example, Morran (1982) noted that "too little self-disclosure will obviously limit a group member's opportunities to develop facilitative relationships. On the other hand, a member who discloses far more than anyone else in the group may frighten other members and thus experience rejection" (p. 220). There is also evidence to suggest that for more seriously impaired patients, who may not be as capable of discriminating between appropriate and inappropriate amounts and types of self-revelation, the encouragement of greater therapeutic openness may be counterproductive (Anchor 1979; Strassberg et al. 1975); therefore, more self-disclosure is not invariably better.

There is also a growing body of empirical literature on the value of interpersonal feedback within group treatments (e.g., Bednar and Kaul 1978; Kaul and Bednar 1986; Kivlighan 1985; Stockton and Morran 1982; Wing 1990). Once again, most reviewers are quite pessimistic about the quality of the research. The major indictment is the general insensitivity of investigators to the multifaceted nature of this concept. Stockton and Morran (1982) commented that little attention has been devoted to factors such as the effects of delayed versus immediate feedback, the impact of differing amounts of feedback, the influence of varying numbers of feedback sources, and the degree to which other members validate the messages conveyed. The clinical literature on this topic provides more enthusiastic endorsement (Yalom 1985, 1986).

Rothke (1989) described interpersonal feedback as a central communication process in which patients share their feelings and perceptions about another individual's behavior. He argued that the importance of feedback is based on its utility in labeling and reducing dysfunctional behaviors and on its facilitation of insight into how one's behavior affects others, the willingness to take greater responsibility for one's actions, and greater comfort in taking interpersonal risks. Yalom (1985, 1986) regarded feedback as the most important dimension of interpersonal work within group psychotherapy, and he provided extensive guidelines on how to optimize its therapeutic potential.

Kivlighan's review (1985) of the empirical literature is most informative. He found that for feedback to have any effect on an individual in group treatment it must be perceived as feedback and accepted as valid, and the group member must be willing to respond to the message. The findings suggest that the acceptance of feedback is influenced by the psychological closeness and level of trust established among group members. Favorable feedback is generally regarded as more credible, desirable, and powerful than negative feedback. Nonetheless, negative feedback may be viewed as quite constructive; this is especially true with a sequence of feedback delivery that has positive messages preceding more critical comments. Moreover, patients who receive a high proportion of both negative and positive personal reactions from comembers and those who both give and receive a high proportion of interpersonal feedback derive greater benefit from group therapy than patients who give and receive less feedback. Flowers et al. (1980) established that group members who adopted the most flexible roles over the course of group development (i.e., sender versus receiver, valence, and rate of delivery) had better coping abilities than those members who were less adaptable.

Two additional observations from Kivlighan's (1985) review have implications for therapists' interventions. The first is the generalized reluctance of people to deliver negative messages, so it seems that group leaders will have to model this behavior and prompt, reinforce, and shape the members' willingness and capacity to engage in constructive confrontation. The second relates to the potentially damaging effect of negative feedback delivered prematurely in the group's development. I have already underscored the importance of establishing a positive and supportive climate early in the life of the group. Because research shows that self-disclosure among members increases levels of group cohesion (e.g., Kirschner et al. 1978), it would appear that more attention should be focused on self-disclosure than feedback as the group is initially crystallizing its norms and refining its understanding of therapeutic work.

Additional leadership interventions are considered in the next section. The research on therapeutic factors, as well as empirical findings on both self-disclosure and feedback, have indicated that although the therapist may play a vital role in influencing the nature of these central processes, it is the quality of the interactions among group members that provides the foundation for effective group treatment. Certainly, group therapists cannot engage in the level of self-disclosure that is possible for group members (except, perhaps, in terms of feelings and reactions to "here-and-now" events), nor is their individual feedback likely to have an impact as consistently as the *consensual validation* communicated by co-members.

Later leadership interventions. From their extensive review of psychotherapy process and outcome research, Orlinsky and Howard (1986) concluded that certain interventions were likely to be correlated with patient improvement. Whereas support, advice, and therapist self-disclosure showed little differential relationship to outcome, confrontation, interpretation, and exploration were frequently effective. Unfortunately, the research on group leadership is rather sparse, so conclusions about specific techniques must be regarded as somewhat tentative. This observation is reflected in the opinions of the international experts, who gave therapist technique rather low ratings in terms of empirical understanding (Table 24–1).

The studies that have been published, however, indicate that Orlinsky and Howard's generalizations (1986), extracted largely from the individual psychotherapy literature, are applicable to group treatments as well. To illustrate, my surveys (Dies 1983b, 1986, 1988) of the leadership research document the value of interpretation as a principal vehicle for therapeutic change. Numerous investigations have shown that interventions "providing concepts for how to understand, explaining, clarifying, interpreting, and providing frameworks for how to change" (Lieberman et al. 1973, p. 238) foster significant levels of patient improvement. Findings suggest that highly abstract analyses by the group psychotherapist are not as valuable as interpretations more closely connected to the experiences of group members within the sessions. In other words, group interventions emphasizing the integration of group process interpretations and the understanding of current outside personal experiences seem more productive (Dies 1983b). Such interpretations more readily promote generalizability to contemporary interpersonal problems than those focused on providing "genetic insight" (i.e., insight into causes and childhood foundations for present conflicts). Because much of this research has been conducted with brief group treatments, it is not clear whether traditional insight would be assigned greater value in longer-term groups.

There is almost no research on therapist confrontation of patients receiving group treatments and only a few studies on the closely related dimension of feedback. Nonetheless, the conclusions about interpersonal feedback offered in the former section would intuitively apply to group leaders as well. From their critique of the individual psychotherapy literature, Beutler et al. (1986) asserted that more effective therapists tend to confront and interpret patient affect more often than do their less helpful counterparts. Moreover, clinicians who do not shy away from demonstrations of anger promote "more realistic and goal-directed expressions of affect on the part of their clients. Indeed, evidence from many sources suggests that rousing patient affect and motivating them to confront their fears enhances both cognitive and behavioral changes" (Beutler et al. 1986, p. 294). Because group members may be reluctant to confront potentially volatile feelings and are disinclined to deliver negative feedback (as noted above), it would appear that the group psychotherapist is uniquely qualified to shoulder this therapeutic responsibility.

Several prominent reviews (e.g., Beutler et al. 1986; Lambert et al. 1986; Orlinsky and Howard 1986) of the psychotherapy research literature have shown that therapist experience and competence play an instrumental role in treatment outcome. Although this topic has not been centrally highlighted in the group literature, it would not be unreasonable to assume that therapist experience and competence affect treatment outcome in a group setting as well, especially in light of the widespread belief that group interventions are inherently more complicated and difficult to master (Dies 1980). Certainly, the positive, open, and active interpersonal qualities emphasized throughout this chapter would be important regardless of therapeutic format, but group treatments pose unique challenges to the clinician. These challenges not only differentiate the group therapist from the practitioner engaged in one-to-one treatments, but also separate the role of the group leader from that of the patients within the group microcosm. Two areas of distinctiveness are particularly noteworthy.

Active structuring of the therapeutic task.   One vital role accentuated during the discussion of pregroup training and early and working phases of group development is the clinician's responsibility for active structuring of the therapeutic task. Before the inauguration of group treatment, the therapist works with patients to establish proper role and outcome expectations and to provide a coherent framework for individual change. This requires a thorough understanding of patient roles, group developmental phenomena, and the core therapeutic ingredients.

Once the group has been launched, the clinician must persistently intervene to establish the therapeutic potential of the group system (e.g., by building positive interpersonal norms, maximizing the potency of early therapeutic factors, and creating opportunities for patients to assume more of the responsibility for intensive interpersonal work). In the earlier phases of group life, the therapist prompts, structures, models, and reinforces. The preponderance of the therapist's interventions are probably more group centered and process oriented than focused on the content of individual group member's concerns. Yalom (1985), for example, provided extensive illustrations of how the clinician employs process illumination, here-and-now focus, and mass group commentary to steer the group toward more constructive interactions. The objective of such interventions is to circumvent obstacles that have stalled the progress of the entire group (e.g., anxiety-laden issues and antitherapeutic norms). Yalom (1985) noted that only the group therapist can effectively implement this role: "Forces prevent members from fully sharing that task with the therapist. One who comments on process sets oneself apart from the other members and is viewed with suspicion as 'not one of us'" (p. 146).

Abundant research evidence has shown that the group therapist is uniquely capable of maintaining the task focus and uniquely informed about how to guide the group process to accommodate the goals of the individual members. For example, Kivlighan and Jauquet (1990) have shown that members' goals become more realistic, interpersonal, and here-and-now oriented over the course of the group's life. Their findings suggest that "group leaders might want to focus on the realistic dimensions during early sessions and then shift their focus to the here-and-now and interpersonal dimensions during middle and late sessions" (p. 217). Given the therapist's designated responsibility to ensure that all members progress toward their individually defined goals and the therapist's specialized knowledge of group developmental phenomena, he or she is in the best position to intervene to manage the group system.

Interpretation and confrontation.   Later in the group's evolution, the therapist's second distinct role becomes more salient, with more of a person-directed stance regarding interpretation and confrontation. Scheidlinger (1987), for example, discussed four interrelated categories of verbal intervention that ostensibly promote self-awareness and insight in individual patients:

1. *Explanation and facilitation,* which represent efforts to move patients "into the role of 'good' patients and the aggregate of strangers into that of 'good' group" (pp. 346–347)
2. *Clarification,* or attempts to understand common experiences that have emerged during group sessions

3. *Confrontation* to direct attention to aspects of interaction, without attempting to uncover the latent meanings
4. *Interpretation* designed to convey an understanding of the underlying or dynamic significance of patients' behaviors or group-level events

Scheidlinger (1987) posited that the latter category is more specifically within the province of the psychotherapist who has "acquired and perfected the skill over many years of professional training and experience" (p. 348). Although clinicians may vary in their views regarding the relative contribution of patients to the interpretation and confrontation during the corrective working through of important personal issues, there is little doubt that the group therapist has a special role in this process.

Conclusions

Throughout this integration of the group psychotherapy research literature, it has been important to caution the reader about the tentative nature of the generalizations. These precautions have been necessary for three basic reasons:

1. The limited empirical foundations
2. The sheer complexity of group interventions
3. The chapter's predominant focus on short-term groups with moderately disturbed outpatient adults

In virtually every review of the research literature, the critics have pointed to the insufficient number of investigations, resulting in only a partial understanding of the phenomenon being considered. I noted, for example, the inadequacies in the literature on group developmental stages, cohesion, self-disclosure, feedback, therapeutic factors, and leadership technique. Investigators have generally explored only a few of the critical issues regarding these multidimensional group processes. The results from the survey of international experts on group psychotherapy research were consistent in showing that our knowledge of therapeutic outcome and process is far from complete. Indeed, there are major gaps in our empirical understanding of every facet of group treatments.

The principal reason for our short-sightedness, of course, is the enormous complexity of group therapy research (Dies 1990a). Although experimental designs and methodology have been refined over the years, it is still feasible to examine only sa very narrow domain of group outcome or process in any given study. Imagine the hundreds, or even thousands, of factors influencing therapeutic change. That we have been able to establish any consistency in our findings is an incredible accomplishment. To discover, for example, that an hour devoted to pregroup training may have a statistically significant, and clinically meaningful, impact on treatment outcome is genuinely astounding! Some might wonder whether my attempts to present a coherent model of group intervention based on empirical findings are entirely delusional, not based on fact, but grounded completely in misinterpretations stemming from a misreading of the research literature. Let's hope that the reader's own experiences are reasonably compatible with the conclusions presented in this chapter.

The choice to focus mainly on short-term, outpatient groups for moderately distressed adults was guided by the results of the survey of international experts on group research and by the nature of publications in the field, which more commonly address these types of group treatments. Clearly, the dimensions of open versus closed groups, context (e.g., inpatient versus private practice), treatment duration (i.e., time-limited versus long-term treatment), and a host of other parameters would shape the nature of the generalizations that are possible. There is widespread recognition, for instance, that brief treatments require the establishment of more modest goals, greater attention to task focus, prompt interventions, and more active participation on the part of the therapist (Dies 1983b, 1986, 1988). Unquestionably, these strategic modifications influence the patients' experience of treatment quite substantially.

The collaborative work among research-oriented clinicians has begun to establish a firm foundation for group interventions. This work will undoubtedly continue and contribute perceptibly to our understanding of how to optimize the uniquely powerful group processes that facilitate therapeutic gain. To assume, however, that we will ever fully comprehend group interventions on the basis of research would be an unreasonable expectation.

References

American Psychiatric Association: Diagnostic and Statistical Manual of Mental Disorders, 3rd Edition, Revised. Washington, DC, American Psychiatric Association, 1987

Anchor KN: High- and low-risk self-disclosure in group psychotherapy. Small Group Behavior 10:279–283, 1979

Bahrey F, McCallum M, Piper WE: Emergent themes and roles in short-term loss groups. International Journal of Group Psychotherapy 41:329–345, 1991

Barlow DH, Hayes, SC, Nelson RO: The Scientist Practitioner: Research and Accountability in Clinical and Educational Settings. New York, Pergamon, 1984

Bednar RL, Kaul TJ: Experiential group research: current perspectives, in Handbook of Psychotherapy and Behavior Change, 2nd Edition. Edited by Garfield SL, Bergin AE. New York, Wiley, 1978, pp 769–815

Bednar RL, Lawlis F: Empirical research in group psychotherapy, in Handbook of Psychotherapy and Behavior Change. Edited by Bergin AE, Garfield SL. New York, Wiley, 1971, pp 812–838

Bednar RL, Melnick J, Kaul TJ: Risk, responsibility, and structure: a conceptual framework for initiating group counseling and psychotherapy. Journal of Counseling Psychology 21:31–37, 1974

Bednar RL, Corey G, Evans NJ, et al: Overcoming the obstacles to the future development of research on group work. Journal for Specialists in Group Work 12:98–111, 1987

Beigel A, Sharfstein SS: Mental health care providers: not the only cause or only cure for rising costs. American Journal of Psychiatry 141:668–672, 1984

Benjamin LS: Principles of prediction using structural analysis of social behavior, in Personality and the Prediction of Behavior. Edited by Zucker RA, Arnoff J, Rabin AJ. New York, Academic Press, 1984, pp 227–241

Bennis WG: A critique of group therapy research. International Journal of Group Psychotherapy 10:63–77, 1960

Bernard HS: Guidelines to minimize premature terminations. International Journal of Group Psychotherapy 39:523–529, 1989

Beutler LE, Crago M, Arizmendi TG: Research on therapist variables in psychotherapy, in Handbook of Psychotherapy and Behavior Change, 3rd Edition. Edited by Garfield SL, Bergin AE. New York, Wiley, 1986, pp 257–310

Bloch S: Therapeutic factors in group psychotherapy, in American Psychiatric Association Annual Review, Vol 5. Edited by Frances AJ, Hales RE. Washington, DC, American Psychiatric Press, 1986, pp 678–698

Bloch S, Crouch E: Therapeutic Factors in Group Psychotherapy. Oxford, Oxford University Press, 1985

Bond GR: Norm regulation in therapy groups, in Advances in Group Psychotherapy: Integrating Research and Practice. Edited by Dies RR, MacKenzie KR. New York, International Universities Press, 1983, pp 171–189

Bonney WC, Randall DA, Cleveland JD: An analysis of client-perceived curative factors in a therapy group of former incest victims. Small Group Behavior 17:303–321, 1986

Brandsma JM, Pattison EM: The outcome of group psychotherapy with alcoholics: an empirical review. Am J Drug Alcohol Abuse 11:151–162, 1985

Burlingame GM, Fuhriman A: Conceptualizing short-term treatment: a comparative review. The Counseling Psychologist 15:557–595, 1990

Burnand G: Group development phases as working through six fundamental human problems. Small Group Research 21:255–273, 1990

Butler T, Fuhriman A: Curative factors in group therapy: a review of recent literature. Small Group Behavior 14:131–142, 1983

Cissna KN: Phases in group development: the negative evidence. Small Group Behavior 15:3–32, 1984

Corazzini JG, Heppner PP: Client-therapist preparation for group therapy: expanding the diagnostic interview. Small Group Behavior 13:219–236, 1982

Corcoran K, Fischer J: Measures for Clinical Practice: A Sourcebook. New York, Free Press, 1987

Dies RR: Group therapist transparency: a critique of theory and research. Int J Group Psychother 27:177–200, 1977

Dies RR: Group psychotherapy: reflections on three decades of research. Journal of Applied Behavioral Science 15:361–373, 1979

Dies RR: Group psychotherapy: training and supervision, in Psychotherapy Supervision. Edited by Hess AK. New York, Wiley, 1980, pp 337–366

Dies RR: Bridging the gap between research and practice in group psychotherapy, in Advances in Group Psychotherapy: Integrating Research and Practice. Edited by Dies RR, MacKenzie KR. New York, International Universities Press, 1983a, pp 1–26

Dies RR: Clinical implications of research on leadership in short-term group psychotherapy, in Advances in Group Psychotherapy: Integrating Research and Practice. Edited by Dies RR, MacKenzie KR. New York, International Universities Press, 1983b, pp 27–78

Dies RR: A multidimensional model for group process research: elaboration and critique. Small Group Behavior 16:427–446, 1985a

Dies RR: Research foundations for the future of group work. Journal for Specialists in Group Work 10:68–73, 1985b

Dies RR: Practical, theoretical, and empirical foundations for group psychotherapy, in The American Psychiatric Association Annual Review, Vol 5. Edited by Frances AJ, Hales RE. Washington, DC, American Psychiatric Press, 1986, pp 659–67

Dies RR: Clinical application of research instruments: editor's introduction. Int J Group Psychother 37:31–37, 1987

Dies RR: Issues in group leadership. Paper presented at the annual meeting of the American Group Psychotherapy Association, New York, February 1988

Dies RR: Reviews of group psychotherapy research. International Association of Group Psychotherapy Newsletter 7:8–11 1989a

Dies RR: Editorial committee report. American Group Psychotherapy Newsletter. 15:7–8, 1989b

Dies RR: Clinician and researcher: mutual growth through dialogue, in Expanding Domains of Psychodynamic Group Therapy. Edited by Tuttman S. Madison, CT, International Universities Press, 1990a, pp 379–408

Dies RR: Evaluation of the journal: a survey of authors and readers. Int J Group Psychother 40:225–230, 1990b

Dies RR, Emery M: Guidelines for authors. Int J Group Psychother 35:457–470, 1985

Dies RR, Riester AE: Research on child group therapy: present status and future directions, in Child Group Psychotherapy: Future Tense. Edited by Riester AE, Kraft I. New York, International Universities Press, 1986, pp 173–220

Dies RR, Teleska PA: Negative outcome in group psychotherapy, in Negative Outcome in Psychotherapy and What to Do About It. Edited by Mays DT, Fanks CM. New York, Springer, 1985, pp 118–141

Drescher S, Burlingame G, Furhiman A: A multidimensional model for group process research: elaboration and critique. Small Group Behavior 16:427–446, 1985

Erickson RC: The question of casualties in inpatient small group psychotherapy. Small Group Behavior 18:443–458, 1987

Evans NJ, Jarvis PA: Group cohesion: a review and reevaluation. Small Group Behavior 11:359–370, 1980

Flowers JV, Kenney BJ, Rotheram MJ: Group therapy cohesion and group member behavior: an experimental study. Small Group Behavior, 1980

Fuhriman A, Burlingame GM: Consistency of matter: a comparative analysis of individual and group process variables. The Counseling Psychologist 18:6–63, 1990

Galloucis M, Kaufman ME: Group therapy with Vietnam veterans: a brief review. Group 12:85–102, 1988

Garfield SL: Research on client variables in psychotherapy, in Handbook of Psychotherapy and Behavior Change, 3rd Edition. Edited by Garfield SL, Bergin AE. New York, Wiley, 1986, pp 213–256

Hartman JJ: Small group methods of personal change. Annu Rev Psychol 30:453–476, 1979

Huston K: A critical assessment of the efficacy of women's groups. Psychotherapy 23:283–290, 1986

Jacobs MK, Goodman G: Psychology and self-help groups: predictions on a partnership. Am Psychol 44:536–545, 1989

Johnson CL: Group counseling with blind people: a critical review of the literature. Journal of Visual Impairment and Blindness 85:202–207, 1989

Kanas N: Group therapy with schizophrenics: a review of the controlled studies. Int J Group Psychother 36:339–351, 1986

Kaul TJ, Bednar RL: Experiential group research: results, questions, and suggestions, in Handbook of Psychotherapy and Behavior Change, 3rd Edition. Edited by Garfield SL, Bergin AE. New York, Wiley, 1986, pp 671–714

Keisler DJ: Interpersonal methods of diagnosis and treatment, in Psychiatry, Vol 1. Edited by Cavenar JO. Philadelphia, PA, Lippincott, 1986, pp 1–23

Kirschner BJ, Dies RR, Brown RA: The effects of the experimental manipulation of self-disclosure on group cohesiveness. J Consult Clin Psychol 46:1171–1177, 1978

Kitchur M, Bell R: Group psychotherapy with preadolescent sexual abuse victims: literature review and description of an inner city group. Int J Group Psychother 38:285–310, 1989

Kivlighan DM: Feedback in group psychotherapy: review and implications. Small Group Behavior 16:373–385, 1985

Kivlighan DM, Jauquet CA: Quality of group member agendas and group session climate. Small Group Research 21:205–219, 1990

Kivlighan DM, Corazzini JG, McGovern TV: Pregroup training. Small Group Behavior 16:500–514, 1985

Klein RH: Some principles of short-term group therapy. Int J Group Psychother 35:309–330, 1985

Korda LJ, Pancrazio JJ: Limiting negative outcome in group practice. Journal for Specialists in Group Work 14:112–120, 1989

Lacoursiere R: The Life Cycle of Groups: Group Developmental Stage Theory. New York, Human Sciences Press, 1980

Lambert MJ, Shapiro DA, Bergin AE: The effectiveness of psychotherapy, in Handbook of Psychotherapy and Behavior Change. Edited by Garfield SL, Bergin AE. New York, Wiley, 1986

Leszcz M: Inpatient groups, in American Psychiatric Association Annual Review, Vol 5. Edited by Frances AJ, Hales RE. Washington, DC, American Psychiatric Press, 1986, pp 729–743

Leszcz M: Group therapy (personality disorders section), in Treatments of Psychiatric Disorders: A Task Force Report of the American Psychiatric Association. Washington, DC, American Psychiatric Association, 1989, pp 2667–2678

Leszcz M: Towards an integrated model of group psychotherapy with the elderly. Int J Group Psychother 40:379–399, 1990

Lewinsohn PM, Clarke GN: Group treatment of depressed individuals: the "Coping with Depression" course. Advances in Behavior Research and Theory 6:99–114, 1984

Liberman R: Reinforcement of cohesiveness in group therapy: behavioral and personality changes. Arch Gen Psychiatry 25:168–177, 1971

Lieberman MA: Comparative analyses of change mechanisms in groups, in Advances in Group Psychotherapy: Integrating Research and Practice. Edited by Dies RR, MacKenzie KR. New York, International Universities Press, 1983, pp 191–213

Lieberman MA: Self-help groups: an overview. Generations 10:45–49, 1985

Lieberman MA: Group properties and outcome: a study of group norms in self-help groups for widows and widowers. Int J Group Psychother 39:191–208, 1989

Lieberman MA: A group therapist perspective on self- help groups. Int J Group Psychother 40:251–278, 1990

Lieberman MA, Yalom ID, Miles MB: Encounter Groups: First Facts. New York, Basic Books, 1973

Livesley WJ, MacKenzie KR: Social roles in psychotherapy groups, in Advances in Group Psychotherapy: Integrating Research and Practice. Edited by Dies RR, MacKenzie KR. New York, International Universities Press, 1983, pp 117–135

Long LD, Cope CS: Curative factors in a male felony offender group. Small Group Behavior 11:389–397, 1980

MacDevitt JW, Sanislow C: Curative factors in offenders' groups. Small Group Behavior 18:72–81, 1987

MacKenzie KR: Therapeutic factors in group psychotherapy: a contemporary view. Group 11:26–34, 1987

MacKenzie KR: Introduction to Time-Limited Group Psychotherapy. Washington, DC, American Psychiatric Press, 1990

MacKenzie KR, Dies RR: CORE Battery: Clinical Outcome Results. New York, American Group Psychotherapy Association, 1982

MacKenzie KR, Livesley WJ: A developmental model for brief group therapy, in Advances in Group Psychotherapy: Integrating Research and Practice. Edited by Dies RR, MacKenzie KR. New York, International Universities Press, 1983, pp 101–116

Mayerson NH: Preparing clients for group therapy: a critical review and theoretical formulation. Clinical Psychology Review 4:191–213, 1984

Melnick J, Woods M: Analysis of group composition research and theory for psychotherapeutic and growth-oriented groups. Journal of Applied Behavioral Science 12:493–512, 1976

Morran DK: Leader and member self-disclosing behavior in counseling groups. Journal for Specialists in Group Work 7:218–223, 1982

Oesterheld JR, McHenna MS, Gould NB: Group psychotherapy of bulimia: a critical review. Int J Group Psychother 37:163–184, 1987

Orlinsky DE, Howard KI: Process and outcome in psychotherapy, in Handbook of Psychotherapy and Behavior Change, 3rd Edition. Edited by Garfield SL, Bergin AE. New York, Wiley, 1986, pp 311–381

Parloff MB, Dies RR: Group psychotherapy outcome research 1966–1975. Int J Group Psychother 27:281–319, 1977

Piper WE, Perrault EL: Pretherapy preparation for group members. Int J Group Psychother 39:17–34, 1989

Roback HB, Smith M: Patient attrition in dynamically oriented treatment groups. Am J Psychiatry 144:426–431, 1987

Robison FF, Morran KD, Hulse-Killacky D: Single-subject research designs for group counselors studying their own group. Journal for Specialists in Group Work 14:93–97, 1989

Rothke S: The role of interpersonal feedback in group psychotherapy. Int J Group Psychother 36:225–240, 1989

Scheidlinger S: On interpretation in group psychotherapy: the need for refinement. Int J Group Psychother 37:339–352, 1987

Schutz WC: On group composition. Journal of Abnormal and Social Psychology 62:275–281, 1961

Shapiro DA, Shapiro D: Meta-analysis of comparative outcome studies: a replication and refinement. Psychol Bull 92:581–604, 1982

Slocum YS: A survey of expectations about group therapy among clinical and nonclinical populations. Int J Group Psychother 37:39–54, 1987

Smith ML, Glass GV, Miller TI: The Benefits of Psychotherapy. Baltimore, MD, Johns Hopkins University Press, 1980

Solomon SD: Individual versus group therapy: current status in the treatment of alcoholism. Adv Alcohol Subst Abuse 2:69–86, 1982

Stockton R, Morran DK: Review and perspective of critical dimensions in therapeutic small group research, in Basic Approaches to Group Psychotherapy and Group Counseling. Edited by Gazda GM. Springfield, IL, Charles C Thomas, 1982, pp 37–85

Strassberg DS, Roback HB, Anchor KN, et al: Self-disclosure in group therapy with schizophrenics. Arch Gen Psychiatry 32:1259–1261, 1975

Subich LM, Coursol DH: Counseling expectations of clients and nonclients for group and individual treatment modes. Journal of Counseling Psychology 32:245–251, 1985

Tillitski CJ: A meta-analysis of estimated effect sizes for group versus individual versus control treatments. Int J Group Psychother 40:215–224, 1990

Tinsley HEA, Bowman SL, Ray SB: Manipulation of expectancies about counseling and psychotherapy: review and analysis of expectancy manipulation strategies and results. Journal of Counseling Psychology 35:99–108, 1988

Toseland RW, Rossiter CM: Group interventions to support family caregivers: a review and analysis. Gerontologist 29:438–448, 1989

Toseland RW, Siporin M: When to recommend group treatment: a review of the clinical and research literature. Int J Group Psychother 36:171–201, 1986

Tuckman BW: Developmental sequence in small groups. Psychol Bull 63:384–399, 1965

Unger R: Selection and composition criteria in group psychotherapy. Journal for Specialists in Group Work 14:151–157, 1989

Vinogradov S, Yalom ID: A Concise Guide to Group Psychotherapy. Washington, DC, American Psychiatric Press, 1990

Waltman DE, Zimpfer DG: Composition, structure, and duration of treatment: interacting variables in counseling groups. Small Group Behavior 19:171–184, 1988

Wetzler S (ed): Measuring Mental Illness: Psychometric Assessment for Clinicians. Washington, DC, American Psychiatric Press, 1989

Wiggins JS, Trapnell P, Phillips N: Psychometric and geometric characteristics of the revised Interpersonal Adjective Scales (IAS-R). Unpublished manuscript, Department of Psychology, University of British Columbia, Vancouver, British Columbia, 1987

Wing KT: Implications of feedback research for group facilitation and the design of experiential learning. Small Group Research 21:113–127, 1990

Winick C, Weiner MF: Professional activities and training of AGPA members: a view over two decades. Int J Group Psychother 36:471–476, 1986

Woods M, Melnick J: A review of group therapy selection criteria. Small Group Behavior 10:155–174, 1979

Yalom ID: The theory and practice of group psychotherapy, 3rd Edition. New York, Basic Books, 1985

Yalom ID: Interpersonal learning, in American Psychiatric Association Annual Review, Vol 5. Edited by Frances AJ, Hales RE. Washington, DC, American Psychiatric Press, 1986, pp 699–713

Zimpfer DG, Carr JJ: Groups for midlife career change: a review. Journal for Specialists in Group Work 14:243–250, 1989

PART VIII

Teaching and Training

CHAPTER 25

Training for Group Psychotherapy

Anne Alonso, Ph.D.

Introduction

Pioneers in group psychotherapy learned how to conduct groups in rather haphazard ways. Beginning in World War II, the clinical world was aware of the need to take care of a large number of patients and of the possibility of doing so capably in groups. Still, for a decade or so afterward, formal training programs did not exist in the United States except for rare experiments, such as the work of the National Training Labs in Bethel, Maine. Group psychotherapists learned mostly by observing one another at work, by reading the literature on group process, and by working at applying what we know about individual therapy to our work with patients in groups. Of necessity, the teachers had little experience and no formal training in group therapy.

In the decades that followed, it became obvious that group therapy was beginning to take its place as a modality that was recognized as a primary treatment option by the established clinical centers. Still, the presence or absence of a mentor tended to be the determining variable that predicted one's career as a group therapist. Gradually, it became clear that more formal training needed to be instituted—training that would allow a clinician to develop the unique skills of a group therapist and to learn the theory to support those skills. Most of this book addresses questions of theory and its application to patient populations and settings. In this chapter I discuss various training models and examine some of the stimuli that catalyze training and some of the factors that constitute an impediment to paying appropriate attention to the training of group psychotherapists in the 1990s.

The professional organizations in each of the major clinical disciplines now acknowledge the need for training in group therapy. However, criteria and models remain fairly nonspecific. For example, the American Medical Association, through the Association of Residency Training Directors, defines the following vague criteria in the *Directory of Graduate Medical Education Programs* (1989):

> Competence in formulating a differential diagnosis and treatment plan for all conditions in the current standard nomenclature, taking into consideration all relevant data. . . . Experience and competence in the major types of therapy including short and long term individual therapy, psychodynamic psychotherapy, family therapy, group therapy, behavior therapy, crisis intervention. (p. 106)

In terms of group therapy, there is certainly general agreement that such a curriculum needs to include some exposure to theory and some supervised clinical experience. Many programs also require the student to have some experiential learning, usually by participating in a training group offered by the department. A very few programs present an opportunity to conduct research in group therapy.

A review of the literature published by Dies (1980) found general agreement about the requirement for four component aspects of training for group psychotherapists: didactic, observational, experiential, and supervisory. The American Group Psychotherapy Association elaborated a specific set of guidelines for the training of group psychotherapists that forms the backdrop for their affiliate societies' training programs across the country. Beyond these general guidelines, there is little specificity or consistency across training settings and programs. They range across a wide terrain and respond to the theoretical philosophy of the setting.

A Model for an Ideal Training Program in Group Therapy

To organize and maintain an ideal training program in group psychotherapy in the current professional climate, several factors must be considered.

Didactic Aspects of Group Training

The abundance of psychological theories and therapeutic techniques presents an interesting challenge for the training of all therapists, and group leaders are no exception. We have not seriously debated the question of whether a trainee needs first to acquire some theoretical sophistication about individual dynamics before learning group dynamics, or whether they are best learned simultaneously. On the one hand, it can be argued that an in-depth knowledge of intrapsychic processes must precede a study of how these processes are expressed in the interpersonal milieu. On the other hand, the trainee's clinical experience first acquaints him or her with a patient's interactive world, from which the intrapsychic life must then be inferred. Given the latter perspective, it becomes important to learn both bodies of theory simultaneously, so that the neophyte clinician can make better sense of internal versus external influences on the patient's dynamics. Another major argument for the latter position has to do with a certain amount of imprinting. If the student is immersed first and only in the dyadic relationship with patients in the study of their intrapsychic life, the chances are that he or she will forever hold this as the primary and most legitimate position. Any other perspective will then be seen as ancillary and inferior. Such a bias will necessarily have a constricting impact on that clinician's future treatment planning and practice.

The basic theories about group development that constitute the didactic core of a training program must also be augmented by studying their applications in a variety of settings and to a particular patient population. These populations may be heterogeneous or homogeneous across demographics, symptom clusters, or diagnoses. Theories range from the more traditional psychodynamic methods (Rutan and Stone 1984, especially Chapters 1, 2, and 3) to cognitive-behavioral models (Lazarus 1968, especially Chapter 23) to humanistic theories (Rogers 1970), and to systems theory (von Bertalanffy 1968), among others. Pressures of cost containment have stimulated clinicians to study short-term treatment models (MacKenzie 1990, especially Chapter 22) and to develop research that assesses and compares those models with more long-term traditional models. A model program for group therapists needs help trainees become familiar with the research and to provide instruction in interpreting the research data that are available. Of course, the opportunity to conduct some research on groups is ideal although difficult to operationalize in the light of current training realities. Didactic teaching must avoid too narrow a perspective by including a range of theories, with some attention to the areas of conflict and agreement among them. This book is organized to facilitate and encourage just this kind of critical integration.

Training by Observation

The observational aspects of training can include participating as a cotherapist in a group led by a senior clinician, studying videotapes of group sessions led by senior clinicians followed by a scholarly discussion of the material, and sitting in as a silent observer with a supervisor or mentor. In some settings, groups led by senior clinicians may be observed "live" through one-way mirrors (Rutan and Alonso 1980).

Training by Experience

Experiential learning via participation in a training group is discussed at length in Chapter 26. Fundamentally, I believe that some kind of experiential learning is crucial; this may include participating in a training group offered by the training institution, joining a personal therapy group as a member, or participating in group experiences at conferences, such as the group experiences offered at the Institute arm of the American Group Psychotherapy Association annual conference.

Supervision of Group Psychotherapy

Supervision may be conducted in a variety of settings. The dyadic supervisory setting has the advantage of simplicity and availability (Coche 1977). Some supervise individually, but this method conflicts with faith in the group as a primary medium for growth and change. Supervision of group therapy is ideally conducted in supervisory groups. This model offers specific opportunities to study and participate in group processes. Keeping in mind that the medium is the message, supervising group therapists in groups clearly demonstrates the power inherent in the model. The supervisory group offers many of the advantages of the therapy group.

Mitigation of shame.   The supervisory group helps to mitigate shame by providing a setting in which exposure is safe and respectful. The movement from novice to expert clinician inevitably leads the trainee along a path littered with stumbling blocks that can challenge the self-esteem of even the most confident student. Although this is true for all aspects of clinical training, in groups the potential for stumbling is increased exponentially because of the multiplicity of individual dynamics interacting in a heated group-as-a-whole context. The patients are afraid of being shamed, but the clinician is also vulnerable to painful exposure before all those patients.

Support.   The supervisory group offers support from peers as well as from the leader. The opportunity to display one's work before peers and a sympathetic expert offers the chance to brave the exposure and to experience one's own and one's colleagues' errors and victories as an ordinary part of the work, which brings the work down to tolerable human scale. The trainee learns both experientially and theoretically how to manage the problems around shame and exposure in his or her group patients.

Opportunity to observe others' experiences.   The supervisory group expands the intellectual and clinical horizons of the members by allowing them to observe the others' experiences in groups. Most group training is severely limited by the constraints of time and opportunity, plus some other nonspecific factors that are discussed later in this chapter. Thus trainees tend to be involved in only one or two groups—a sparse accumulation of experience by any standards. By participating actively in a supervision group, one hears and is vicariously caught up in the groups presented by the other members in the supervisory hour.

Encouragement of competition.   The supervisory group encourages healthy competition that stimulates experimentation and dialogue around theory and technique. Because no two clinicians are identical in their application of clinical theory or the technique that flows from that theory, the supervisory group often becomes a heated arena for dialogue, for subtle and not-so-subtle one-upmanship among the members, and for challenges to the supervisor's stance. Out of this intellectual ferment, students often will take risks that bring about unexpected results, both for better and worse. The ensuing discussions can provide a fertile ground for new learning for students and supervisor alike.

Expansion of empathic capacity.   The supervisory group is an effective method for expanding the empathic capacity of each leader because one listens to how one's peers understand one's patient group and how they interpret it. Every clinician is talented in a certain range of empathic connections and limited in other dimensions as well. Some of the limits to empathy have to do with the fear and inexperience that a novice leader will bring to the difficult work of group treatment. However, one's colleagues are apt to be in tune with the clinical issues in a different range of empathy, and their view of the group can open the therapist's eyes to a greater awareness of the universe of internal experience of the group and its members.

Relief of projective-identification problems. The supervisory group is a way of relieving the therapist in the throes of unconscious projective identification. The problem of projective identifications in the therapy group is not necessarily related to the level of calm or experience of the clinician. One of the most powerful curative forces in a therapy group is the opportunity for each member to temporarily disown the more noxious aspects of the self by eliciting them in another. That other is a willing participant in this process in exchange for like favors. Each unconsciously splits off that unacceptable part of himself or herself, thereby reducing each person's anxiety. At best, this allows the work of analysis to proceed, until each is ready to reown the split-off parts of his or her own personality. The whole therapy group also can join in a groupwide projective identification with the leader, who may end up feeling the disowned aspects of one or more members as his or her own and react unwittingly from that frame of reference. Of course, when this happens the leader's neutrality and, along with it, his or her capacity for empathy for those members caught in the projective identifications with the clinician are compromised. In a parallel process, the supervisory group will replicate this dilemma. Free of the force field of the therapy group's projective identifications, the colleagues and supervisor can help the clinician separate his or her own boundaries from those of the members. In fact, the members of the supervisory group may selectively be able to empathize with the therapy group members in a way that broadens the leader's empathic range for the patients.

An ideal model for a group therapy training program integrates all of the above factors as follows:

The training program should have a minimum duration of 2 years.

1. *Didactic:* Weekly seminar, 1.5 hours in duration, for integrative study of theory and techniques. (See Appendix 25–A for a sample bibliography for such a seminar.)
2. *Clinical experience:* Conduct one group for the entire 2 years, plus several time-limited groups, including inpatient and outpatient experiences.
3. *Supervision:* Supervisory group for 1.5 hours per week for 2 years.

4. *Experiential:* Participation in a training group for 2 years. Exposure to other, briefer training experiences such as participating in two or more American Group Psychotherapy Association Institutes.

The above model represents an ideal case. It may be necessary in any given program to develop compromises. For example, two 45-minute supervisory sessions a week or a 1-year training experience may be what is feasible given the scarcity of resources.

The Mental Health Climate as It Impinges on Group Training

As always in a time of scarcity of resources, a treatment that promises to deliver first-class health care efficiently and parsimoniously is welcome in clinics and managed health care settings, as well as in the private practitioner's consultation room. Thus group therapy is emerging as a highly desirable option. At the same time it is still viewed as a supplemental or second-class treatment option by many of the more traditionally trained clinicians who are the directors of these health delivery systems. This hidden devaluation of the modality emerges from a variety of sources. Most psychotherapists first learned how to treat patients individually, and they spent vastly more time training in individual therapy than in group therapy. Thus senior clinicians still tend to value the dyadic model as "first class" out of a bias unmodified by personal experience. More often than not, their own treatment was dyadic in nature. Some of them may have experienced painful times in their training groups, and the memory has led them to avoid group models. This bias may now clash with their current intellectual appreciation of the usefulness of group therapy as a primary treatment for psychological distress. They give lip service to the practice of group therapy with insufficient conviction and enthusiasm. Of course, their bias is not lost on the trainees, who may collude in the avoidance by failing to put together large enough and cohesive enough groups for a successful training opportunity or by relegating group treatment to very impaired patients only. The system may collude further by selecting out the "best" patients for individual treatment. The most successful group training programs are those in which the chief of the entire service is perceived as an enthusiastic practitioner of group therapy.

Another complicating factor relates to the rotation of leadership of groups due to the limited availability of clinicians in training. Because trainees in most clinics conduct groups with severely ill patients and because they regularly must abandon these groups as they graduate, the groups themselves never get far beyond the earliest stages of cohesion before they are again traumatized by the loss of yet another leader. This results in frequent dropouts from the groups, which dishearten the leader, who may become further convinced that the method is not effective. Thus a vicious circle is established. One way of mitigating this effect is to place the trainee in a cotherapist dyad with a staff person who will remain with the group over the long haul and who will carry the history of the group from one generation of leaders-in-training to another.

Supervision is an underrated process in the best of times, and in times of scarcity, the availability of supervisory resources may be diminished in favor of the billable hour (Alonso 1985). Supervisors may be disheartened in such times, and they may feel devalued by the system. If this devaluing of the supervisory experience is not counterbalanced by attention to the intellectual stimulation and morale of the group supervisors, the sense of subtle (or not-so-subtle) burnout will permeate the learning environment in group therapy and other psychotherapies.

The increased reliance on biological treatments may tempt the trainee away from investment in psychotherapy in favor of learning the biological at the expense of the psychological. It is encouraging, however, to see the emergence of research that demonstrates the synergy of psychological and biological interventions, such as that demonstrating the benefits for breast cancer patients treated in support groups (Spiegel et al. 1989). The media are reporting the arguments for and against the validity of such research data, but the fact is that ideal training integrates both psychological and biological interventions. It is obvious that the care of emotional distress is prohibitively expensive for many. The clinician who wishes to serve patients beyond the prosperous few has never had a better incentive for learning how to conduct expert group psychotherapy.

Teaching and Learning About Group Therapy Beyond the Formal Training Years

It is often difficult for a professional helper to acknowledge his or her own need for help and support, let alone to ask for such. Opportunities for continued learning in group therapy are explored elsewhere in this book and include membership in professional organizations such as the American Group Psychotherapy Association, peer group discussions, journals, membership in experiential learning groups, and conducting research in the area of group therapy. Supervisors of group therapy would also derive benefit from collegial study of teaching methods to utilize with their trainees. As we are pressed to provide group treatment, we may serendipitously find ourselves in a golden age of evolving techniques and theories that provide exciting elaborations of the practice of group psychotherapy.

References

Alonso A: The Quiet Profession: Supervisors of Psychotherapy. New York, Macmillan, 1985

Coche E: Supervision in the training of group therapists, in Supervision, Consultation, and Staff Training in the Helping Professions. Edited by Kaslow FW. San Francisco, CA, Jossey-Bass, 1977, pp 219–231

Dies R: Group psychotherapy: training and supervision, in Psychotherapy Supervision. Edited by Hess AK. New York, John Wiley, 1980, pp 337–362

Lazarus AA: Behavior therapy in groups, in Basic Approaches to Group Psychotherapy and Group Counseling. Edited by Gazda GM. Springfield, IL, Charles C Thomas, 1968, pp 149–175

MacKenzie KR: Introduction to Time-Limited Group Psychotherapy. Washington, DC, American Psychiatric Press, 1990

Rogers CR: On Encounter Groups. New York, Harper & Row, 1970

Rutan JS, Alonso A: Sequential cotherapy of groups for training and clinical care. Group 4:40–50, 1980

Rutan JS, Stone W: Psychodynamic Group Psychotherapy. Lexington, MA, DC Heath, 1984

Spiegel D, Blom JR, Kraemer HC, et al: Effect of psychosocial treatment on survival of patients with metastatic breast cancer. Lancet ii:888–891, 1989

von Bertalanffy L: General Systems Theory: Foundations, Development, Applications. New York, George Braziller, 1968

Appendix 25–A

Sample Bibliography

Alonso A, Rutan JS: Uses and abuses of transference interpretations in groups, in Progress in Group and Family Therapy. Edited by Aronson ML, Wolberg LW. New York, Brunner/Mazel, 1983, pp 23–30

Alonso A, Rutan JS: The treatment of shame and the restoration of self respect in groups. Int J Group Psychother 38:3–14, 1988

Arsenian J, Semrad EV, Shapiro D: An analysis of integral functions in small groups. Int J Group Psychother 12:421–434, 1962

Bach GR: Intensive Group Psychotherapy. New York, Ronald Press, 1954

Bader BR, Bader LJ, Budman S, et al: Pre-group preparation model for long-term group psychotherapy in a private practice setting. Group 5:43–50, 1981

Bion WR: Experiences in Groups. New York, Basic Books, 1960

Borriello JF: Leadership in the therapist centered group-as-a-whole approach. Int J Group Psychother 26:149–162, 1976

Christ J: Contrasting the charismatic and reflective leader, in The Leader in the Group. Edited by Liff ZA. New York, Jason Aronson, 1975, pp 104–113

Durkin H: The Group in Depth. New York, International Universities Press, 1964

Ezriel H: Psychoanalytic group therapy, in Group Therapy: 1973. Edited by Wolberg LR, Schwartz EK. New York, Stratton Intercontinental Medical Books, 1973, pp 183–210

Foulkes SH: Introduction to Group-Analytic Psychotherapy. London, Heinemann, 1948

Foulkes SH, Anthony EJ: Group Psychotherapy: The Psychoanalytic Approach, 2nd Edition. Baltimore, MD, Penguin Books, 1965

Freud S: Group psychology and the analysis of the ego (1921), in The Standard Edition of the Complete Psychological Works of Sigmund Freud, Vol 18. Translated and edited by Strachey J. London, Hogarth Press, 1955, pp 67–143

Glatzer HT: Handling transference resistance in group therapy. Psychoanal Rev 40:36–43, 1953

Glatzer HT: The working alliance in analytic group psychotherapy. Int J Group Psychother 28:147–161, 1978

Grunebaum H, Kates W: Whom to refer for group psychotherapy. Am J Psychiatry 132:130–133, 1977

Kadis AL, Krasner JD, Winick C, et al: A Practicum of Group Psychotherapy. New York, Harper & Row, 1963

Kauff PF: Diversity in analytic group psychotherapy: the relationship between theoretical concepts and technique. Int J Group Psychother 29:51–66, 1979

LeBon G: The Crowd: A Study of the Popular Mind. New York, Ronald Press, 1957

Malan DH, Balfour FHG, Hood VG, et al: Group psychotherapy: a long term follow-up study. Arch Gen Psychiatry 33:1303–1315, 1976

McDougall W: The Group Mind. New York, GP Putnam, 1920

Pines M: The frame of reference of group psychotherapy. Int J Group Psychother 31:275–285, 1981

Rice AK: Individual, group, and intragroup processes. Human Relations 22:565–584, 1969

Rutan JS, Alonso A: Some guidelines for group therapists. Group 1:4–13, 1978

Rutan JS, Alonso A: Group therapy, individual therapy, or both? Int J Group Psychother 32:267–282, 1982

Rutan JS, Rice CA: The charismatic leader: asset or liability? Psychotherapy and Training: Theory Research Practice 18:487–492, 1981

Scheidlinger S: On the concept of mother-group. Int J Group Psychother 24:417–428, 1974

Slavson SR: Analytic Group Psychotherapy. New York, Columbia University Press, 1950

Stone WN: The curative fantasy in group psychotherapy, in Group Therapy (monograph No. 10). New York, The Washington Square Press, 1983

Stone WN, Gustafson JP: Technique in group psychotherapy of narcissistic and borderline patients. Int J Group Psychother 32:29–47, 1984

von Bertalanffy L: General system theory and psychiatry, in American Handbook of Psychiatry. Edited by Arieti S. New York, Basic Books, 1966, pp 705–721

Wolf A, Schwartz E: Psychoanalysis in Groups. New York, Grune & Stratton, 1962

Wong N: Clinical considerations in group treatment of narcissistic disorders. Int J Group Psychother 29:325–345, 1979

Yalom ID: The Theory and Practice of Group Psychotherapy. 2nd Edition. New York, Basic Books, 1975

Zetzel E: Current concepts of transference. Int J Psychoanal 37:369–376, 1956

CHAPTER 26

Process Groups for Training Psychiatric Residents

Hillel I. Swiller, M.D.
Enid A. Lang, M.D.
David A. Halperin, M.D.

Definition

A *process group* is a group that studies its own behavior in order for it its members to learn about group dynamics, individual dynamics, and interpersonal communications. Process groups usually exist as part of a training program for mental health professionals. Generally they are led by experienced group therapists and work in confidence. When such a group functions well, it has the added benefit of being a source of support to its members during what can be a difficult time—learning to work with the mentally ill.

Models other than the one developed at the Mount Sinai School of Medicine and described in this chapter were reported by several authors (Jensen 1983; Salvendy and Stewart 1983; Willenbring and Spensley 1983). Some aspects of this model were described in a recent publication (Lang et al. 1989). This chapter is intended to be a comprehensive overview of the value of, problems with, and technique for such a group as explored and developed by us and our colleagues during the past 15 years. This model has been developed in work with psychiatric residents

We would like to thank Drs. Herman Alpert, Daniel Birger, Lawrence Bloom, Sylvia Flescher, Philip Luloff, Gail Meisel, Fred Sander, Morton Seigel, Allen Terdiman, James Welch, and the late Richard Bralove. This work was begun under and inspired by the leadership of the late Aaron Stein.

and is reported in that fashion, but with minor modifications it is applicable to the training of any mental health professionals.

Value of the Process Group

Value for Psychiatric Residents

Few professional experiences are as stressful as the psychiatric residency. Intimate contact with psychotic patients generates anxiety and depression in everyone, but especially in the beginner. To feel ignorant, powerless, and under relentless scrutiny—much of it hostile—is enormously difficult, especially when the beginner feels deep bonds with the first patients whom he or she treats. Yet this is the role of the psychiatric resident. Moreover, new psychiatric residents have finished their medical training, where ambiguities were minimized, and entered a field of great ambiguity. Most importantly, they find themselves in the uncomfortable position of being assessed not only on the basis of what they know—a familiar experience for a medical school graduate—but also on the basis of who they are. For example, their capacity for empathy, minimally improved by hard work, is open to critical evaluation. Clearly, responsible support is called for. In addition, this is a time when residents must cope with becoming adults in their personal lives. They may be marrying, separating, and bearing or raising children, and they may be dealing with decisions about these matters. They may also be caring for aging parents.

The process group offers residents support by helping them understand the universality of their experience. When it functions well, the group fosters esprit de corps in the residency cohort, enabling individual members to better withstand the pressures of training. Another meaningful dimension of support is the relationship with the process group leaders.

The process group is a unique opportunity. It offers residents the chance to learn experientially about some of the most difficult and important areas in psychiatry. By studying their own behavior as a group, they can learn in unusual depth about group dynamics, individual dynamics, and interpersonal communications.

Value for the Faculty and Administration

The process group provides the best possible teaching in group dynamics. In an age of increasing cost accountability, administrations increasingly value group therapy as a treatment modality. Here the residents learn through first-hand experience. The process group is also useful in achieving other teaching goals. It is of great value for instruction in both interpersonal communications and intrapsychic dynamics. In each of these areas, teaching is enriched by transcending the strictly intellectual. Concepts such as resistance and defense are taught most powerfully when part of the teaching is experiential.

People work better when they feel understood and supported. People work better when they have greater understanding of the stresses they must meet.

Value for the Process Group Leaders

The psychiatric residents' process group provides the group leaders with a unique opportunity to work with highly motivated, intelligent, and healthy group members. These groups often work far more rapidly and in greater depth than all but the most highly functioning patient groups. For leaders this represents both a challenge and an extraordinary opportunity to learn and to sharpen their skills. When combined with peer supervision, leadership of process groups provides one of the best continuing-education tools available to senior clinicians.

Objections to Process Group

Objections by Residents

Many residents' major objection to process groups is their fear of self-exposure to the leaders, to the departmental administration through the leaders, and to their peers. This fear is best dealt with directly by ensuring the leaders' confidential relationship with the group. Leaders should make no reports to the administration about the group and should have no administrative or teaching relationship with the group members. If the small size of the faculty makes this difficult, it is far better to bring in outside leaders for the group than to compromise the leaders' obligation for confidentiality.

The issue of exposure to one's peers is a far more complicated one. The reality is that residents have ongoing collegial and competitive relationships with each other. Regardless of contention for chief residencies, for fellowships, and for jobs, they must continue to work together. What makes for appropriate self-revelation in such a context forms a theme that runs through the life of every residents' process group. There is no simple answer. Addressing this issue at different times throughout the life of the group is an important learning experience.

Occasionally, process group members find that the experience is distressing in ways that can be neither adequately addressed nor contained by the group. These group members have the right to discontinue their participation in the group with no penalty in their training. A very few leave with an animosity toward training groups (and, by extension, toward group therapy), which persists. This is unfortunate but must be seen in an appropriate perspective: rigorous training in any modality is not for everyone. People leave residencies in internal medicine and in surgery. If the proportion of group members who drop out remains small, it must be seen as inevitable in the context of training. (Obviously, a substantial number of dropouts is another matter.)

Objections by Faculty and Administration

The misuse of the process group as a revolutionary commissariat is invariably a major concern of the departmental administration. Will the residents use the group solely to discuss their grievances and to project their hostility outward and onto the administration? Process groups can be misused in this way. Clearly if this misuse persists, it represents a failure of group leadership. Experienced leaders will recognize this tendency as a group resistance and will encourage the members to learn from this group dynamic as from any other.

The administration may be concerned that the process group will precipitate a psychotic decompensation in a marginally healthy resident. This concern is a responsible one, but it is based on a misunderstanding of process group dynamics. Group therapy can be stressful. Far more often, however, it is supportive. Fragile residents are much more apt to draw strength from a process group. There are many regressive situations that a resident experiences during psychiatric training. Those that take place in the process group are the only ones that the resident experiences in the immediate presence of a senior clinician. Leaders will act to prevent scapegoating or other undue peer pressures. The stressed resident always has the option of avoiding the group; this choice should be respected by leaders and administration alike. The reason that process groups can be unfairly held responsible for resident difficulties is that in the relatively public atmosphere, a resident's difficulties may first come to inescapable notice. This in no way means that they developed there. In fact, an asset of the process group is that it may help to identify those residents in need of help earlier than might otherwise be possible. Some may be directed to early personal therapy. Others who find emotionally regressive situations deeply disturbing may wisely reevaluate their choice of the field.

Differences Between a Process Group and a Psychotherapy Group

The leaders of a process group do not have a mandate to do psychotherapy. The parameters of difference between the two kinds of groups include time, membership, subgrouping, and termination.

Time

In a therapy group, the therapist sets the time and length of the group meetings. In a process group, the administration sets both the length and time of the group sessions. In addition, a therapy group may run for an indeterminate length of time, with members leaving as they improve. The time that a process group runs is usually limited by the completion of the training program. Incidentally, it has been our experience that the optimal period for the residents to be in a process group is the full 3 years of the training program, beginning the first week of the first year of the residency and ending in the last week of the third year of the residency. However, many programs offer a much shorter group experience.

Membership

In a therapy group, the therapist selects the patients to be in a group; in a process group, membership is determined by presence in a resident cohort, chosen by the administration. All members of the cohort are invited to attend.

Subgrouping

In psychotherapy groups there is a strict rule forbidding socialization outside the group. In a process group the members must work together all the time. Because the members have extragroup relations, self-disclosure is not always indicated.

Termination

Termination of a patient from a therapy group is an individual event that ends the member's participation in the group, but not necessarily the status of patienthood. Termination in a process group occurs for all members at the same time and is marked by the transition to a position of equality or collegiality between the leaders and the members.

Contract

The contract the leader makes with a process group is complicated by the involvement of a third party—the administration. As in most significant relationships, an unclear contract is a prescription for trouble. It is essential that all three parties to the process group contract be clear about the agreement. The administration should agree that the process group is an important part of the teaching program, as well as agreeing to provide a place and a time to meet. This is not as simple as it sounds. In a training program members of the faculty invariably contend for trainees' time. Encroachment on the time of the training group can easily become a problem. The administration must further agree that the leaders' relationship with the group is confidential. Administration personnel should neither expect nor receive any reports on residents' work in the group. Although the administration may wish to receive occasional reports about group attendance (partly to help evaluate the function of the group), it should be understood that such reports will be limited to the number of residents attending and will not include information about specific residents. The administration must agree that the leaders will provide no evaluations of the work, talents, or limitations of specific group members.

The leaders agree that it is their task to help the group study its own behavior. Through this study the leaders agree that they will help the members increase their knowledge of group and individual dynamics and of interpersonal communications. The leaders agree that they will keep the proceedings of the group confidential and will have no other administrative or instructional role in the work of the members of the group. The members of the group agree that they will participate in the work of the group. Seen from one perspective, the contract forms the boundaries of the group, and it therefore will be a subject of many discussions within the group. Especially early in the group's development, boundary issues will be prominent, with topics such as confidentiality addressed over and over. This work on the contract is stage appropriate and may be useful early in the group but may become a resistance at a later time.

Teaching Through the Process Group

Group Dynamics

The group has the agreed-on task of studying its own behavior, and yet obstacles to this work continually arise. Unconscious dependent, aggressive, and erotic wishes arise in the group as they do everywhere. These wishes, and the defensive responses to them, dominate the group unless they are recognized and acknowledged. By inviting the group to consider this phenomenon of resistance to self-study and encouraging the group to investigate the nature of the specific mechanisms of resistance, the leaders enable the group to learn the essence of group dynamics both experientially and intellectually. This invitation to address resistance must be supplemented—particularly early in the group's development—by the leaders' providing information to overcome the group's ignorance. It should be noted that the process group usually does not address unconscious strivings in their most primitive aspects. Such work generally requires psychoanalytic data not available to the group. Primitive wishes are addressed at the appropriate level of derivatives. For example, it is generally more relevant to address the competitive feeling in regard to becoming a chief resident than to spend a great deal of time on unadulterated patricidal wishes. The latter discussion may represent a resistance on the part of the leaders. One deals with the material at the level where affect is both available and prominent.

Boundaries

The group can learn a lot about itself if the leaders help members with an investigation of the group's boundaries, including the boundaries of time and place of the meetings. For example, the residents might resent that the process group is scheduled to meet from 1 to 2 P.M., leaving them no time to eat lunch. Could the process group leaders please shift the time of the meeting? It can be pointed out that the group is testing many boundaries with that request: they are testing their power over the leaders, they are testing the leaders' clout with the administration in their ability to change a fixed schedule, and they are evaluating the level of concern that the leaders have for the group, that is, do the leaders care if they are fed? The leaders must function as gatekeepers of the boundaries by seeing that the designated room is available on time, by being on time, and by closing the door at the starting time of the meeting. Any failure of the leaders as boundary keepers will appear in the themes of the process group. For example, if the leaders have been ineffective in getting the previous users of the meeting room out of the space on time, the group will see the leaders as impotent. As a consequence a group member might supplant the role of the leaders by closing the door. Although such behavior in a psychotherapy group might be interpreted in terms of the group member's oedipal strivings, in a process group the member's behavior can be fruitfully explored in terms of boundary issues.

The boundary of confidentiality remains an important issue for the group throughout its beginning phase. If a training program has a tradition of process groups, new residents come to the first meeting of the group with some information about what happens in process groups from residents in other years. What the residents have learned forms an unspoken group "myth" and must be explored by the leaders with the group. Another boundary that the group explores for its entire life is the boundary of content or appropriateness. Residents wonder what can be said by the leaders, or more importantly, by the residents themselves. Occasionally, residents who are most outspoken about their feelings about themselves or other group members leave the process group or even the training program. When this happens, the leaders have to discuss the member's leaving or absence in terms of the boundaries or norms set by the rest of the group.

Another boundary to be studied is the group composition. Group composition includes who is present and absent at a particular session as well as who is in the resident cohort that makes up the process group. The exploration of this boundary is especially relevant when an impaired resident has been included in the training cohort. Group process leaders will find an exploration of boundaries with the residents to be very instructive and revealing, as well as being a nonjudgmental vehicle for handling the many emotionally charged issues that may arise within the group.

Individual Dynamics

The study of psychodynamics is incomplete without introspective reflection. Leaders do not focus the group's attention on any individual's specific dynamics. Although the process group is primarily concerned with group issues, learning about individual dynamics invariably takes place.

It is worth noting at this point that honest, affectively charged interaction combined with thoughtful reflection on oneself produces personal change and growth. Psychotherapy is not a goal of the process group, but one should not shy away from the reality that personal growth may accompany a process group experience. One may with justice call this a psychotherapeutic outcome of what has been entered on as a learning experience. Most process groups will address this apparent contradiction at some time or other. Trainees must recognize that it is a basic demand of the field (not just of the process group) that the endeavor to do psychotherapy with others requires the clinician to accept all relevant opportunities for personal growth.

Interpersonal Communication

In the process group each member is offered unusually candid feedback regarding his or her style of interpersonal communication. Members are told here, as they are told almost nowhere else, by a group of intelligent, motivated, and trained observers what works, what doesn't, and why. Additionally, all members observe one another and have the opportunity to study alternative styles in depth. Members can and do attempt to incorporate aspects of each other's style into their own repertoire.

Support

The stresses of training and life events call for supportive remarks, such as "it must be hard for you to discuss these things with people you're not sure you trust." Depending on their individual style, leaders could point out the universal aspects of a problem that the group or its members are having. In some cases a personal anecdote about the leaders is helpful. Whatever techniques are employed, enough warmth must be provided to sustain, in Winnicott's terms, "good enough" leaders maintaining an adequate "holding environment." The process group can do work only in an environment that engenders trust. Thus the qualifications of process group leaders should include a certain level of personal warmth and confidence, in addition to a deep understanding of groups. Indeed, one of the most supportive tasks of group leaders is to be good role models.

The humanness of the leaders, as expressed through humor and self-candor, helps the residents deal with authority figures. The termination stage of the process group provides opportunities for the residents to establish collegiality with the leaders without abandoning the task of the group understanding itself.

Differences Between and Similarities of Process Groups and Psychotherapy Groups

Because process groups and therapy groups share certain characteristics, it is important to explicitly delineate their differences. First and foremost, they have different reasons for existing. The therapy group exists to provide therapy for its members; the process group exists as an educational tool. Members join the former to relieve some element of suffering; members join the latter to increase their learning.

Generally speaking, the leader of a therapy group selects (or at least participates in the selection of) the group members and chooses the time and place of the meetings. The ongoing therapy group is open ended; members join and leave the group as individuals. In the process group, leaders have no voice in member selection and little influence as to time and place, and the group is closed, with all members starting and completing their work together. The leaders thus have far less discretion in the formation and boundaries of the process group than of the therapy group, and the membership has different expectations.

Members of a therapy group have agreed to participate in psychotherapy and therefore have ostensibly agreed to a greater degree of self-revelation and self-exploration than members of a process group. Of course, not all members of therapy groups prove willing to uphold this aspect of their contract, and with such members the work is often unsuccessful. Conversely, some members of process groups are willing to move quite deeply into self-exploration, if not into self-revelation, and for such members the process group experience may be particularly helpful.

One cannot truly learn about psychodynamics without learning about oneself, and one rarely learns profound things about oneself without consequent change and growth. Although it is not the goal of a process group to provide its members with therapy, some members will find the experience therapeutic. The leaders of the process group should not explore individual dynamics with the rigor that they would in a therapy group, but they must be willing to acknowledge that the distinction between the two types of groups is not always perfectly clear. The boundary between therapy and education is not always easily drawn.

Subgrouping has very different meanings in the two types of groups. In psychodynamic therapy groups, subgrouping is invariably a resistance. In the process group, subgrouping is primarily an outgrowth of the out-of-group work relationships among the members. Resistance elements of subgrouping within the boundaries of the process group should be addressed, but the phenomenon of subgrouping itself must be respected as natural and productive.

Techniques of Leadership

The techniques for leadership of a process group follow ineluctably from an awareness of the contract and of the similarities and differences between process groups and psychotherapy groups. The leaders direct their attention toward group dynamics while maintaining an awareness of the frame of the group established by its goal (self-study) and its boundaries (membership, time, place, confidentiality, and content). As the group proceeds, unconscious wishes arise (dependent, aggressive, and erotic) that are defended against by the full range of group and individual resistances. At any given moment the leaders assess the level of productive work, and if it is satisfactory, they remain silent. If the work is unsatisfactory, the leaders invite the group to consider that fact and help them—to the required degree—to identify and overcome the current resistance.

Early in the group's development, the leaders may have to be fairly active; as the group matures, more and more of this work will be done by the members themselves. The ability to do increasing amounts of the work is one excellent measure of the learning that the group provides for its members.

At times, in response to an assessment of the stresses (primarily professional but also personal) that the group is encountering, the leaders may choose to promote supportiveness and nurturing within the group rather than focus exclusively on learning. Again, as the group matures, more and more of this support and nurturing may be provided by the members themselves.

Generally it is best for the leaders not to model self-revelation but to serve as a model of abstinence, tolerant acceptance of strong affect, and personal restraint. The leaders' natural countertransference wish to be liked by younger colleagues needs to be kept in mind. The temptation is ever present to be likable rather than useful. The leaders' task is to be useful.

Coleadership and Peer Supervision

For administrative purposes, coleadership is often employed in early stages of residency training. It should be clear, however, that coleadership introduces significant complications and is best carried out by experienced leaders. Groups with coleaders have a great deal of splitting, and leaders themselves do a good deal of unconscious competing. In some ways, it is easier to lead any psychodynamic group (psychotherapy group or process group) alone. Nonetheless, there are distinct advantages to coleadership of the process group.

Perhaps the most important benefit of coleading a process group is the opportunity for the leaders themselves to grow and learn. These tasks are best accomplished in a context that combines coleadership and peer supervision. This combination provides the leaders with a maximum opportunity for productive critical scrutiny. The leaders' understanding of group dynamics and technique are consistently refined by the two interdigitating levels of collegial cooperation. Little will be lost through the operation of one's own ignorance or countertransference. Through the leaders' examination of their own work in this setting, insight and skill are enriched to a degree not usually available to senior clinicians.

It should be noted that the peer supervisory group is best run as just that: a peer supervisory group. It should not be conducted as a leaderless process group. Process elements within the supervisory group are discussed only when a group resistance prevents the supervisory group from carrying out its task. Its task is not self-study; its task is the study of its members' work as process group leaders. The supervisory group addresses—as necessary and appropriate—the process between the coleaders. The combination of process and nonprocess supervision is an essential part of what makes this experience so invaluable to experienced clinicians.

Conclusions

This model of psychiatric residents' process groups utilizes self-study for the purpose of teaching about group and individual dynamics and about interpersonal communication. With minor modifications, the model presented here is applicable to trainees in all the mental health professions. It provides intellectual and experiential learning and support for the members. By doing so, these groups help faculty and administrators as well as students to achieve their goals. They also provide a unique continuing-education opportunity for their leaders.

References

Jensen PS: The Transition to Residency Seminar. Journal of Psychiatric Education 7:261–267, 1983

Lang HA, Halperin DA, Swiller HI: Process groups for the training of psychiatrists, in Group Psychodynamics: New Paradigms and New Perspectives. Edited by Halperin DA. Chicago, IL, Year Book Medical Publishers, 1989, pp 209–225

Salvendy JT, Stewart MF: Periodic T-groups for psychiatric residents. Journal of Psychiatric Education 7:287–295, 1983

Willenbring ML, Spensley J: The support group in psychiatric residency: how can we best help our residents. Journal of Psychiatric Education 7:268–273, 1983

Winnicott DW: The theory of the parent-infant relationship. Int J Psychoanal 41:585–595, 1960

CHAPTER 27

How to Run a Group Psychotherapy Workshop

Lawrence J. Bader, Ph.D.

Purpose

There are at least five reasons why clinicians would do well to learn about ways of understanding and conducting a workshop. First, clinicians have a wealth of theoretical and practical knowledge gathered from their training, their supervision, and their work experiences that could be shared with colleagues less knowledgeable than themselves. Second, leading workshops provides practitioners with an opportunity to extend their clinical practice to an educational rather than a clinical setting. This diversification could be a stimulating alternative for the practitioner, while simultaneously serving a practical need to expand sources of economic remuneration in an increasingly competitive and continuously changing health care field. Third, preparing and giving a workshop help workshop leaders to sharpen their ideas about groups in a way that everyday practice of clinical work does not. Fourth, by offering a workshop for colleagues, clinicians demonstrate their competence to peers, which is gratifying to the leader sand helpful in developing a wider professional network. Last, a well-run workshop offers group psychotherapists an opportunity to communicate in a skilled way about a content area in group psychotherapy, thereby providing further opportunities for members of the health care professions to continue their professional education.

With the above reasons in mind, I developed this chapter to describe both in theory and in practice an easily understood applied approach to organizing and conducting a workshop. This approach has a proven track record that can be translated to any workshop size or theme. The rest of the chapter is organized into six sections. In the first section, I identify my assumptions about workshops. In the second section, I define, with examples, concepts that I believe bear directly on conducting a workshop. In the third section, I highlight pitfalls to be avoided. In the fourth section, I discuss workshop errors and workshop failures. In the fifth section, I develop a generic workshop model. And last, I offer a summary of this chapter.

Assumptions

In preparing for a workshop, I make four assumptions that help me distinguish it from other group-related learning events.

First, a workshop is not primarily a cognitive experience, as represented by a seminar offered within an educational or training setting. A seminar is usually an intellectually stimulating experience with the seminar leader providing information, questions, and guidance for a discussion that is usually kept on a cognitive rather than an emotional plane. Usually a seminar involves a body of knowledge and grappling with ideas, as in a seminar entitled "Theories of Group Psychotherapy." Intellectual mastery is the goal.

Second, I assume that a workshop as a learning experience differs from group therapy; whereas group therapy focuses on personal unhealthy and healthy patterns of thought, feeling, and action, a workshop is usually work related for the participant. It builds on his or her health and on his or her desire to learn and to apply this learning to the work setting (Ladd 1986).

Third, I assume that a useful workshop blends theory, experience, and application in a way that presents participants with a conceptual framework, provides them with an opportunity to experience one or more of the concepts, and then offers them a chance to apply both concepts and experience to real-life work situations (Hill 1982).

Fourth, I assume that good workshop design is based on the clinician's understanding of small-group and large-group dynamics; it draws on the practitioner's knowledge of small-group theory and on his or her skill in putting people together in a useful way. Thus organizing and conducting a workshop constitute a nonclinical use of a clinician's knowledge and experience of group dynamics.

With these assumptions, I now turn to theoretical concepts that I have found useful in organizing and conducting my workshops.

Relevant Concepts

There are a handful of concepts that I have found to be extremely useful in helping me to understand the theory of organizing and conducting a workshop. These concepts are derived from a variety of disciplines, but they are mostly related to the theory and practice of small-group behavior. In this section I identify each concept, offer a simple definition, and provide examples to help demonstrate its relevance in conducting workshops. Although I have found these concepts to be useful, I am aware that different concepts could be helpful to others. However, for me, the following concepts have stood the test of time:

- Boundary
- Phase
- Content-process
- Feedback
- Management of disturbance

Boundary

According to Singer et al. (1975), a boundary distinguishes in from out. I have found this concept to be more useful than any other when I am developing clinical or nonclinical group events. The clinical relevance of boundaries was noted by Rice and Rutan (1981) in their discussion of systemic considerations for developing groups on an inpatient service. Because a boundary distinguishes in from out, boundaries have wide-ranging implications for decisions made by workshop leaders. For example, who is included in the workshop, in what numbers, and for what time period are all boundary management decisions. In addition, when preparing for a workshop, leaders need to decide which material to include in which sequence and for how much time. These, too, are boundary management decisions.

Including too few or too many participants with material that does not meet their needs often results in workshop failure. For example, it is difficult if not impossible to conduct a workshop with fewer than three individuals because too few individuals limit the information shared and restrict the excitement that is brought into a small-group discussion of applying the concepts to back-home work situations. It is equally difficult to conduct a workshop with a large group (e.g., 100 members) without the aid of adjunct discussion leaders to help guide the small-group discussions in ways to apply the learning. This is not to suggest that a large group cannot discuss an issue, but rather to suggest that for the event to be called a workshop, the discussion needs to be effectively guided back to the work environment of each individual participant.

Phase

A phase in a group's development offers the practitioner guidelines with which to understand the sequence of events over time in a group. Tuckman (1965) reported that by understanding phases, the practitioner develops a way to observe a group event and develops interventions that are mindful of each individual and of group development. Workshops follow the beginning, middle, and end phases of group development, which offer the practitioner general guidelines for action.

In the beginning phase, when participants need to orient themselves to the work of the learning event and to the membership in the learning event, feelings of dependency are common. Thus the workshop leader needs to acquaint the membership with the proposed activities in a way that takes into account member strength and vulnerability. Tasks that promote getting acquainted are specific to that phase. In the beginning phase, confrontations of members by the workshop leader can cause undue harm and severely retard and perhaps destroy the workshop's development. I have known of workshop leaders to ruin a potentially robust workshop by their inattentiveness to the early-phase work of inclusion, orientation, and safety.

At the other end of the temporal spectrum, the phase-specific task of termination occurs at the end of the workshop (Lawler 1980). Termination is an important event, often neglected by workshop leaders. If a workshop is going well, leaders may be reluctant to end it; if it is going poorly, they may feel guilty about ending it. In both cases, and in other circumstances, insufficient time spent in ending a workshop deprives members and leaders of a meaningful experience of assessing gains, noting missed opportunities, and experiencing and expressing feelings connected to ending. Group therapists are familiar with the process of endings because they are usually schooled in developmental theory and phases of group development and because they have had experiences with endings of short-term or long-term therapy groups.

I recommend that a workshop leader devote enough time for a three-part sequence of termination. First, provide participants with time to privately reflect on their experience. Second, encourage each member to complete, with examples, a written questionnaire inquiring about the usefulness of the workshop. And third, have the entire membership meet as a large group to discuss their learning and their misgivings about the workshop. This three-part termination 1) provides workshop members with an individual sense of their experience; 2) gives them an opportunity to put their thoughts and feelings in written form, a process that often helps to clarify their experience; and 3) offers them a chance to vent feelings and to exchange perspectives with other workshop members.

Content-Process

Process consultation as described by Schein (1969) is a form of organizational consultation designed to offer feedback to leader-managers about how they work compared with what they do. Thus content refers to the substance of the communication between people and can be identified and measured by the words that are used, whereas the process of communication refers to the patterns of both verbal and nonverbal behavior between those who are communicating. In developing a workshop, the content refers to the body of knowledge to be learned, whereas the process refers to the sequence of learning events. Whereas the content refers to words that are spoken, the process involves the participants' treatment of one another, the handling of conflict, and the overall atmosphere in which the workshop evolves. For example, an atmosphere that promotes excessive confrontation and a high level of stress would probably work less well than one that fosters a balance of support and challenge.

Balance between content and process is also important. Major errors in workshop conduct are committed by workshop leaders who focus their entire workshop on content with little or no chance for discussion or application. Alternatively, a common error made by group therapists in their initial workshop involves an assumption about the conduct of a group event. Many group therapists assume that only a therapy group model using experience-based learning is desirable. The idea that a guided experience within a previously established conceptual framework could provide useful learning is often overlooked.

I have also known of experienced and competent clinicians who, although knowledgeable about their specialty area, have given little thought to the process of the workshop. It appears that they assume that a workshop consists of either a large group discussion of mutual concerns among workshop participants or a consultation from the workshop leader to the participants in the area of the leader's expertise. By following the guidelines offered in this chapter, a clinician can bring the same degree of competence to bear in leading a workshop that he or she brings to his or her clinical specialty. The leader simply needs to manage the boundaries of time, focus, role, and member interest and then bring the discussion back to the work environment of the participants, a place to which the learning from the workshop event needs to be applied.

Feedback

Feedback is a concept that has been around for a long time. Based on work in physics, it was adapted by the National Training Labs and by group leaders and group therapists over the years (Egan 1976). It is usually meant to define a process whereby one person gives information to another person about the thoughts, feelings, or actions that the other person needs to correct, according to the individual giving the feedback. Guidelines for effective feedback include, but are not limited to, the following: the importance of making the feedback descriptive rather than judgmental, specific rather than general, in the present rather than postponed, given with permission rather than as a surprise, and given in an area in which the recipient has the power to effect change. In their focus on helping individuals improve the quality of their lives, group therapists have expanded the definition of feedback to move beyond a correction of behavior that is off-center to include all communications about any aspect of an experience from the observer's perspective.

Providing feedback before, during, and after a workshop is critical to the success of this event. Information that is available before a workshop begins gives the workshop leader clues about the needs and interests of participants and about the relevance of this workshop offering. For example, a large turnout by members who freely chose to attend usually means that the content or the leader drew the participants. On the other hand, registration by only a few participants suggests that the workshop planners should review their thinking about the place this particular workshop occupies in that context of professional education.

Feedback during the workshop can offer the workshop leader guidelines on the workshop's progress. The workshop leader's ability to accurately read the many sources of feedback throughout the entire workshop often ensures the overall success of the event. Feedback that is critical in content and constructive in tone is more easily responded to than feedback that is hostile and designed to hurt. The former often refers to mistakes made by the leader that can be corrected without too much difficulty. For example, as I was conducting a workshop my anxiety led me to forget about offering the participants a break for stretching and refreshments. About 2 hours into the workshop, when a number of members inquired about the location of the bathroom, I became more mindful of their needs and suggested the timeliness of a 10-minute break.

On the other hand, when critical feedback is given in an angry tone, or with a bitter edge or said sarcastically, the leader may respond defensively and consider the feedback to be either irrelevant or too important. If the workshop leader considers the feedback to be irrelevant, he or she runs the risk of discounting important information. I believe that workshop participants are always right in that they are responding to their perception, which is valid for them. A common error made by group therapists is to consider critical feedback as coming from the distortions of the workshop participant. In this way workshop participants are responded to as members of a therapy group, rather than as participants in an educational experience.

On the other hand, there is a danger of taking the critical feedback too seriously. I have known workshop leaders who, devastated by critical feedback, became remorseful and defensive rather than receiving the feedback as an opportunity to acknowledge a possible error and to use this error as a source of professional development. In this situation a colleague, coleader, or someone connected to the workshop can be very helpful in permitting the leader to register the criticism and to use it constructively.

Management of Disturbance

Management of disturbance is a term that I learned from Ruth Cohen (personal communication, March 1972), a trained psychoanalyst and superb workshop leader. The concept refers to a situation in which the workshop's development is disturbed because one of the members becomes distraught and is not able to participate in the conduct of the workshop. When this happens, Cohen suggests that the member's reactions need to be responded to in a way that is respectful to that member, to all members, and to the workshop's development. According to Cohen, and confirmed by my experience, disturbances need an immediate response in which the distraught, discouraged, or disgruntled member is acknowledged and efforts are made to integrate the member into the mainstream of the workshop. As a last resort, the workshop leader needs to feel secure in exercising his or her judgment about removing a member who does not seem willing or able to participate.

For example, I was once part of a problem-solving group that critiqued previously held workshops. One problem presented to us by a workshop leader involved confusion about his responses to a continuously critical and chronically disruptive workshop member. Many members of my team proposed that the workshop leader could have treated the member as if he were part of a therapy group. I disagreed, noting the differences in boundaries between a therapy group and a workshop, and in contrast with my colleagues, suggested that "all was not grist for the mill." In this case, I felt that the "mill and the grist did not match."

The general guideline that I follow is to make every effort to help the member presenting the disturbance to participate in what I consider to be the workshop event. However, in keeping with my view that a workshop leader needs to manage the boundaries of the workshop, including the boundary of membership, I believe that the leader has the power to exclude members and needs to feel confident in exercising such rightful authority. Then, after the exclusion, attention needs to be paid to the other members, some of whom may feel relief and some of whom may unrealistically fear that they may be the next to go.

Pitfalls

In this section I review some of the major pitfalls to be mindful of as workshops are planned and carried out. I believe that all pitfalls can be understood by using the previously discussed concept of boundary management. I have identified a handful of common leader-centered pitfalls:

- Confusion about the differences between a workshop, group therapy, and a seminar
- Mismanagement of time
- Incorrect sequencing of learning events
- Attempting to please participants, coupled with an inability to stay with the planned focus
- Inflexibility

Lack of Differentiation Between a Workshop, Group Therapy, and a Seminar

This confusion is understandable if a practitioner's postgraduate training in group therapy did not include an understanding of the process of organizing and conducting a workshop using groupdynamic principles. Recall the previously discussed instance in which a workshop consultant, who was also trained as a group therapist, would have had the workshop leader treat the workshop participant as a group therapy member. Although the participant may have needed therapy, he or she nevertheless signed up for an event consistent with a workshop and inconsistent with therapy. To treat the distraught member as if he or she were part of a therapy group is disrespectful to the other workshop members, who have signed up for an educational rather than a clinical event.

Stressful circumstances that come from dissatisfied and angry workshop participants can be managed best by remembering the boundary that you and they occupy and by acting accordingly. A useful guideline under those difficult circumstances is to support the member who is critical and then try to find ways to help him or her stay within the workshop learning task. It is equally possible for a workshop leader to forget the part of the workshop that has the experiential and the applied components and to focus exclusively on the conceptual part, particularly if the leader wishes to impart a body of knowledge in a way that he or she was originally taught in his or her graduate education.

Mismanagement of Time

Determining how much time to allow for which task is a major responsibility of the workshop leader. Both boundary and phase concepts inform the workshop leader about the proper use of time. For example, sufficient time needs to be taken at the beginning of a workshop to allow the leaders to address the work of the first phase, which is to become acquainted. Too little time to discuss goals, expectations, and feelings could plunge the participants into the workshop without sufficient orientation. Too much time in the first phase could delay the forward motion of the workshop. For example, once when I gave a 3-hour workshop for 25 participants, I asked each participant to take 5 minutes to introduce himself or herself and, therefore, took too much time for this initial task. This left insufficient time for the rest of the work, thereby frustrating many of the members.

Incorrect Budget and Sequence of Learning Events

A few years ago, a colleague consulted me about conducting a workshop. She expressed serious concern about not having enough to say in the 3 hours allotted to her. When our discussion made it clear to her that she was not required to talk for all 3 hours, she proceeded to develop a sequence of learning events that began with a didactic presentation and went on to small-group discussion and large-group reporting. She was greatly relieved and went on to conduct a very successful workshop.

The Need to Respond to Workshop Participants

This need can reflect a flexible response to new information and can lead to a well-run workshop, or it can lead to a loss of focus and a poorly run workshop. I recall a workshop participant who could not respond to my instructions to talk about a particular theme in a small group of five or six other people. Her feedback to me suggested that her reaction was more extreme than the situation warranted. On the other hand, her humiliation was real, and her willingness to relate her current state in the workshop to past experiences in school was courageous. A brief discussion with her in her small group, which was unplanned but necessary, kept her working within the boundary of the workshop. I felt that if I did not respond to her, I would have left her with unnecessary pain and might have lost her as a participant, along with the others.

In a group, where tremendous personal pain has an impact on the ties among people, a distraught workshop participant can significantly damage himself or herself and also place a heavy burden on the group. I have also encountered situations in which a member's inquiry could have diverted me from my focus with the large or small group. Although I supported the basis for the question and the question itself, I reserved the right to suggest the time in which the question could best be answered.

From problems presented to me by dissatisfied workshop participants or by frustrated workshop leaders, it seemed to me that often workshop leaders trap themselves by their eagerness to respond to each question and forget the overall purpose and sequence of the workshop. This results in a mismanagement of boundaries related to time, task, role, and sequence of learning events. The situation moves downhill rapidly when workshop participants lose confidence in their leader, fearing a loss of potential learning from the event. Thus by paying too much attention to one member's question, a leader risks losing a significant portion of the members, who may distance themselves from involvement in the learning event. That is why the concept of boundaries is so critical and requires leaders to continually ask themselves "What and who is in or out at this time?"

Inflexibly Responding to Workshop Size

Workshop leaders need to design a workshop that addresses the number of participants. For example, it is possible to conduct workshops for large groups of people over a longer period of time if the sequence of learning events is planned well and if the leader engages other colleagues to help with the planning and implementation. On the other hand, a small number of participants usually requires more intimate participation on the part of the workshop leader and could lead to more self-disclosure on his or her part.

Learning From Errors

Errors are common occurrences in leading workshops. For example, an error is made when a leader loses perspective and conducts something other than a workshop, or when he or she mismanages the time for one or more of the learning sequences. Finally, an error may be made if the legitimate needs of the workshop participants are either ignored or dismissed. All workshop leaders, whether new in the field or experienced, would do well to note that every error described and every pitfall detailed are familiar to the most seasoned of workshop leaders. My colleagues and I have made all of the above errors, as well as many others. For me, the question is not whether I will make an error, but rather when I do, will I be able to correct it within the workshop and learn from it so I may improves future workshops?

For the balance of this section, I first address short-term corrections within the workshop and, second, look at ways to ensure long-term gains.

Within-Workshop Corrections

When I have followed the guidelines for remaining open to critical feedback, I have been able to quickly correct an error in time to repair potential damage. Recall my example of mismanaging the boundaries of time and my delay in giving the participants a much-needed break.

Recently, as I began to answer questions from workshop participants, a workshop member spoke up, asking me to move on with my planned presentation and not become lost in the details. My quick review of the situation revealed that the critique was justified; my anxiety had contributed to a detour from my purpose in an effort to please a few vocal members. After I acknowledged the situation, I said that the questions for discussion were excellent but would best be raised at a later time.

In all, within-workshop corrections are easy to make if the leader is open to changes in a way that respects the workshop's purpose and the members' interests. However, there are occasions when something goes wrong and a workshop fails. By that I mean that more than just a handful of participants believe that the workshop was, at best, unsatisfactory. When this occurs (and if you are leading workshops it will occur), I offer a sequence of activities that could help. First, register the criticism rather than deny it. Second, assume that there is a great deal to be derived from the criticism. Third, try to appreciate the data on which the criticism was based. In this way you can evaluate the merits of the criticism rather than become defensive about it. It is possible that you were unaware of the problem or that you were aware of it but did not know how to correct it in time. In either case, the data give you what you need to make corrections for the future. Fourth, try not to take the criticism too personally; you will recover faster if you put it into a larger perspective. And finally, try to lead another workshop as soon as possible, putting into practice what you have learned.

A Generic Workshop Model

By using the previously identified assumptions, I now offer a model that is applicable to any workshop theme with one or more leaders for any length of time. I chose a 3-hour workshop model for several reasons. First, I am most familiar with this model, and it is often common at large professional meetings. Second, the American Group Psychotherapy Association presents this model to its workshop leaders in an effort to orient them to one useful model of workshop practice (M. Block, personal communication, 1989). It should be noted, however, that this workshop model represents only one way, and not the only way, to think about and conduct a workshop.

To reiterate, the model's major concept is boundaries, and it rests on the assumption that an effective workshop usefully blends theory, experience, and application. In the example I describe, I start with theory, then move to experience, and end with application. Although I believe that all three are necessary and sufficient ingredients of an effective workshop, either the experimental or the theoretical component can come first, followed by the other and capped off by application. However, I am convinced that a workshop is not complete without application to back-home work situations, an experimental involvement of the participants, and a conceptual framework to draw on. In short, it needs to tap all that makes us human—our thoughts, our feelings, and our behavior.

In offering a 3-hour workshop, I divide the time into six parts to reflect the relative amount of time needed for each of the six segments in proportion to the total time allotted for the entire workshop event. Thus I begin the workshop in an effort to manage the boundary of time. For example, I spend about 10% of the total time in acquainting members with each other, with me, and with the workshop content. This helps prepare participants for the events to come.

To begin the process of getting acquainted, I review the purpose of the workshop, its outline, and the context in which it is given. Then I ask participants to identify themselves by name and work environment and ask for a statement of purpose in taking the workshop. In this beginning phase, I provide an opportunity for all members to participate, while at the same time providing myself with information about the members. This information can point both to potential and to pitfalls. After each member talks, I try to say something about his or her potential contribution to the workshop; I also try to help those members for whom I believe there would be potential pitfalls to find ways to connect meaningfully to the workshop or to leave the workshop before it becomes a negative experience.

This process of getting acquainted, which is part of the first phase of the workshop, is particularly important in light of the absence of contact among the workshop members and the leader before its beginning. In contrast to a group therapy situation, where the group leader interviews potential new members and decides to include or exclude them from the group, the workshop leader is presented with the membership in the first moments of the workshop. They've included themselves and were not included by the workshop leader.

Introductions for a 3-hour workshop could take 20 minutes. Then, I review the sequence of learning for the workshop, followed by a presentation of relevant concepts connected to the theme. During this presentation, which usually takes 30% of the workshop time, my goal is to help members learn and relearn concepts with which they can work. I respond only to questions that help clarify the concept, and I discourage questions or discussion that could divert me from it.

After my presentation and before a 10-minute break, I encourage members to make notes capturing their reaction to the concepts presented. During this time, as they complete their note-taking, I organize the composition of the application groups. For example, for a 25-person workshop, I usually organize the membership into five groups of 5 people each and direct them to take 50 minutes to work on the theme of applying the previously presented concepts. I try to compose the groups by considering information shared by individual members in the first phase of orientation. More specifically, I try to put members together whom I believe can identify with each other, share equitably in conversation, and in a brief 50 minutes, learn from each other.

During the small-group discussion, I visit each group as a consultant to ensure that the members understand their task, work on the theme, help each other, and overcome obstacles. At the end of the small-group discussion, I have used 75% of the workshop time, and I am ready for the next part. This involves a discussion with the whole group and an exchange of any learning that has occurred. After this discussion, 10% of the time usually remains for a critique of the workshop and for saying goodbye.

Summary

In this chapter, I have demonstrated how clinicians who are knowledgeable and skilled in the area of group therapy may expand their clinical work from group therapy to the nonclinical activity of conducting a workshop. I have linked a move in this direction to the practitioner's need for developing skills that can be used in other contexts, to his or her desire to be of use to colleagues by providing a forum for group therapy training, and, finally, to an interest in widening the basis for monetary remuneration in an ever-changing health care environment. In organizing this chapter, I have noted my assumptions about workshops, with an emphasis on the differences between sa workshop, a seminar, and group psychotherapy. I have identified five concepts that have been useful in my thinking through and planning a workshop, and I have assigned a special place to boundary management. I have tried to speak to the pitfalls that can beset a workshop leader and have made suggestions for ways to overcome them. I have also described ways to learn from workshop errors and from workshop failures. Finally, I have offered a generic model that is flexible in sequence and adaptable to any workshop theme in any clinical area, to large or small groups, and to time periods from half a day to a week or more. I hope that this presentation has provided readers with a useful conceptual model that will support reflection, good feeling, and action.

References

Egan G: Confrontation. Group and Organizational Studies 11:223–243, 1976

Hill BJ: An analysis of conflict resolution techniques. Journal of Conflict Resolution 26:109–138, 1982

Ladd C: Rethinking the workshop. Training and Development Journal 40:5–12, 1986

Lawler MH: Termination in a work group: four models of analysis and intervention. Group 4:3–27, 1980

Rice C, Rutan JS: Boundary maintenance in inpatient therapy groups. Int J Group Psychother 31:297–310, 1981

Schein E: Process Consultation. New York, Addison-Wesley, 1969

Singer DL, Astrachan M, Gould W, et al: Boundary management in psychological work with groups. Journal of Applied Behavioral Science 11:137–176, 1975

Tuckman BW: Developmental sequence in small groups. Psycho Bull 63:384–399, 1965

Index

Page numbers printed in **boldface** refer to tables or figures.

I

L

M